THE LSE COMPANION TO HEALTH POLICY

The LSE Companion to Health Policy

Edited by

Alistair McGuire

Professor of Health Economics, LSE, UK

Joan Costa-Font

Reader in Political Economy, LSE, UK

Edward Elgar
Cheltenham, UK • Northampton, MA, USA

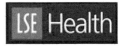

Published by
Edward Elgar Publishing Limited
The Lypiatts
15 Lansdown Road
Cheltenham
Glos GL50 2JA
UK

Edward Elgar Publishing, Inc.
William Pratt House
9 Dewey Court
Northampton
Massachusetts 01060
USA

A catalogue record for this book
is available from the British Library

Library of Congress Control Number: 2012930622

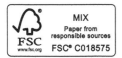

MIX
Paper from
responsible sources
FSC® C018575

ISBN 978 1 78100 423 4 (cased)

Typeset by Servis Filmsetting Ltd, Stockport, Cheshire
Printed and bound by MPG Books Group, UK

Contents

Contributors

Sara Allin, Assistant Professor, School of Public Policy and Governance, University of Toronto, and Senior Researcher, Canadian Institute for Health Information.

R. Gwyn Bevan, Professor of Management Science, Department of Management, The London School of Economics and Political Science, United Kingdom.

Rebecca Butterfield, Visiting Researcher, Personal Social Services Research Unit (PSSRU), LSE Health and Social Care, The London School of Economics and Political Science, United Kingdom.

Catherine Campbell, Professor, Institute of Social Psychology, The London School of Economics and Political Science, London, United Kingdom, and External Professor and Fellow of HIVAN (the Centre for HIV/AIDS Networking), University of KwaZulu-Natal, Durban, South Africa.

Adelina Comas-Herrera, Research Fellow, Personal Social Services Research Unit (PSSRU), LSE Health and Social Care, The London School of Economics and Political Science, United Kingdom.

Zack Cooper, Research Economist, Centre for Economic Performance, The London School of Economics and Political Science, United Kingdom.

Joan Costa-Font, Reader, Department of Social Policy, LSE Health, and European Institute, The London School of Economics and Political Science, United Kingdom.

Mariachiara Di Cesare, Research Associate in Population Health, School of Public Health, Imperial College London, United Kingdom.

Heba A. Elgazzar, Economist, Human Development Department, World Bank, Washington, DC, USA, and Associate Researcher, Personal Social Services Research Unit (PSSRU), LSE Health and Social Care, London School of Economics and Political Science, London, United Kingdom.

José-Luis Fernández, Deputy Director and Principal Research Fellow, Personal Social Services Research Unit (PSSRU), LSE Health and Social Care, The London School of Economics and Political Science, United Kingdom.

Andrew Gibbs, Researcher, Health Economics and HIV/AIDS Research Division (HEARD), University of KwaZulu-Natal, Durban, South Africa.

Catherine Henderson, Research Officer, LSE Health and Social Care, The London School of Economics and Political Science, United Kingdom.

Cristina Hernández-Quevedo, Research Fellow, European Observatory on Health Systems and Policies, LSE Health, The London School of Economics and Political Science, United Kingdom.

Lucia Kossarova, doctoral student, LSE Health, The London School of Economics and Political Science, United Kingdom.

Cristina Masseria, Research Fellow, European Observatory on Health Systems and Policies, World Health Organization (WHO), LSE Health, The London School of Economics and Political Science, United Kingdom.

Alistair McGuire, Professor of Health Economics, Department of Social Policy and LSE Health, The London School of Economics and Political Science, United Kingdom.

Philipa Mladovsky, Research Fellow, European Observatory on Health Systems and Policies, LSE Health, The London School of Economics and Political Science, United Kingdom.

Alec Morton, Lecturer in Management Science, Department of Management, The London School of Economics and Political Science, United Kingdom.

Michael Murphy, Professor of Demography, Department of Social Policy, The London School of Economics and Political Science, United Kingdom.

Irene Papanicolas, Research Officer, LSE Health, The London School of Economics and Political Science, United Kingdom.

Maria Raikou, Research Fellow in Health Economics, LSE Health, The London School of Economics and Political Science, United Kingdom.

Caroline Rudisill, Lecturer in Health Economics, Department of Social Policy, The London School of Economics and Political Science, United Kingdom

Victoria Serra-Sastre, Lecturer, Department of Economics, City University London, United Kingdom.

Charitini Stavropoulou, Lecturer in Health Care Management, Department of Health Care Management and Policy, University of Surrey, Guildford, United Kingdom.

Nebibe Varol, Research Associate, LSE Health, The London School of Economics and Political Science, United Kingdom.

Joshua M. Wiener, Director, Aging, Disability and Long-Term Care, RTI International, Washington, DC, USA.

Raphael Wittenberg, Senior Research Fellow, Personal Social Services Research Unit (PSSRU), LSE Health and Social Care, London School of Economics and Political Science, United Kingdom.

Valentina Zigante, doctoral student, European Institute, The London School of Economics and Political Science, United Kingdom.

Acknowledgements

The editors are grateful to the LSE Health, LSE Santander Fund and the Xarxa de Recerca en Economia i Politques Publiques (XREPP) and CAEPS Centre of the Univeristy of Barcelona for their financial and logistic support in organising the workshop that allowed the idea of the book to flourish and become a reality. We are especially grateful to Anna Maresso for her editing work and to the authors for their patience in amending and improving their text to meet the quality standards of this textbook.

Introduction
Alistair McGuire and Joan Costa-Font

Health policy attempts to explore the range of aims and objectives pursued in financing, producing and distributing health care to any given population. The analysis of health policy covers the implementation of specific policies as they attempt to target the delivery of health care to different individuals, assesses the equity and efficiency of this process and evaluates the outcomes as a means of increasing the health of specific populations. As such, health policy is a wide-ranging subject covering many academic disciplines, employing many different methodologies and, given the importance of the specific institutions financing, producing and delivering health care, tends to be country or even population specific. For these reasons the range of analytical coverage is vast.

What most studies in health policy have in common is an interest in applying theory to improve practice. That the theory underlying health policy attempts to model a complex interplay of individual, community and society-wide behaviours means, not surprisingly, that the field encompasses many different ideas and analytical approaches, and advocates different practices depending on which of many analytical stances are adopted. It is a difficult area of study subject to many biases and flaws.

Yet most health policy analysts would support the broad principle that policy ought to be evidence based. The aim of the chapters in this book is to bring to bear some evidence on a range of central areas within health policy. There is no doubt that the range of areas covered is not comprehensive, but we have attempted to incorporate the most important ones. Consequently the text is broken into six parts covering Quality, Access and Inequalities; Supply and Health Care Markets; Insurance and Expenditures; Pharmaceuticals and New Technologies; Ageing and Long-term Care; and Behaviour and Health Production.

In the section on Quality, Access and Inequalities, Hernández-Quevedo and Costa-Font review the various explanations of why health inequalities exist, analysing measurement issues and empirical evidence along the way. They highlight the persistence of health inequalities across different countries. In discussing the persistence of such inequalities despite the major policy efforts directed towards alleviating them, they highlight that the policy responses are inhibited for various reasons. Most importantly, they explore the difficulties in accurately measuring the different aspects of health inequality, including problems arising from limited data and those relating to the self-reporting of health status and the biases inherent in such subjective measures issues. They conclude that, without sound data it is difficult to target policy responses and incentivizing individual behaviour.

This is clearly illustrated in a practical manner in the following chapter by Gibbs and Campbell, who focus on a specific attempt to strengthen community participation in primary health care – an objective that has been the focus of health policy in a number of low-income countries where problems of ensuring supply in the face of low funding levels and of access dominate. The authors look at a case study located in Southern

Africa, highlighting the practical difficulties of widening primary health care participation in areas where the goals of health policy are constrained by traditional hierarchies and values. The case study highlights the importance of ensuring that providers are motivated before access can be assured, and emphasises the role of monetary incentives in furthering participation generally.

This theme is taken up by Elgazzar, who considers the case of health policy as it attempts to widen access in middle-income countries generally. The argument is that middle-income countries face challenges distinct from those of low-income countries. While ability to pay for health care and lack of safety nets remain common issues in low- and middle-income countries, Elgazzar argues that there is growing income availability, while the diseases faced are increasingly different. Middle-income countries are increasingly facing similar diseases, cardiovascular disease and diabetes being examples common in the wealthier countries of the world. This changing disease pattern requires changes in the institutional delivery of health care in middle-income countries, and the chapter questions the ability of institutions to adapt rapidly to changing disease patterns. The persistence of health inequalities in middle-income countries is also discussed, where, developing the theme of earlier chapters, the role of traditional (social) influences is emphasised, although it is argued that these are exacerbated by the prominence given to responding to the preferences of a growing middle class.

The final chapter in this section develops further the issue relating to measurement problems, and here the case of measuring the performance of the primary care sector is examined. Effective health policy can only be developed if the effects can be adequately assessed, and this requires building on sound data. Kossarova notes that, while attention has been increasingly devoted to measuring the performance of the health sector in responding to the needs of chronic care, there has been less attention devoted to measuring the performance of ambulatory or outpatient care. She finds that similar problems arise in this area of care, including a difficulty in measuring quality of health care partly stemming from adequately defining the different dimensions of care. She argues that these problems are not insurmountable and considers one way forward through the use of avoidable mortality as a measure of performance.

Part II considers the growing importance of seeing health policy within the context of market-based incentives. In a number of countries a separation between institutions funding health care and institutions providing health care has been increasingly formalised. On occasion this has been coupled with attempts to improve the expression of patient preferences through motivating patient choices across providers of care. Zigante, Costa-Font and Cooper review the recent European literature in this area and argue that there is increasing evidence to support the role of competition among providers and of patient choice in improving both the efficiency of the delivery of health care and equity of access. They argue that the responsiveness of health care systems to patients' wants is enhanced through the introduction of policies that enhance choice and competition at the patient level.

Of course such policies do not generally rely on a price mechanism to allocate health care resources. Most systems are dominated by some other form of rationing process, the most common being waiting times. Morton and Bevan in Chapter 6 examine the reasons behind the use of waiting times as a rationing device. They argue that different health care systems justify waiting times in different ways – ways that are consistent with their own institutions and objectives. They do not think that these various explanations are conceptually inconsistent, and suggest a conceptual framework to categorise waiting times. They also argue that the various policies aimed at manipulating waiting times are shaped by the specific institutional context giving rise to waiting times experienced by any given health care system.

In the last chapter in this section Allin and Masseria examine a specific indicator relating to access to health care. They argue that the issue of self-reported unmet need is an important leading indicator of access. They discuss the various problems associated with defining such subjective measures of health needs by examining a specific data set. In highlighting measurement issues in particular, they argue that any single indicator of health system performance is rarely capable of adequately capturing all dimensions of care. They conclude that any comprehensive assessment of health policy requires an array of performance measures.

Part III opens with an examination by McGuire, Serra-Sastre and Raikou of the reasons why health care expenditure has been rising globally. In examining the trends in health care expenditure across high-income countries, they emphasise the role of technology adoption and diffusion. The chapter concludes with a discussion of whether future cost containment is necessary or indeed will prove effective. Emphasis is given to supply-side measures, such as the recent introduction of diagnosis-related group (DRG) hospital reimbursement and health technology assessment across a number of countries.

This theme is picked up by Papanicolas, who examines the effectiveness of performance payment structures. In reviewing the literature, she finds that, while such policies are increasingly common forms of payment structure in a number of countries, there is limited evaluation of the variety of schemes in place. While theory and intuition suggest that such payment mechanisms should lead to increased efficiency in the delivery of care, this is one of many areas in health policy where the actual evidence to support this policy is seen to be rather weaker than actually perceived.

The section concludes with a consideration of social protection in low- and middle-income countries by Mladovsky. They review the four principal mechanisms for financing health care in low- and middle-income countries, tax-based NHS systems, social health insurance, private health insurance and community financing, suggesting that no single model is likely to provide all the answers. Each mechanism is associated with strengths, but also serious weaknesses that limit the likelihood of its achieving successful social health protection in many country contexts.

Part IV considers the role of new health care technology and, in particular, pharmaceuticals in delivering health care. Given the importance, noted earlier, of health care technology in driving health expenditures, Serra-Sastre and McGuire highlight the lack of knowledge about the process of adoption and diffusion of new technology in this sector. Some explanatory factors are exposed; for example the structure of health insurance, hospital size and market competition have been shown to speed technology take-up. However, the general conclusion is that more evidence is required on how new health care technologies diffuse, how this might be regulated and what is the specific impact on health care expenditure.

Varol, Costa-Font and McGuire pick up on the role that regulatory responses might have in technology diffusion, specifically considering the case of pharmaceuticals. They investigate how the regulatory environment impinges on the launch strategies of pharmaceuticals in the main OECD markets during the period 1960–2008. The general finding is that regulation does inhibit diffusion. Thus there is always a trade-off between regulating new technology for safety and efficacy reasons, and the timing of access to new medicines.

In Part V Murphy examines the impact of proximity to death on health care costs. He notes that health care costs rise significantly in the final year of life, a finding that holds consistently across time and health care systems. Given increasing life expectancy in a number of countries, he examines the literature to determine whether the impact on aggregate health care costs can be determined. While the evidence is mixed, he argues that there is a tendency towards health status improvement in the elderly that may push back the health care costs, such that the last year of life remains the most important determinant, but he warns that this may be accompanied by increasing social care costs.

Expanding on this theme, Henderson reviews the literature on the health and social care divide within the UK. As well as analysing the reasons for this divide, she discusses the consequences for the users of health and social care services and for the wider public. She then considers potential remedies proposed to overcome this divide by examining the international and UK-specific evidence.

The theme of how to pay for long-term social care is further analysed by Comas-Herrera and colleagues. Having discussed the various options available for individuals to finance long-term care, they conclude that none is optimal and all require substantial government intervention. Whether this is forthcoming will depend not only on health policy objectives but also on the ability of the government to raise adequate funds to cover this expenditure. They also note that these are likely to be safety-net levels of expenditure and that there will be evolving equity problems as the wealthier extend access to possible private insurance finance.

In Part VI Di Cesare and Murphy then turn to examine the use of historical time series to present consistent data that allow policy makers to examine trends in improvement in health. They do so by examining trends in mortality over time in England and Wales. They point out that even with high-quality data such as these, there are still inconsistencies over time. They examine means of smoothing such inconsistencies, noting that considerable effort must be undertaken to do so. The general point is that if data on mortality require such attention, it is likely that even greater attention to detail must be paid to other data trends for these to be useful for policy making.

Rudisill then considers the importance of individual understanding of risk with respect to health interventions. To the extent that health policy relies to a large extent on motivating individuals to change behaviour, if individuals do not understand the importance or quantitative influence of risk on behaviour, policy will undoubtedly be limited. Having first examined various conceptual means of examining risk preferences, she concludes by outlining the policy implications for what risk research can tell us about health-related behaviours and decision making.

The final chapter by Stavropoulou examines a central institution common to all health systems: the doctor–patient relationship. Reviewing the literature on this relationship, she contends that attention has been devoted to the physician's role. She argues that increasing attention to the patient's role in this relationship is warranted. This seems particularly pertinent at a time when patients have greater access to information than ever before.

In common with the general coverage of health policy, the text covers a wide range of conceptual and practical issues from a number of different perspectives. While we can only introduce the reader to the vast literature that analyses the complexities of health policy, it is hoped that this will stimulate the appetite for further reading in this area.

PART I

QUALITY, ACCESS AND INEQUALITIES

1 Inequalities in health: why do we care? How do we care? What can we do about them?
Cristina Hernández-Quevedo and Joan Costa-Font

1. INTRODUCTION

A widely accepted governmental goal in Western countries is that individuals should enjoy good health, through ensuring equitable access to health irrespective of each individual's social position. This takes place primarily by lowering (and ideally removing) barriers to health care access so as to reduce the socioeconomic vector in health access and financing, and thus achieve health equity standards. The World Health Organization performance framework, introduced in *The World Health Report* (2000), establishes that the main goals of a health care system are: health attainment, by ensuring access to care; responsiveness to population needs from health care services; and a fair distribution of financing. To accomplish health equity goals, health systems typically design programmes and institutions that attempt to lower existing barriers to health care, primarily those affecting its financing and general access – and to a lesser extent preventive programmes. Fairness in health financing is addressed by providing comprehensive coverage and limiting the use of direct payments. Similarly, barriers to health care access are normally addressed through programmes that improve the delivery of health care and prevention, although public programmes are seldom capable of dealing with pre-existing unequal conditions. Equity in health, however, has been considered an undesirable policy objective because it would impose many restrictions on individuals' choice of how to live their lives (Oliver and Mossialos, 2004). Hence interest focuses on the differences of levels of health outcomes across individuals with different socioeconomic characteristics, such as income, job status, education or geographical area, with the desirable policy objective of attaining a less unequal distribution of health outcomes.

Widespread evidence consistently points towards the existence of a socioeconomic gradient in health. Several competing explanations have been offered to explain this empirical behaviour. Hence, in most countries, despite public health system coverage being in place, significant inequalities in health and health care remain pervasive over time (Marmot, 2000). Empirical methods to identify and measure the extent of income-related dispersion of health status have evolved widely to incorporate advances of regression-based decompositions. Finally, given that health is a multidimensional concept, different measures of health arguably measure different dimensions of health as a construct. Indeed, in the UK, for instance, the so-called widening mortality gap between professional and unskilled manual men is well acknowledged (House of Commons Health Committee, 2009). This has motivated policy actions to make sure that future health improvements are shared by the population. However, in order to justify policy actions, the right evidence on the right data must be provided. This is the underlying rationale of this chapter: to assist the debate by organising it and to evaluate the state of the art.

In particular, this chapter will attempt to explain the origins of inequalities in health, along with the key findings. Measurement issues, evidence, policy debates and ways forward are also discussed. We attempt to provide an overview of the state of the art of the literature on health inequalities. We draw upon and bring together advances from the economics, social science and epidemiological literature to suggest ways forward and policy implications.

First, the sources of a social gradient in health are outlined in Section 2; Section 3 follows with measurement of inequalities in health outcomes; Section 4 discusses data requirements; Section 5 covers policy implications; and Section 6 concludes with ways forward.

2. SOURCES OF A SOCIAL GRADIENT IN HEALTH

The reduction of inequalities in health and in the access to health services is one of the main objectives of any health care system. Economists have developed empirical methods that allow us to quantify the degree of inequality in the distribution of health measures and health care utilisation, and to compare inequalities over time and space, identifying those factors that lead to inequalities, thus providing some evidence to policy makers. Figure 1.1 summarises different sources of health inequalities. Indeed, an income gradient in health needs might arise due to an income gradient in prevention (1), in the use of health care (2), in the finance of health care, or might have a direct effect (4), or an alternative might well be the result of institutional barriers to access (5), among other sources. The empirical evidence is vast and cannot be summarised in a chapter; generally speaking, this chapter will cover some of the relationships summarised in Figure 1.1.

Economic and social hierarchies in society influence individuals' health status, which

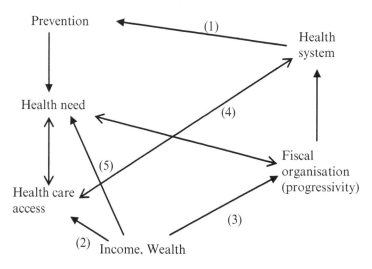

Source: Author's elaboration.

Figure 1.1   Sources of health inequalities

means that more affluent individuals along with those with higher social participation and position in a society influence access to health production inputs. Income and economic affluence influence individuals' budget restrictions; moreover, sources of income determine access to enabling inputs such as education, which, in turn, affect health.

Most of this association is dynamic, influenced by unobserved factors; often we barely observe changes over time. The *Marmot Review* (Marmot, 2009, p. 3) established that inequalities in health result from a combination of material goods, social status and participation, as well as education and housing, as follows: 'Inequalities in social determinants closely relate to health inequalities – the more unequal income distribution, educational outcomes, and housing quality are, for instance, the more unequal health is.'

The review refers to the so-called absolute hypothesis, where absolute income and material condition are argued to affect health. Parallel to this, Wilkinson (1996, 1997) developed an alternative explanation for health inequalities based on the effect that inequalities in income exert on the health status of individuals.

Longitudinal studies seem to point towards evidence for the 'absolute-income hypothesis' (Gerdtham and Johannesson, 2004); the explanations are not mutually exclusive and suggest that to reduce inequalities in health, it may be important to design interventions that address both psychosocial and purely material health production determinants.

None the less, not all inequalities in health are determined by socioeconomic position (Le Grand, 1987), which implies that inequalities should be clearly distinguished from inequities. Even when they are, not all of the causes of social inequalities in health can be 'avoided' by (usually short-term) public policy interventions in individual health production processes. Some inequalities are not under individual or public authority control – for instance inequalities resulting from the depreciation of health capital over time; the same would apply to biologically driven gender differences in health (Wagstaff et al., 1991), or environmental or generic features.

The health economic and policy literature has documented that inequalities favouring the better-off exist in all European countries, both with respect to the use of health care and with respect to the distribution of health itself, and that the degree of inequality is particularly associated with education, income and job status (Hernández-Quevedo et al., 2006, 2008). Although health deteriorates with age and is a function of the socioeconomic status of the individual, the exact nature of this union is complex and controversial. An important source of debate is the association between health and socioeconomic status, in particular health and education (see Grossman, 2000; Smith, 2004); and health and income or wealth (see, e.g., Smith, 1999, 2004). A positive relationship between health and socioeconomic status is widely documented across many societies and periods (see, e.g., Smith, 1999; Deaton, 2003). But the causal mechanisms underlying this relationship are complex and controversial. Socioeconomic status can influence health through the direct influence of material deprivation on the health production function and on the access to health care, or of education on the take-up and compliance with medical treatments; health may influence socioeconomic status through the impact of health shocks on labour market outcomes, such as unemployment, early retirement (Bound, 1991; Disney et al., 2006) and earnings (Contoyannis and Rice, 2001). In addition, it has been argued that this association between health and socioeconomic status could be due to 'third factors', such as time preference rates, that do not imply any causal relationship (Hernández-Quevedo et al., 2008).

3.   MEASUREMENT BASICS

Inequality is in itself a measure of relative dispersion that can be identified visually by comparing extremes on a distribution, but it confronts severe difficulties when it comes to finding ways to compare two country distributions over time and space. One way to measure the intensity of this dispersion of individuals' health status, along with societal income distribution, is by exploring income-related inequality indices over time and over different health dimensions, and its potential origins, including health care use and health care payments, among other health system barriers. This information is a key tenet of health system evaluation in respect of one of the key health policy goals, along with efficiency and quality, especially in Western countries where individuals are inequality averse. Methods based on concentration curves and concentration indices have been extensively used to measure inequalities and inequities in health (Wagstaff and van Doorslaer, 2000). The main advantages of the concentration indices are the following: they capture the socioeconomic dimension of inequalities in health and the information of the whole distribution; they can be represented graphically through the concentration curve; and they allow checks of dominance (Wagstaff et al., 1991).

The concentration index (CI) is derived from the concentration curve (CC). This is illustrated in Figure 1.2 for a measure of ill health. The sample of interest is ranked by socioeconomic status. If individuals are ranked by income level, the horizontal axis begins with the poorest individual and progresses through the income distribution up to the richest individual. This relative income rank is then plotted against the cumulative

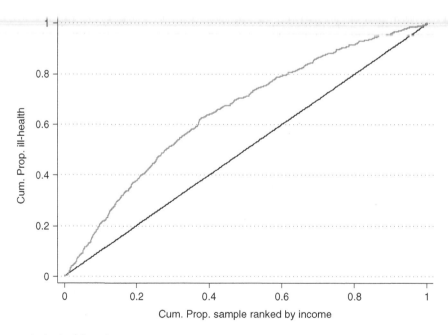

Source: Author's elaboration.

Figure 1.2   Concentration curve for ill health

proportion of ill health on the vertical axis. Along the 45-degree line, the line of perfect equality, the population shares of illness are proportional to income (e.g. the poorest 20 per cent of individuals experience 20 per cent of the illness in the population). Figure 1.2 shows a 'pro-poor' distribution of ill health, where the poorest 20 per cent of income earners experience more than 20 per cent of illnesses. The size of inequality can be summarised by the health concentration index, which is given by twice the area between the concentration curve and the 45-degree line.

There are various ways of expressing the CI algebraically. The one that is mostly used in the literature for its convenience is:

$$\text{CI} = \frac{2}{\mu}\sum_{i=1}^{N}(h_i - \mu)\left(R_i - \frac{1}{2}\right) = \frac{2}{\mu}\text{cov}(h_i, R_i) \tag{1.1}$$

This shows that the value of the CI is a measure of association between individual health (h_i) and the individual's relative rank (R_i), scaled by the mean of health in the population (μ). The whole expression is multiplied by 2, to ensure that the CI ranges between -1 and $+1$. Equation (1.1) indicates that the CI is a measure of the degree of association between an individual's level of health and their relative position in the income distribution. It is important to highlight that a value of CI = 0 does not mean absence of inequality, but an absence of the socioeconomic gradient in the distribution – that is, an absence of inequality associated with the socioeconomic characteristics.

The CI has been recently redesigned by Erreygers (2009) in order to overcome several of its limitations and, for example, to allow for comparisons of populations with different levels of mean health, which was problematic using the CI defined in expression (1.1) (Wagstaff, 2005). Extensions of this index, such as the Index of Health Achievement (Wagstaff, 2002), allow the incorporation of the trade-off between equity and efficiency (measured as the prevalence of ill health in the population). Moreover, some steps have been taken to show that the CI could be calculated following a longitudinal dimension, hence taking into account the history of the individual (Jones and López-Nicolás, 2004). Further, the CI can be decomposed into the contributions of individual factors to income-related health inequality, in which each contribution is the product of the sensitivity of health with respect to that factor and the degree of income-related inequality in that particular factor (Wagstaff et al., 2003).[1]

4.   DATA REQUIREMENTS

4.1   Health Measures

Health variables
When analysing equity in outcomes at the individual level, different health outcome measures have been used in the literature, from subjective measures of health such as self-assessed health (e.g. Nummela et al., 2007) and quasi-objective indicators of health status such as the SF-36 physical functioning score (e.g. Marmot et al., 2005), indicators of specific illnesses such as coronary heart disease (e.g. Hemmingsson and Lundberg, 2005), limiting longstanding illness (e.g. Eikemo et al., 2008), body mass index (e.g.

BOX 1.1   HEALTH MEASURES EMPLOYED

- Subjective health
    - Self-reported health
        - Adaptation effects
        - Ordered effects
        - Combination with quality of life
    - Visual analogue scale
    - Quality of life (SF-36 etc.)
- Objective health
    - Morbidity
    - Lifestyles
        - Smoking
        - Obesity

Kopp and Rethelyi, 2004), and mental health problems (García-Álvarez et al., 2007), to more objective measures of health such as biological markers (Johnston et al., 2007). At an aggregated level, health population variables have been used such as life expectancy (Regidor et al., 2003), quality-adjusted life years (e.g. Gerdtham and Johannesson, 2000; Burström et al., 2005) and disability-free life expectancy (Matthews et al., 2006). Given the data requirements for the analysis of socioeconomic inequalities in such population health measures, most of the literature on socioeconomic inequality is based on individual health indicators.

Box 1.1 summarises different health measures classified into different groups including objective and subjective variables. Equity for these outcomes has been studied according to social class (Kelleher et al., 2003), self-reported education (Silventoinen et al., 2005) and disposable household income (Nummela et al., 2007), mainly.

Self-assessed health is the most common subjective measure of individual health, providing an ordinal ranking of perceived health status that is generally available in socioeconomic surveys at both national and international level. The usual health question asks the respondent to rate their general health, sometimes including a time reference (individuals are asked to rate their health in the last 12 months) or an age benchmark (respondents are asked about their current health compared to that of individuals of their own age). Five categories are usually available for the respondent, ranging from very good or excellent to poor or very poor.

Self-assessed health in the literature has been used in studies on the relationship between health and socioeconomic status (Adams et al., 2003; Benzeval et al., 2000; Deaton and Paxson, 1998; Ettner, 1996; Frijters et al., 2005; Salas, 2002; Smith, 1999), the relationship between health and lifestyles (Kenkel, 1995; Contoyannis and Jones, 2004) and the analysis of socioeconomic inequalities in self-assessed health (van Doorslaer et al., 1997). Some interesting results have been found: it is a powerful predictor of subsequent mortality (Idler and Kasl, 1995; Idler and Benyamini, 1997); its predictive power does not vary across socioeconomic groups (Burström and Fredlund, 2001); it is a good predictor of subsequent use of medical care (van Doorslaer et al., 2000) and a good predictor of inequalities in mortality (van Doorslaer and Gerdtham, 2003). Together with the self-reported measure of health, more objective measures are included in the general surveys to identify those individuals who are hampered in daily activity or suffering a variety of chronic conditions.

This subjective measure of health has caused debate in the literature concerning its validity. It has been argued that perceived health does not correspond to actual health (see Bound, 1991), while other researchers have regarded this variable as a valid indicator of true health (see Butler et al., 1987). As a self-reported subjective measure of health, self-assessed health may be prone to measurement error.

Reporting bias
Reporting bias has been a concern in the literature and can be defined as the differential reporting of health across individuals or groups of individuals with the same health status. The systematic use of different threshold levels by sub-groups of a population reflects the existence of reporting bias. This source of measurement error has been termed 'state-dependent reporting bias' (Kerkhofs and Lindeboom, 1995), 'scale of reference bias' (Groot, 2000) and 'response category cut-point shift' (Sadana et al., 2000; Murray et al., 2001). This occurs if sub-groups of the population use systematically different cut-point levels when reporting their self-assessed health, despite having the same level of 'true health'. These differences may be influenced by, among other things, age, gender, education, income, language and personal experience of illness. Basically, it means that different groups appear to interpret the question within their own specific context and therefore use different reference points when they are responding to the same question. It has been shown by Bago d'Uva et al. (2008) that correcting for reporting differences generally increases education-related inequalities in health.

Various approaches have been developed to correct for reporting bias in the literature. The first is to condition on a set of objective indicators of health and argue that any remaining variation in self-assessed health reflects reporting bias. For example, Lindeboom and van Doorslaer (2004) use Canadian data and the McMaster Health Utility Index as their quasi-objective measure of health, finding some evidence of reporting bias by age and gender, but not for income. However, this approach relies on having a sufficiently comprehensive set of objective indicators to capture all the variation in true health. The second approach uses health vignettes such as those currently included in the World Health Survey (Kapteyn et al., 2004; Murray et al., 2001; Bago d'Uva et al., 2008). The third examines biological markers of disease risk in the countries considered for comparison. Studies such as Banks et al. (2006) combine self-reported data with biological data, which could result in less ambiguous results. Also Johnston et al. (2007) report that the income gradient appears significant when using an objective measure of hypertension measured by a nurse rather than the self-reported measure of hypertension included in the Household Survey of England.

Objective measures such as physicians' assessments or hospital stays are best for comparative purposes, because individuals tend to evaluate their own health relative to that of their peers. If one group is characterised by a lower level of objective health, subjective assessments made in reference to different peer groups will mask this differential.

However, the availability of objective measures of health, such as biomarkers, is limited. First, their availability is restricted to very specific national surveys. At the

European level, neither the European Community Household Panel Survey (ECHP) nor the European Union Survey of Income and Leaving Conditions (EU-SILC) include objective measures, only self-reports. Only the Survey of Health, Ageing and Retirement in Europe (SHARE) and the forthcoming European Health Interview Survey include objective (e.g. walking speed, grip strength) and quasi-objective (e.g. activities of daily living, symptoms) measures of health. At national level, only few countries include objective measures, such as Finland (blood tests and anthropometric tests – FINRISK), Germany (anthropometric measures – National Health Interview and Examination Survey; urine and blood samples – German Health Survey for Children and Adolescents) and the UK – English Longitudinal Study of Ageing (ELSA) and Health Survey of England (HSE).

Together with their limited availability, biomarkers may still be subject to bias and are not included in longitudinal data. The main methodological challenge lies with the standardisation of data collection, as variations may arise from different methods of collection. For example, a person's blood pressure may vary according to the time of day it is taken. In fact, information on the details of objective health data collection is not often provided. This measurement error is particularly problematic if it is correlated with sociodemographic characteristics, hence biasing estimates of social inequalities. Collecting biological data also tends to reduce survey response rates, which limits the sample size and their representativeness (Masseria et al., 2007). The limitation of biological markers to cross-sectional data is an important disadvantage since longitudinal data allow the exploration of the dynamic relationship between health, socioeconomic status and access to health care (Hernández-Quevedo et al., 2008).

4.2   Measuring the Socioeconomic Gradient

Box 1.2 describes different potential sources of a socioeconomic gradient that might well differ across the individual's life cycle (e.g. those early in the cycle rely more on their wealth than on income). Normally, studies employ a measure of income but fail to account for measures of wealth in computing the socioeconomic position ranking to then estimate a concentration index. Normally, income data employed are current income, although a few studies have managed to disentangle the effect of permanent income. Similarly, in measuring the effect of wealth, different sources of wealth such as savings and housing wealth traditionally exert different effects in that some are more liquid and easy to transform into income. Finally, other important factors that are associated with income and not all studies control for are knowledge and social environment.

4.3   Data Sets

The main data sets analysed to measure equity in health at the European level are the Statistics on Income and Living Conditions (EU-SILC) and the European Community Household Panel (ECHP), both provided by Eurostat, which are general socioeconomic data sets that favour cross-country analysis, together with health national surveys such as the British Household Panel Survey. The World Health Survey also includes a self-reported measure of health and health in eight domains, such as mobility, self-care, pain and discomfort, cognition, interpersonal activities, vision, sleep and energy,

---

BOX 1.2   SOURCES OF THE SOCIOECONOMIC VECTOR

- Current income $(Y = Y_p + Y_e)$
  - Permanent income (Y_p)
  - Non-permanent income (Y_e)
- Wealth $(W = S + H + F)$
  - Savings wealth (S)
  - Housing wealth (H)
  - Financial wealth (F)
  - Inherited wealth (I)
- Knowledge (K)
  - Education
  - Ability
    Informal knowledge
  - Health knowledge
- Environmental effects (E)
  - Personal environment (individual effects)
    - Marriage
  - Neighbourhood effects (contextual effects)
  - Peer effects (endogenous effects)
    - Social interactions

---

and affect. This, together with information on sociodemographic characteristics of the individual (age, sex, height, weight, education, employment status, main occupation and ethnicity), allows analysing the level of equity in health for health care. Further, the Commonwealth Fund International Health Policy Survey is one of the main cross-national surveys beyond Europe that collects information on socioeconomic inequalities in health. In addition, the SHARE data are used for measuring equity in health for the elderly (Dalstra et al., 2006). However, the lack of data sets that provide a longitudinal perspective shows the limitations of the current evidence on inequalities in health and the policies related to policy making, if policy makers are interested in the health history of the individual. One of the areas where there is a limited record is that of environmental influence in health production. To date, limited or no evidence has been recorded on how sensitive inequalities are to the inclusion of environmental effects.

4.4   Recent Key Findings from the Literature

International studies on the socioeconomic determinants of health are a helpful tool to identify the patterns of socioeconomic health inequalities in Europe. Cross-country analysis of both education and income-related inequalities in health outcomes have been provided in the literature at European level, and are referenced in this section.

Large education-related inequalities in self-assessed health have been observed at the European level, finding that large socioeconomic inequalities in self-reported health status still persist at the European level (Kunst et al., 2005). Besides, education-related inequalities have been found in Europe in common chronic diseases: high inequalities favouring the better-off are observed for stroke, diseases of the nervous system, diabetes and arthritis (Dalstra et al., 2005). The size of these socioeconomic differences in chronic diseases has been found to decrease with age. Moreover, countries in the Scandinavian welfare regime have been placed less favourably regarding education-related inequalities in health than those in the Anglo-Saxon and Eastern European regimes, with only Sweden showing relatively small education-related inequalities in health (Eikemo et al., 2008).

In terms of income-related inequalities in health, it has been shown at the European level that an increase in income is associated with improvements in self-assessed health status at the individual level (Mackenbach et al., 2005). Adult socioeconomic status (SES) shows stronger association with self-rated health than childhood SES. There are both gender and national differences in the association between childhood and adulthood SES (Hyde et al., 2006). Besides, quality of life is associated with socioeconomic position, but the associations vary by country (Knesebeck et al., 2007). Socioeconomic differences in self-assessed health status have also been found in Eastern European countries such as Russia, Estonia, Lithuania, Latvia, Hungary, Poland and the Czech Republic. The main findings, which identify education and material deprivation as important determinants of health status, are not dissimilar from those in the EU-15 (Bobak et al., 2000).

Using longitudinal data, Hernández-Quevedo et al. (2006) found evidence of long-run income inequalities for the eight waves covered by the ECHP (1994–2001) in health limitations in daily activity in 14 EU member states, with health limitations concentrated in those individuals at the bottom of the income distribution. The study also found that downwardly income-mobile individuals are more likely to suffer any limitation in daily activity due to their health status than upwardly mobile individuals. Earlier evidence has shown similar findings for the EU (van Doorslaer et al., 1997; van Doorslaer and Koolman, 2004).

Other studies have analysed inequalities in other health outcomes, such as obesity, smoking or screening. According to the latest literature on obesity, the prevalence of obese individuals in the EU-15 varies with age, education, SES, marital status and smoking behaviour. Individuals in lower socioeconomic groups are more likely to be obese, as well as those individuals with low educational attainments (Costa-Font and Gil, 2008). Regarding smoking, education and income are strong predictors of smoking in Finland, Denmark, Ireland, the UK, Belgium, Germany, Austria, Italy, Spain, Portugal and Greece (Huisman et al., 2005). Evidence of education-related inequalities in smoking prevalence has also been found in Estonia, Latvia, Lithuania and Finland (Helasoja et al., 2006).

Current research still suffers from major shortcomings, including: (i) limited understanding of the factors explaining the health production process and sources of inequalities, including the role of mental conditions along with cognitive biases in measuring self-reported health; (ii) crude measures of health outcomes and health care use, though increasing availability of genetic markers and more 'objective' measures of health allow to account for this; and, finally, (iii) inadequate identification of what stands behind measures of socioeconomic position, namely different income sources and measures of wealth and social environmental controls. The effects of the latter differ across the life cycle.

5.   POLICY IMPLICATIONS AND ACTIONS

5.1   The Role of the World Health Organization and the European Union

There is a growing role for reducing socioeconomic inequalities in health in the agenda of the EU member states, given the enlargement of the EU and the ageing population. Together with the governments from the new member states, international organisations such as the World Health Organization and the EU have played an important role in providing a framework and the principles to encourage action in many countries.

The World Health Organization, in the Health For All Policy Framework for the WHO European Region, has provided a set of quantitative objectives known as 'Health21', which should be achieved by 2020. Several countries that are concerned with inequalities in health, but that do not have a national agenda in this regard, have followed their recommendations (e.g. the Czech Republic, Latvia, Lithuania). The 'Health21' document highlighted the need to pay attention to reducing differences in health status between and within member states. The policy framework set out a number of proposed targets, such as: by the year 2020, the health gap between socioeconomic groups within countries should be reduced by at least one-quarter in all member states, by substantially improving the level of health of disadvantaged groups. In particular: the gap in life expectancy between socioeconomic groups should be reduced by at least 25 per cent. Moreover, the creation of the Commission on Social Determinants of Health by the World Health Organization can be highlighted. Its final report (WHO, 2008) recognises the poor health of the poor, the social gradient in health within countries and the existence of health inequities between countries, and provides a guide to measures to achieve equity in health.

EU member states have also recently committed themselves to set up national action plans to combat poverty and social exclusion. As a key component of this process, Atkinson et al. (2002) set out recommendations for the development of indicators of social inclusion in the EU. These were developed in response to the 2000 Lisbon European Council meeting's resolution to 'promote a better understanding of social exclusion through continued dialogue and exchanges of information and best practice, on the basis of commonly agreed indicators'. At the special European summit in Lisbon in March 2000, social policy was explicitly introduced for the first time as a distinct focus of attention for European cooperation. It was agreed that common objectives for eradication of poverty and social exclusion would be adopted, that national policies would be designed to meet these, and that progress would be monitored. As a result of this trend towards European social policy harmonisation, cross-country comparative information on social inequalities and exclusion (in terms of health or other dimensions) has gained additional relevance in Europe.

However, there is heterogeneity in the approaches considered by the EU member states when tackling inequalities in health and equity in health care systems. There are countries with legislative commitments, approving laws with specific references to health inequalities (e.g. Greece, Germany); countries with general goals, presenting evidence of commitment to health equity but not setting quantitative targets (e.g. Denmark, France, Hungary, Italy, Norway, Poland, the Slovak Republic, Sweden); and, finally, those countries that include quantitative targets, either specified by international organisations such as the World Health Organization (the Czech Republic, Latvia, Lithuania) or by their own national policy (Ireland, the UK, Finland, the Netherlands) (see Dahlgren and Whitehead, 2006).

5.2   Potential Policy Actions

The Social Determinants of Health Commission (WHO, 2008) concludes that action on the social determinants of health must involve the whole of government, civil society and local communities, business and international agencies. In fact, policies and programmes should include all key sectors of society, not just the health sector. Three broad sets of recommendations are suggested to close the gap in health inequities. These are: improv-ing daily living conditions, that is, housing, early child development, health care and social protection; tackling the unequal distribution of resources; and, finally, measuring and understanding the problem.

None the less, a focus on many potential areas may lead to a reduction of health inequalities. Among these are the following:

- *Health-related behaviours* (smoking, alcohol consumption, diet, obesity), which call for actions to tackle inequalities in health prevention. It is not clear what measures should be employed, although current developments along the lines of libertarian paternalism are currently being taken into consideration to ground policy actions.
- *Psychosocial factors* (psychosocial stressors) along with the extent to which stress and anxiety have a specific social gradient consistent with theories of relative income inequality (Wilkinson, 1998). If anxiety and stress are more prevalent among lower-income groups due to tighter lifestyle restrictions, it is conceivable that an income gradient might arise in physical health given the interaction of mental and physical health co-morbidities.
- *Environmental determinants* (social support, social integration), particularly the extent to which individuals' information updating and personal and social support are driven by a specific income vector. If access to health information is subject to an income gradient, then more affluent individuals will inevitably have better access to health production factors, which translates into better health.
- *Material factors* (housing conditions, working conditions, financial problems), and generally speaking the existence of income inequalities and a socioeconomic vector in the access to other merit goods such as housing.
- *Access to health care* (access to good-quality services). The organisation of the health system can determine the extent to which individuals have access to health care in the event of need and, especially, what percentage of their income will be needed for health care.
- *Attitudes towards the distribution of health and health care.* Most European coun- tries have explicit public health policies addressing some or all of these areas. However, countries might well differ in their aversion to health inequalities, which might explain why some have higher inequalities than others. On the other hand, lower aversion to health inequalities implies that health inequality will rank as less

of a policy priority in governmental decision making, and that individuals and political institutions will not use this evidence in health care discussions.

Other more recent policy debates refer to whether the population-based approach or the vulnerable populations approaches are complementary or contradictory. While some authors argue that focusing on vulnerable populations as a target for public health interventions should be a complement to the population-based approach, other authors, such as Rose et al. (2008), argue that there are problems when designing policies that focus on the vulnerable: first, the definition of being vulnerable requires setting an arbitrary cut-off point; and second, it may be that the level of the intervention should be the whole of the society.

Finally, it is important not to dismiss the theoretical debate on the source of health inequalities – in particular, the absolute-income hypothesis suggesting that income itself is the direct determinant of health distribution, or the relative-income hypothesis that would indicate instead that the hierarchy of individuals in the income distribution affects mental health, which in turn influences income (Wilkinson, 1998). However, recent evidence from Gerdtham and Johannesson (2004) suggests that the former seems to hold.

6.   KEY CHALLENGES

In understanding the existing evidence suggesting that inequalities are persistent over time, we might need to develop further evidence on what the underlying sources of health inequalities are, and whether attitudes towards inequalities in health vary over time. Regarding sources of health inequalities, it is important to mention that inequalities might result from changes in the distribution and are sensitive to improvement at the extremes, namely the relatively richer (poor) becoming less (more) healthy, or due to distributional changes in the middle. Whether one or the other takes place, it might well be the result of different factors mentioned in this chapter. Evidence seems to suggest some success in overcoming the first source of inequality, with poorer population cohorts getting healthier. However, some persistence remains in many countries where welfare states are more established, which have achieved some diminishing returns in health production (Preston, 1975). The latter suggests that health inequalities might arguably be the result of limited distribution variation in the middle of the health distribution. More recent evidence by van Ourti et al. (2009) suggests that economic growth might be a source of health inequalities if income elasticity of health increases over income quintiles. Evidence from the majority of European countries suggests no variation in income elasticities, which is argued to explain the stability of health inequalities.

Some of the challenges in developing effective strategies in many countries centre on the limited availability of data on health and health inequalities, lack of political will and fiscal pressures limiting the resources available for implementing strategies. Overall, more needs to be done across the EU in developing coherent and effective strategies to reduce health inequalities. Furthermore, although some tools have been developed, there is a need to greatly increase the evidence base of which policies are achieving a reduction in inequalities, as pioneered in the Netherlands at local level, and to communicate this research at an international level.

One of the biggest challenges for policy makers is to assess the impact of their policies on health inequalities: plenty of good-quality evidence to guide policy; new and more consistent data for comparative national-level analysis; and well-designed evaluative studies would be ideal, particularly those taking advantage of natural experiments (changes in employment opportunities, housing provision or cigarette pricing for example).

NOTE

1. A detailed guide of the calculation of the CI and its latest extensions can be found in O'Donnell et al. (2008).

REFERENCES

Adams, P., M.D. Hurd, D. McFadden, A. Merrill and T. Ribeiro (2003), 'Healthy, wealthy and wise. Tests for direct causal paths between health and socioeconomic status', *Journal of Econometrics*, **112**, 3–56.

Atkinson, A., B. Cantillon, E. Marlier and B. Nolan (2002), *Social Indicators: The EU and Social Inclusion*, Oxford: Oxford University Press.

Bago d'Uva, T., E. van Doorslaer, M. Lindeboom and O. O'Donnell (2008), 'Does reporting heterogeneity bias the measurement of health disparities?', *Health Economics*, **17**(3), 351–75.

Banks, J., M. Marmot, Z. Oldfield and J.P. Smith (2006), 'Disease and disadvantage in the United States and England', *Journal of the American Medical Association*, **295**(17), 2037–45.

Benzeval, M., J. Taylor and K. Judge (2000), 'Evidence on the relationship between low income and poor health: is the government doing enough?', *Fiscal Studies*, **21**, 375–99.

Bobak, M., H. Pikhart, R. Rose, C. Hertzman, M. Marmot (2000), 'Socioeconomic factors, material inequalities, and perceived control in self-rated health: cross-sectional data from seven post-communist countries', *Social Science & Medicine*, **51**, 1343–50.

Bound, J. (1991), 'Self-reported versus objective measures of health in retirement models', *Journal of Human Resources*, **26**, 106–38.

Burström, B. and P. Fredlund (2001), 'Self-rated health: is it as good a predictor of subsequent mortality among adults in lower as well as in higher social classes?', *Journal of Epidemiology and Community Health*, **55**, 836–40.

Burström, K., M. Johannesson and F. Diderichsen (2005), 'Increasing socio-economic inequalities in life expectancy and QALYs in Sweden 1980–1997', *Health Economics*, **14**(8), 831–50.

Butler, J.S., R.V. Burkhauser, J.M. Mitchell and T.P. Pincus (1987), 'Measurement error in self-reported health variables', *The Review of Economics and Statistics*, **69**(4), 644–50.

Contoyannis, P. and A. Jones (2004), 'Socio-economic status, health and lifestyle', *Journal of Health Economics*, **23**, 965–95.

Contoyannis, P. and N. Rice (2001), 'The impact of health on wages: evidence from the British Household Panel Survey', *Empirical Economics*, **26**, 599–622.

Costa-Font, Joan and J. Gil (2008), 'What lies behind socio-economic inequalities in obesity in Spain: a decomposition approach', *Food Policy*, **33**(1), 61–73.

Dahlgren, G. and M. Whitehead (2006), *European Strategies for Tackling Social Inequities in Health: Levelling up. Part 2*, Copenhagen: WHO Regional Office for Europe.

Dalstra, J.A., A.E. Kunst, C. Borrell, E. Breeze, E. Cambois, G. Costa, J.J.M. Geurts, E. Lahelma, V.H. Oyen, N.K. Rasmuszen, E. Reejidor, T. Spadea and J.P. Mackenbach (2005), 'Socioeconomic differences in the prevalence of common chronic diseases: an overview of eight European countries', *International Journal of Epidemiology*, **34**(2), 316–26.

Dalstra, J., A. Kunst and J. Mackenback (2006), 'A comparative appraisal of the relationship of education, income and housing tenure with less than good health among the elderly in Europe', *Social Science and Medicine*, **62**, 2046–60.

Deaton, A.S. (2003), 'Health, inequality, and economic development', *Journal of Economic Literature*, **XLI**, 113–58.

Deaton, A.S. and C.H. Paxson (1998), 'Aging and inequality in income and health', *The American Economic Review*, **88**, 248–53.

Disney, R., C. Emmerson and M. Wakefield (2006), 'Ill-health and retirement in Britain: a panel data-based analysis', *Journal of Health Economics*, **25**, 621–49.

Eikemo, T.A., M. Huisman, C. Bambra and A.E. Kunst (2008), 'Health inequalities according to educational level in different welfare regimes: a comparison of 23 European countries', *Sociology of Health & Illness*, **30**(4), 565–82.

Erreygers, G. (2009), 'Correcting the Concentration Index', *Journal of Health Economics*, **28**(2), 504–15.

Ettner, S.L. (1996), 'New evidence on the relationship between income and health', *Journal of Health Economics*, **15**, 67–85.

Frijters, P., J.P. Haisken-DeNew and M.A. Shields (2005), 'The causal effect of income on health: evidence from German reunification', *Journal of Health Economics*, **24**, 997–1017.

García-Álvarez, A., L. Serra-Majem, L. Ribas-Barba, C. Castell, M. Foz, R. Uauy, A. Plasencia and L. Salleras (2007), 'Obesity and overweight trends in Catalonia, Spain (1992–2003): gender and socioeconomic determinants', *Public Health Nutrition*, **10**(11A), 1368–78.

Gerdtham, U.-G. and M. Johannesson (2000), 'Income-related inequality in life-years and quality-adjusted life-years in Sweden', *Journal of Health Economics*, **19**, 1007–26.

Gerdtham, U.-G. and M. Johannesson (2004), 'Absolute income, relative income, income inequality and mortality', *Journal of Human Resources*, **39**(1), 228–44.

Groot, W. (2000), 'Adaptation and scale of reference bias in self-assessments of quality of life', *Journal of Health Economics*, **19**(3), 403–20.

Grossman, M. (2000), 'The human capital model', in A.J. Culyer and J.P. Newhouse (eds), *Handbook of Health Economics*, Amsterdam: Elsevier, pp. 347–408.

Helasoja, V. et al. (2006), 'Trends in the magnitude of educational inequalities in health in Estonia, Latvia, Lithuania and Finland during 1994–2004', *Public Health*, **120**(9), 841–53.

Hemmingsson, T. and I. Lundberg (2005), 'How far are socioeconomic differences in coronary heart disease hospitalisation, all-cause mortality and cardiovascular mortality among adult Swedish males attributable to negative childhood circumstances and behaviour in adolescence?', *International Journal of Epidemiology*, **34**(2), 260–67.

Hernández-Quevedo, C., A.M. Jones, Á. López-Nicolás and N. Rice (2006), 'Socioeconomic inequalities in health: a comparative longitudinal analysis using the European Community Household Panel', *Social Science and Medicine*, **63**(5), 1246–61.

Hernández-Quevedo, C., A.M. Jones and N. Rice (2008), 'Persistence in health limitations: a European comparative analysis', *Journal of Health Economics*, **27**(6), 1472–88.

House of Commons Health Committee (2009), *Health Inequalities. Third Report of Session 2008–2009*, London: The Stationery Office Limited.

Huisman, M., A.E. Kunst and J.P. Mackenbach (2005), 'Educational inequalities in smoking among men and women aged 16 years and older in 11 European countries', *Tobacco Control*, **14**, 106–13.

Hyde, M., H. Jakub, M. Melchior, F. van Oort and S. Weyers (2006), 'Comparison of the effects of low childhood socioeconomic position and low adulthood socioeconomic position on self-rated health in four European studies', *Journal of Epidemiology and Community Health*, **60**, 882–6.

Idler, E.L. and Y. Benyamini (1997), 'Self-rated health and mortality: a review of twenty-seven community studies', *Journal of Health and Social Behavior*, **38**(1), 21–37.

Idler, E.L. and S.V. Kasl (1995), 'Self-ratings of health: do they also predict change in functional ability?', *Journal of Gerontology*, **50B**, S344–S353.

Johnston, D.W., C. Propper and M.A. Shields (2007), 'Comparing subjective and objective measures of health: evidence from hypertension for the income/health gradient', IZA Discussion Paper No. 2737, Bonn: Institute for the Study of Labour.

Jones, A.M. and Á. López-Nicolás (2004), 'Measurement and explanation of socioeconomic inequality in health with longitudinal data', *Health Economics*, **13**, 1015–30.

Kapteyn, A., J.P. Smith and A. van Soest (2004), 'Self-reported work disability in the US and the Netherlands', RAND Labor and Population Working Paper, Santa Monica, CA: RAND Corporation.

Kelleher, C.C., S. Friel, S.N. Gabhainn et al. (2003), 'Socio-demographic predictors of self-rated health in the Republic of Ireland: findings from the National Survey on Lifestyle, Attitudes and Nutrition (SLAN)', *Social Science and Medicine*, **57**(3), 477–86.

Kenkel, D. (1995), 'Should you eat breakfast? Estimates form health production functions', *Health Economics*, **4**, 15–29.

Kerkhofs, M. and M. Lindeboom (1995), 'Subjective health measures and state dependent reporting errors', *Health Economics*, **4**, 221–35.

Knesebeck, O., M. Wahrendorf, M. Hyde and J. Siegrist (2007), 'Socio-economic position and quality of life among older people in 10 European countries: results of the SHARE Study', *Ageing and Society*, **27**, 269–84.

Kopp, M.S. and J. Rethelyi (2004), 'Where psychology meets physiology: chronic stress and premature mortality – the Central-Eastern European health paradox', *Brain Research Bulletin*, **62**(5), 351–67.

Kunst, A.E. et al. (2005), 'Trends in socioeconomic inequalities in self-assessed health in 10 European countries', *International Journal of Epidemiology*, **34**(2), 295–305.

Le Grand, J. (1987), 'Inequalities in health: some international comparisons', *European Economic Review*, **31**, 182–91.

Lindeboom, M. and E. van Doorslaer (2004), 'Cut-point shift and index shift in self-reported health', *Journal of Health Economics*, **23**, 1083–99.

Mackenbach, J.P., P. Martikainen, C.W.N. Looman, J.A.A. Dalstra, A.E. Kunst, E. Lahelma and members of the SedHA working group (2005), 'The shape of the relationship between income and self-assessed health: an international study', *International Journal of Epidemiology*, **34**, 286–93.

Marmot, M. (2000), 'Inequalities in health: causes and policy implications', in A.R.S. Tarlov (ed.), *The Society and Population Health Reader: A State and Community Perspective*, New York: The New Press, pp. 293–309.

Marmot, M. (2002), 'The influence of income on health: views of an epidemiologist', *Health Affairs*, **21**(2), 31–46.

Marmot, M. (2009), *Marmot Review: First Phase Report*, June. Strategic review of health inequalities in England post 2010, London: Department of Health.

Marmot, M. et al. (2005), 'Social determinants of health inequalities', *Lancet*, **365**, 1099–104.

Masseria, C., S. Allin, C. Sorenson, I. Papanicolas and E. Mossialos (2007), 'What are the methodological issues related to measuring health and drawing comparisons across countries? A research note', Methodological note, Brussels: DG Employment and Social Affairs, European Observatory on the Social Situation and Demography.

Matthews, R.J., C. Jagger and R.M. Hancock (2006), 'Does socioeconomic advantage lead to a longer, healthier old age?', *Social Science and Medicine*, **62**, 2489–99.

Murray, C.J.L., A. Tandon, J. Salomon and C.D. Mathers (2001), 'Enhancing cross-population comparability of survey results', GPE Discussion Paper No. 35, Geneva: WHO/EIP.

Nummela, O.P., T.T. Sulander, H.S. Heinonen et al. (2007), 'Self-rated health and indicators of SES among the ageing in three types of communities', *Scandinavian Journal of Public Health*, **35**(1), 39–47.

O'Donnell, O., E. van Doorslaer, A. Wagstaff and M. Lindelow (2008), *Analyzing Health Equity Using Household Survey Data: A Guide to Techniques and their Implementation*, Washington, DC: The World Bank.

Oliver, A. and E. Mossialos (2004), 'Equity of access to health care: outlining the foundation for action', *Journal of Epidemiology and Community Health*, **58**(8), 655–8.

Preston, S.H. (1975), 'The changing relation between mortality and level of economic development', *Population Studies*, **29**(2), 231–48.

Regidor, E., M.E. Calle, P. Navarro et al. (2003), 'Trends in the association between average income, poverty and income inequality and life expectancy in Spain', *Social Science & Medicine*, **56**(5), 961–71.

Rose, G., K.-T. Khaw and M. Marmot (2008), *Rose's Strategy of Preventive Medicine*, Oxford: Oxford University Press.

Sadana, R., C.D. Mathers, A.D. Lopez, C.J.L. Murray and K. Iburg (2000), 'Comparative analysis of more than 50 household surveys on health status', GPE Discussion Paper No. 15, EIP/GPE/EBD, Geneva: World Health Organization.

Salas, C. (2002), 'On the empirical association between poor health and low socioeconomic status at old age', *Health Economics*, **11**, 207–20.

Silventoinen, K., J. Pankow, P. Jousilahti, G. Hu and J. Tuomilehto (2005), 'Educational inequalities in the metabolic syndrome and coronary heart disease among middle-aged men and women', *International Journal of Epidemiology*, **34**(2), 327–34.

Smith, J.P. (1999), 'Healthy bodies and thick wallets', *Journal of Economic Perspectives*, **13**, 145–66.

Smith, J.P. (2004), 'Unravelling the SES health connection', *Aging, Health and Public Policy: Demographic and Economic Perspectives*, **30**, 108–32.

van Doorslaer, E. et al. (1997), 'Income-related inequalities in health: some international comparisons', *Journal of Health Economics*, **16**(1), 93–112.

van Doorslaer, E., et al. (2000), 'Equity in the delivery of health care in Europe and the US', *Journal of Health Economics*, **19**, 553–83.

van Doorslaer, E. and X. Koolman (2004), 'Explaining the differences in income-related health inequalities across European countries', *Health Economics*, **13**, 609–28.

van Doorslaer, E. and U.-G. Gerdtham (2003), 'Does inequality in self-assessed health predict inequality in survival by income? Evidence from Swedish data', *Social Science and Medicine*, **57**, 1621–9.

van Ourti, T., E. van Doorslaer and X. Koolman (2009), 'The effect of income growth and inequality on health inequality: theory and empirical evidence from the European Panel', *Journal of Health Economics*, **28**(3), 525–39.

Wagstaff, A. (2002), 'Inequality aversion, health inequalities and health achievement', *Journal of Health Economics*, **21**, 627–41.

Wagstaff, A. (2005), 'The bounds of the Concentration Index when the variable of interest is binary, with an application to immunization inequality', *Health Economics*, **14**(4), 429–32.

Wagstaff, A. and E. van Doorslaer (2000), 'Measuring and testing for inequity in the delivery of health care', *Journal of Human Resources*, **35**, 716–33.

Wagstaff, A., P. Paci and E. van Doorslaer (1991), 'On the measurement of inequalities in health', *Social Science & Medicine*, **33**(5), 545–7.

Wagstaff, A., E. van Doorslaer and N. Watanabe (2003), 'On decomposing the causes of health sector inequalities with an application to malnutrition inequalities in Vietnam', *Journal of Econometrics*, **112**, 207–23.

Wilkinson, R. (1996), *Unhealthy Societies: The Affliction of Inequality*, London: Routledge.

Wilkinson, R. (1997), 'Health inequalities: relative or absolute material standards', *British Medical Journal*, **314**(7080), 591–5.

Wilkinson, R. (1998), 'Low relative income affects mortality', *British Medical Journal*, **316**(7144), 1611–12.

World Health Organization (2000), *The World Health Report: Health Systems: Improving Performance*, Geneva: World Health Organization.

World Health Organization Health Commission on the Social Determinants of Health (2008), 'Closing the gap in a generation: health equity through action on the social determinants of health', Final report on the Commission on the Social Determinants of Health, Geneva: World Health Organization.

2 Strengthening community participation in primary health care: experiences from South Africa
Andrew Gibbs and Catherine Campbell

1. INTRODUCTION

The thirtieth anniversary of the Alma-Ata Declaration (WHO, 1978) generated renewed interest in the role of primary health care (PHC) in achieving universal health and reducing health inequalities (Chan, 2008; McCoy et al., 2008; WHO, 2008). However, profound challenges remain in implementing this approach, particularly in poor countries, which experience the poorest health outcomes and face numerous challenges in delivering health services. This has led to growing calls to analyse the barriers that need tackling to implement PHC more effectively to achieve Alma-Ata's goals.

In this chapter we use a case study to focus on a central pillar of PHC – the participation of communities in efforts to improve their health. This aspect of PHC has typically been poorly implemented (Lawn et al., 2008). Yet without proper community involvement, programmes have little chance of succeeding (Campbell, 2003). This case study emerges from the authors' three-year involvement in documenting the efforts of a university-based NGO (HIVAN) to support the Entabeni Project in KwaZulu-Natal, South Africa – a project seeking to strengthen the work of health volunteers providing home-based care for people living with HIV/AIDS (PLWHA), as well as providing health advice to AIDS-affected households in a remote rural area.

HIVAN was invited to work in partnership with the volunteers after undertaking research into community responses to AIDS in Entabeni. The research highlighted the existence of the volunteers, as well as the difficulties they faced. HIVAN's role was one of external change agent (ECA) – helping the community to access the training and support they needed to operate more effectively. In the Entabeni Project 'community participation' was understood in terms of strengthening the participation of this group of volunteers in local HIV/AIDS management. The volunteers' work constituted a 'bottom-up' project, initiated and staffed by local people (mostly unemployed and poorly educated women) in response to the desperate suffering of people dying of AIDS, often with little or no access to any formal health care. These health volunteers were referred to as 'community health workers' in line with international trends (Campbell and Scott, 2011).

The project sought to improve the level and quality of community participation in the delivery of health care, to improve the reach and quality of PHC services in the community and to form the basis for a wider social development agenda. These two aims were actioned via three goals: (i) training the volunteers to improve the care they provided; (ii) helping volunteers to mobilise greater community support for their work; and (iii) building external support for the volunteers.

This chapter provides an overview of the achievements and challenges the project faced to generate debate about challenges in implementing community participation and highlighting possible strategies to overcome these.

2.   THE ALMA-ATA DECLARATION AND COMMUNITY PARTICIPATION

In 1978, 134 countries signed the Alma-Ata Declaration, recognising the need for primary health care. Community participation was accorded a central role in realising the aims of the Declaration, which emphasised the need for 'maximum community and individual self-reliance and participation in the planning, organisation, operation and control of primary health care' (WHO, 1978, p. 2).

Alongside promoting PHC, the Declaration provided a new political approach to health, reframing health from a biomedical perspective to include an emphasis on health promotion and recognition of how social inequalities shape ill health. In reframing the causes of ill health, the Declaration also reframed solutions to include a social justice approach to health promotion, recognising that health could only be achieved through a combination of top-down interventions and local responses and the central role that PHC should play.

From a top-down perspective health promotion was broadened beyond medical interventions to include tackling social determinants of health, including 'intersectoral collaboration', based on the assumption that health could only be achieved through coordinated action of the health sector and non-health sectors.

The Declaration also emphasised the need to support local responses to ill health. For health systems, this included decentralisation from national health systems to district health systems, allowing decisions about channelling resources to be made locally and supporting a PHC agenda. Alongside this, a strong emphasis was placed on the need for communities to actively participate in responses to ill health. Such participation by communities was seen as a precondition for tackling some causes of ill health and extending the reach of PHC into hard-to-reach communities.

Since the Declaration, community health workers (CHWs) have been given a key role in achieving community participation in the delivery of PHC. The functions of CHW programmes are conceptualised in one of two ways. Their role is sometimes conceptualised as *target oriented*, working to achieve specific health outcomes through their ability to 'reach' inaccessible communities. It is sometimes conceptualised as *empowerment oriented*, viewing CHW programmes as springboards for (a) general community strengthening for prevention and health-enhancing social development; and (b) the empowerment of health vulnerable groups such as youth and women (Rifkin, 1996). Successful programmes typically rely on community embeddedness (Campbell and Scott, 2011; Bhattacharyya et al., 2001).

Since Alma-Ata various efforts to implement PHC through CHW programmes have led to great successes. In urban Mexico one CHW programme achieved universal immunisation through CHWs being able to target individual households and to provide a flexible service (Walker and Jan, 2005). Explaining how CHW programmes have improved maternal, newborn and child health, Rosato et al. (2008) emphasise CHWs' role in engaging in non-health activities such as improved economic well-being and literacy in their communities. Despite many successful programmes, however, PHC has not been globally instituted and health inequalities continue to rise (CSDH, 2008).

The anniversary of Alma-Ata has led to global calls to 'revitalise primary health care', from politicians and civil society. Politicians view global health and social inequalities as a global security threat (*World Health Report* – WHO, 2008). Furthermore, the Millennium Development Goals – in particular Goal 4, Reduce Child Mortality; Goal 5, Improve Maternal Mortality; and Goal 6, Combat HIV/AIDS, Malaria and Other Diseases – are unlikely to be achieved without significant health system reform (Lawn et al., 2008; Chopra et al., 2009). Meanwhile civil society activists see a return to PHC as a potential pathway to social justice in the context of global health inequalities (McCoy et al., 2008).

There is currently significant international commitment to the approach advocated by the Declaration, as a result of the WHO's Commission on the Social Determinants of Health report (CSDH, 2008). The report echoes the Declaration's emphasis on the social causes of ill health and the need for community participation and empowerment, along-side intersectoral collaboration, in tackling ill health (CSDH, 2008).

3.   HOMING IN ON SOUTH AFRICA

Africa is the continent that has made the least progress in achieving health improvements since Alma-Ata (Schaay and Sanders, 2008). In South Africa health has deteriorated recently. It is one of only 12 countries globally where under-five child mortality has risen since 1990 (Coovadia et al., 2009). Life expectancy at birth in 2009 declined nearly 14 years compared to 1994; from 63 to 50 years for men and from 68 to 54 years for women (Chopra et al., 2009).

Since 1994, South Africa has placed PHC at the centre of its health policies (Barron and Roma-Reardon, 2008). The National Health Plan of 1994 emphasised the need to develop a cohesive, unified health system, based on a district-level system. The Plan removed user fees for PHC and introduced a wave of construction of PHC facilities. Recently, South Africa recommitted itself to PHC in the 2008 Birchwood Declaration, emphasising health as a human right and calling for a doubling of funding to PHC, alongside the need for better alignment between the health and non-health sectors to achieve health improvements (South African Department of Health, 2008).

Despite some successes in South Africa in relation to Alma-Ata and PHC, there is widespread recognition that there is a long way to go (Barron and Roma-Reardon, 2008). In discussions about the barriers to achieving these goals, key obstacles repeatedly emphasised are (i) HIV/AIDS and (ii) HCW shortages (Schaay and Sanders, 2008). Sub-Saharan Africa is disproportionately affected by HIV/AIDS, accounting for 67 per cent of the global AIDS burden (UNAIDS, 2008). South Africa is central to this epidemic, with an adult HIV-prevalence rate of 18.1 per cent (ages 15–49) (UNAIDS, 2008). The impact of HIV/AIDS has undermined the provision of PHC in South Africa, placing additional burdens on health care facilities (Cleary et al., 2008) and reduced the health care workforce – estimates of HIV-prevalence in this sector are 11 per cent (Connelly et al., 2007).

There is also a human resources shortage for the delivery of health. Globally it is estimated that 57 countries have severe human resources shortages, with a deficit of 2.4 million doctors, nurses and midwives (Schaay and Sanders, 2008). Since 1994 in South Africa the number of registered professional nurses has declined from 251 to 110.4 per 100 000, while the number of doctors has remained constant at 25 per 100 000 (Lehmann, 2008). Declining numbers of health professionals (relative to population) undermine the ability of health systems to provide and expand the scope and reach of PHC.

The South African government's policy response to these crises has been to implement a CHW policy (Clarke et al., 2008). CHWs are allocated multiple roles in South Africa, from home-based care for PLWHA through to counselling people undertaking HIV tests, and adherence support for anti-retroviral medication. This has led to the implementation of a formal CHW system, alongside numerous voluntary groups providing a mixture of services. However, policy implementation has been patchy and many informal groups receive little or no support from the government (Clarke et al., 2008).

In this chapter we contribute to generating debate on PHC implementation through a case study of a project that sought to focus on one aspect of the Alma-Ata Declaration that has been identified as particularly poorly implemented – community participation (Lawn et al., 2008). Recognising that community participation is crucial for achieving PHC (WHO, 1978), for tackling HIV/AIDS (Campbell, 2003) and for addressing the health worker shortage (Schaay and Sanders, 2008), but acknowledging that it is incredibly difficult to achieve, we seek to advance understandings of barriers and opportunities to meaningful participation.

4.   CASE STUDY: ENTABENI PROJECT

Entabeni is a remote rural community in KwaZulu-Natal Province in South Africa. Thirty kilometres from the nearest hospital and urban centre, residents make a living either through smallholder farming or migrating to urban centres. About 35 per cent of pregnant women are HIV-positive (Barron et al., 2006). The community is governed through two overlapping forms of authority, the local elected municipality and the *Inkosi* (traditional chief) who inherited his role.

The Entabeni Project was a community-led project seeking to increase the accessibility and quality of home-based care for PLWHA through promoting community participation. The Project emerged after research into community responses to HIV in Entabeni, by the Centre for HIV/AIDS Networking (HIVAN), identified the CHWs' provision of home-based care as a mainstay of the HIV response in Entabeni. The CHWs would walk many kilometres to provide basic care to PLWHA. They would assist families with tasks such as bathing and caring for dying patients, and advise them on accessing health and welfare services and grants. At times they would push patients in wheelbarrows to local roads to get them to clinics (Campbell et al., 2008).

HIVAN organised research feedback sessions to groups in Entabeni, including women, church leaders, local ward leaders, school learners, traditional healers, out-of-school young people, teachers, members of a sewing group, and a local development group (Campbell et al., 2012). Research was also fed back to the area's *Inkosi*. The outcome of these sessions was that HIVAN was asked to work with the CHWs to strengthen their efforts (Campbell et al., 2012). Over three years, HIVAN raised funding to support the Project's work, and a senior HIVAN researcher with 20 years of community development work experience took on the role of external change agent (ECA) (Nair and Campbell, 2008). The ECA's role was to assist the volunteers in accessing the training and support they needed to maximise the effectiveness of their work, and to advise on project management. Over the three years the ECA aimed to transfer full responsibility for the enhanced Project to the CHWs, supported by external public sector and NGO agencies.

The Project's central goal was to improve the quality of community participation in the spirit of the Alma-Ata Declaration (WHO, 1978), as well as the South African government's National Strategic Plan on HIV (South African Department of Health, 2007). Through strengthening the role of the CHWs, the Project sought to achieve both 'target-oriented' objectives such as improving people's access to care and support, particularly those living with HIV/AIDS, and 'empowerment-oriented' objectives. The latter were to be achieved through using the CHWs as a springboard for general community development, and advancing the empowerment of vulnerable groups such as youth and women (Rifkin, 1996). In order to achieve these, three goals were identified: (1) skills development and confidence building of CHWs; (2) building local community support for the CHWs; and (3) building external support for the CHWs.

Various aspects of the Project have already been written up (Campbell et al., 2007, 2008, 2009a, 2009b, 2012; Campbell, 2010). In this chapter, we draw on this material to discuss the Project's successes and challenges in achieving each of the three goals outlined above. We use this as a basis for a discussion of the barriers and facilitators to strengthening community participation in the provision of PHC, and of potential lessons for future participatory programmes.

Goal 1: Building Skills and Confidence of CHWs

The Project's goal of training CHWs in providing AIDS-related care was relatively easy to achieve and very successful (Campbell et al., 2009a). The CHWs were highly motivated, seizing any opportunity to improve their skills. The ECA linked this previously isolated and network-poor group to numerous external organisations willing to provide training. Training included: home nursing skills to optimise the care and comfort of those with AIDS-related illnesses in the absence of formal medical support; how to implement peer education for increased HIV awareness among young people; how best to support people in gaining access to social grants; and skills in financial management and leadership of small projects.

Such training dramatically improved the standard of care for PLWHA. It also inspired and motivated some of the CHWs to take control of aspects of the Project, including staffing an outreach centre that provided counselling services and information on accessing social grants. In addition, some CHWs also took it upon themselves to provide training on HIV/AIDS to school children.

In spite of CHWs taking control of limited Project activities, they did not progress to participating actively in overall project management and decision making. Leadership of the Project and CHW group remained tightly in the hands of an older man – Mr M – who had been integral to setting up the group. Even after three years, and despite many interventions by the ECA to challenge Mr M's dominance, the CHWs (mostly women) remained nervous of challenging the leadership of Mr M (an older man, supported by the *Inkosi*).

Goal 2: Building Internal Community Support for CHWs

HIVAN's research on community responses identified a key barrier to the effectiveness of the CHWs as the limited support they received from key grassroots community groups within Entabeni (Campbell et al., 2008). The Project worked extensively to develop internal community support for the CHWs among key leaders in Entabeni (including both church leaders and the *Inkosi*) and two other groups, young people and men.

As a group, church leaders were important to involve given their large following in Entabeni, particularly among women who made up the majority of their congregation and the majority of CHWs. They were initially reluctant to become engaged in the Project, often framing HIV/AIDS as a form of divine retribution, and were unwilling to allow the CHWs to talk about condoms or AIDS explicitly in church (Campbell et al., 2007; Campbell et al., 2005).

To develop support from church leaders, the Project ECA arranged a series of training sessions for them, during which they discussed HIV/AIDS. These were particularly successful and over time church leaders became highly supportive of the CHWs, allowing discussions about HIV in church services and inviting the AIDS trainer back repeatedly to talk about HIV to their congregations.

The other key leader in Entabeni was the *Inkosi* (traditional chief), who ruled the community. The supreme community gatekeeper, it was he who allowed HIVAN to conduct research and later to work with the CHWs. He tended to keep a distance from the Project, but occasionally referred positively to the CHWs' work at high-profile community events, giving an important boost to their status.

However, his autocratic patriarchal leadership style, favouring the authority of older men, was at variance with the Project's goal of using the CHWs' growing confidence in their health skills as the starting point for their increased participation in local leadership and decision making (Campbell, 2010). Furthermore, the *Inkosi* was a strong advocate of polygamy and very opposed to the use of condoms by his subjects – ideas that ran contrary to those the CHWs were promoting.

The Project also looked to engage two key local constituencies, men and young people. Neither group was represented among the volunteers, who were typically middle-aged women. Mobilising men was seen as crucial given their dominance in the public and private domains. Husbands and boyfriends often complained that their wife's or girlfriend's involvement in the Project was a waste of time, and threatened to stop it. Additionally, given that polygamy or having multiple girlfriends was widespread among men, women felt very vulnerable to HIV but unable to negotiate condom use in the face of reluctant partners. The Project struggled to get men to attend specific AIDS awareness training events. However, those men that became actively involved tended to be those who managed to secure the Project's limited number of paid leadership positions. Given that most CHWs were women, and a central aim had been to provide these women with opportunities for leadership, this was ironic.

The second group the Project attempted to involve were young people. Given the high levels of unemployment and limited opportunities in Entabeni, project involvement had originally been seen as an ideal opportunity for advancing young people's skills and employability. Yet despite many young people expressing interest, only five became active participants, the rest leaving shortly after receiving training to look for jobs in local towns (Gibbs et al., 2010).

Overall the Project's aim of developing support for the CHWs from within the community met with mixed success. There was some support from church leaders. While the *Inkosi* allowed the CHWs to do their work, his leadership style contradicted the project ethos. In addition two key groups – men and young people – failed to become meaningfully involved in the work of the CHWs despite many efforts to recruit them.

Goal 3: Building External Support for CHWs

Successful CHW programmes require external organisations to play a significant role in supporting, managing and providing materials (Campbell and Scott, 2011). As such, the Project worked extensively to strengthen links between the CHWs and public sector agencies (Department of Health, Municipality and Department of Welfare) and two NGOs (a missionary NGO and a counselling NGO). HIVAN's initial research highlighted only very limited and sporadic support for the work of the CHWs from external organisations. The rural nature of the community – 30 kilometres from the nearest town – meant that access was difficult. Additionally, Entabeni straddled bureaucratic borders, and community residents often struggled from one government office to the next after being told that they did not fall into that office's area of concern. Despite these difficulties, all external partners approached by the ECA in the early stages of the Project expressed a willingness to support the Project's work (Nair and Campbell, 2008).

In South Africa the Department of Health is formally responsible for managing and supporting CHWs, although in practice such support is often minimal. The ECA worked long and hard to get the regional DoH to action their formal responsibilities to the CHWs. Of particular importance was a nurse, based at the Entabeni Primary Care Clinic, who was directly responsible for providing day-to-day support to CHWs in her clinic's catchment. The nurse was overworked, however, providing support to many different CHWs groups over a large area, and lacked specific training in community liaison to enable her to work effectively. The nurse's main input to the Project was organising occasional training for the CHWs. Despite providing little support, the nurse required the CHWs to provide written reports on their work – incredibly difficult given that many CHWs were barely literate – and instead of giving feedback on what they had written, the nurse simply filed them for 'future reference'.

The Department of Health paid a small stipend for Mr M, the leader of the CHWs, via the District Health Office. The HIVAN ECA encouraged Mr M to visit the Office and discuss problems the group was facing to see what additional support they could provide. When Mr M reached the Office the staff member he spoke to was shocked that a CHW had approached her directly, rather than using the formal communication channels. She refused to discuss problems, saying that he was wasting the Department's money by being away from his work and threatened to 'dock' his pay for 'wasting' a day.

In meetings with the ECA, officials from the District Health Office acknowledged that the CHWs were eligible for home-based care kits and, importantly, stipends. Given the hard work the CHWs did for no pay, in conditions of extreme poverty, a small stipend would have been highly welcome. This promised stipend failed to materialise, however. For two years, HIVAN raised international funding for a nominal stipend, hoping that a sustainable stipend would eventually be made available from the District Health Office, but this was not to be. The uncertainty and disappointment around the ECA's failure to secure stipends led to much disillusionment among the CHWs, some of whom left in frustration.

In its early stages, the Department of Welfare was also keen to become involved in the Project, seeing it as an opportunity to extend the reach of its social grants to a previously remote and inaccessible community. HIVAN's early research had pointed to the difficulties many community members experienced in accessing these grants (Campbell et al., 2008). A senior manager at the Department of Welfare promised support for the Project, and promised to instruct the area's formally designated social worker to visit the community to advise people on grants. However, this promise did not materialise. When the ECA visited him at his office in a town some distance from Entabeni, he said he was doing several people's work due to staff shortages, and lacked the capacity to support people in such a remote place.

The final government organisation the Project approached was the local municipality, which is formally charged with supporting the extension of health and social development services into under-served areas. A senior official at the municipality was very supportive of the Project in principle, seeing it as a possible 'pilot scheme' fitting closely into his work at the municipality. His initial enthusiasm soon dissipated. Attempts to reach him by phone were deflected by his secretary, saying that he was 'drowning in work'.

Alongside formal government structures, a range of small-scale NGOs operated in and around Entabeni. Two NGOs, a missionary NGO and a NGO that specialised in providing counselling, provided much support to the Project.

The missionary NGO was effectively a single person who coordinated a group of local people setting up a crèche, vegetable gardens and craft projects. The missionary emphasised that her work needed to be located in the community and worked incredibly slowly to ensure that the people she worked with had ownership of activities. From the beginning of the Project, she committed herself to becoming involved, and provided small sums of financial support and significant advice. However, she was constantly under financial pressure and limited by her inability to speak the local language fluently.

The other NGO that became involved was a local branch of a national NGO specialising in counselling. The Director saw the Project as an opportunity to expand her organisation's reach into a remote area previously out of her reach. She participated actively in the Project, listening carefully during meetings and providing resources to support activities. Her NGO provided CHW training of various sorts, and supported the setting up of an 'outreach centre' to provide a base for the CHWs. However, this NGO is poorly funded. At various stages it was unable to get to Entabeni because of a lack of funds to transport its staff.

As the descriptive account of the Entabeni Project has made clear, over the three years it was very successful in achieving Goal 1 – providing training and building the confidence of the CHWs. But its efforts to build internal and external support for the CHWs – Goals 2 and 3 – had more mixed results.

5.   ANALYTICAL DISCUSSION

In this section we provide an analytical discussion of how successes and weaknesses in achieving each of the goals has supported or undermined the Project's 'target-oriented' and 'empowerment-oriented' objectives.

Goal 1: Building Skills and Confidence of CHWs

As discussed above, the Project was very successful in achieving its 'target-oriented' objectives, namely developing the skills of the CHWs. However, the CHWs never played a significant role in the Project's leadership, undermining the Project's empowerment objectives. The major barrier was Mr M, the group's leader, as well as the reluctance of the CHWs to challenge him, despite their frustration with the quality and style of his leadership of their volunteer team. Mr M continued to dominate the CHW group after three years, despite extensive efforts from HIVAN's ECA to encourage him to delegate some of his authority to the female CHWs, and to develop a more democratic leadership style. CHWs remained fearful of him, unwilling to challenge his authority, and Mr M appointed men to the small number of paid leadership positions that were available (Campbell et al., 2009b).

Goal 2: Building Internal Community Support for the CHWs

Throughout the Project a central goal was to build active support for the CHWs from within the community. While there was some passive acknowledgement of their worth from some quarters, this seldom translated into active support for their work. A central reason for limited community support was the Project's failure to mobilise the involvement of men and young people. Three forms of stigma undermined their participation: the continued stigmatisation of AIDS, which the Project failed to seriously challenge; the stigmatisation of caring, which was dismissed as women's work; and the stigmatisation of volunteering. In relation to the last, men and young people often laughed at female volunteers who would 'work for nothing', saying that there was no dignity in unpaid work. Given the Project's inability to secure a sustainable stipend, there was little that could be done to challenge the perception that caregiving and volunteering were insignificant activities (Campbell and Cornish, 2010).

The Project also failed to resonate with what young people wanted out of life. Research seeking to understand the disappointing levels of youth participation in the Project suggested that young people looked forward to a future of paid work in the urban areas rather than conducting unpaid and arduous work in a remote rural community (Gibbs et al., 2010). In addition, whilst the 'target-oriented' aspects of the Project got some support from the *Inkosi*, both through his allowing the project to happen and through his praise for the CHWs' work in public speeches, his authoritarian and patriarchal style was at variance with the Project's 'empowerment-oriented' dimensions.

Goal 3: Building External Support for CHWs

The ECA devoted a substantial proportion of time to developing external support for the CHWs, both from public sector agencies formally charged with supporting Entabeni, and from relevant NGOs. Overall, the public sector failed to provide the support that was envisaged. Two small NGOs were the Project's main external support.

The public sector representatives the Project worked with were typically overworked, demoralised by the sheer size of the problems they were tackling, and lacked the specific skills and motivation needed to support community participation. Bureaucratic structures remained rigid and top-down, unable to respond to requests from CHWs. This meant that CHWs did not receive regular health care supplies from the government, or close management and supervision from primary health care nurses – limiting their ability to deliver services.

The NGOs were better able to provide the close support that was needed to support the CHWs' role in community participation. Small and under-funded, they were not burdened by bureaucracy or excessive workloads, and were often able to be instantly responsive to the CHWs' needs.

The Project's ECA – an experienced and well-networked social worker employed by HIVAN – played a key role in efforts to broker relationships both within the community and external to the community. She also provided a strong focal point for project activities and put great time and effort into supporting and motivating the CHWs, and worked tirelessly in driving forward every aspect of the Project. In a community that placed little emphasis on the role of women, she was often placed in conflict with men who wielded significant authority, however. Furthermore, as an NGO employee on a three-year contract, she lacked the institutional leverage and clout to press public sector agencies to deliver on their verbal commitments to supporting the CHWs.

Finally, despite numerous promises by the Department of Health to provide stipends, these never materialised. The lack of stipends limited the Project's ability to engage men and young people, and caused great distress and disillusionment among the volunteers.

6.   ACTIONABLE LESSONS FROM THE CASE STUDY

We have provided a case study of the immensity of the challenges facing those seeking to strengthen community participation in health care in Entabeni. The Project was very successful in its 'target-oriented' objective of delivering services in a remote, rural area. Yet it struggled to develop the role of CHWs beyond that of simply being 'an extra pair of hands' providing often unpaid services in the context of an overburdened formal health sector (Walt, 1990). The Project failed to achieve its 'empowerment-oriented' objectives of using involvement in HIV/AIDS work as a springboard for the wider social development of female participants. The case study provides us with space to reflect on what can be learnt for actionable 'good practice' in strengthening community participation and what are some 'additional lessons learnt' that need to be taken into account.

Good Practice Demonstrated by the Entabeni Project

The Project provides concrete examples of how projects supporting CHWs can be successful, particularly in achieving 'target-oriented' objectives.

Active involvement of community members in project design, inception and running
Successful CHW projects need to be embedded in communities (Campbell and Scott, 2011). The Entabeni Project was conceptualised and run as a community-led project, with a central role played by local residents in shaping and determining the direction of the Project. Whilst the ECA was heavily involved in all aspects of the Project, she saw her role as one of facilitating volunteer empowerment to strengthen their work and eventually take control of the project – rather than having any stake in exercising any control over project activities in her own right.

Training for CHWs was both medically and socially oriented
The training provided by the Project responded directly to requests from the CHWs. This included home nursing skills (e.g. dealing with bedsores), psychological counselling skills, peer education skills, project management skills and so on. As such, this work was consistent with the Alma-Ata focus on the need to combine a wide range of skills building that goes beyond narrowly conceived physical care.

External change agents (ECAs) are crucial for mobilising support in marginalised communities
The Project also demonstrated the important role an ECA needs to play in mobilising and implementing CHW programmes in marginalised communities. Given the barriers such programmes face, a strong ECA, working to facilitate rather than impose a programme strengthening community participation, opens up opportunities for the brokering of relationships and development of networks that CHWs themselves could not have developed without significant outside support.

Outstanding Challenges

While the Project was successful in its 'targeted-oriented' objectives, it was much less successful in its 'empowerment-oriented' objectives. Of particular importance was the Project's inability to develop intersectoral collaborations between the CHWs and groups internal and external to Entabeni. Given the value placed on intersectoral collaboration in achieving health goals and strengthening community participation (UNAIDS, 2008; South African Department of Health, 2007), this case study provides a series of lessons for similar projects.

Payment of CHWs
A key barrier to project progress was the lack of stipends for the CHWs. Ensuring sustainable and meaningful payment for CHWs is necessary for programme success (Campbell and Scott, 2011). Payments increase retention, and build recognition among community members of the valuable work of CHWs in delivering health services. Furthermore, the promise of payment is likely to draw in a wider range of local groups – particularly men and young people – into projects.

Strong public sector support for CHWs
A key factor identified in ensuring successful CHW programmes is strong public sector support for CHWs (Campbell and Scott, 2011). However, this can only occur when there

are adequate staff in public sector organisations, who have the time, skills, motivation and responsibility for providing this. The Project was crucially hampered by the weak support for the CHWs from the regional health and welfare agencies formally charged with supporting health and social development in Entabeni.

Provide training to public sector employees in community participation
Formal health and social development policy allocates public sector employees an increasing role in facilitating community participation in the delivery of health services. However, as the Entabeni Project has shown, they often lack the necessary training to play this role. Public sector employees therefore need specific training and skills to develop this new area of competence.

Ensure public sector management buy-in
Despite public sector management recognition of the need for greater involvement of communities in service delivery in the Project, incentive structures were not in place to support those charged with implementing this. Management needs to ensure that there are incentives – such as performance measures and job descriptions – that encourage public sector employees to engage in supporting communities.

Greater focus on human resource constraints outside the health sector
While there is significant focus on the human resource crisis in the health sector, there needs to be a similar focus on how human resource constraints in other public sector organisations undermine the types of intersectoral collaboration and support CHWs; their programmes would need to make an optimal contribution to tackling health inequalities.

Programmes wanting to achieve both 'target-oriented' and 'empowerment-oriented' outcomes need to be long term
The Entabeni Project was conceptualised as a three-year project. However, as became increasingly apparent, the challenge of building local capacity through which marginalised women can begin to resist, or at least ameliorate the impacts of, long-term social and economic inequalities cannot be met in three years. Strengthening community participation to achieve 'empowerment-oriented' project outcomes is a long-term process requiring considerable investment from external organisations and ECAs.

7. CONCLUSION

The failure of health systems to tackle health disparities and the emergence of new issues such as HIV/AIDS and the lack of human resources for health have led to resurgent interest in the Alma-Ata Declaration. Not only does it offer a strong framework for understanding ill health, including recognition of the social determinants of health, but it also outlines a strategy for achieving this, emphasising the need for PHC, closely linked into community participation and intersectoral collaboration.

Effective PHC can only be achieved with substantial community participation. After Alma-Ata, community participation became formalised through CHW programmes, with two objectives – targeted-oriented objectives and empowerment-oriented objectives (Rifkin, 1996). Our case study project sought to achieve both these objectives through strengthening community participation. In reporting on the experiences of the Entabeni Project, we have sought to generate debate about the complexity of achieving such objectives. Whilst the Project was highly successful at achieving its target-oriented objectives of improving the access to and quality of care provided by the CHWs, it was much less successful at achieving its wider empowerment objectives.

We conclude by suggesting that strengthening community participation to achieve both objectives requires the development of incentives to engage in and/or support community participation, drawn from our discussion above. The framework of incentives needed to strengthen community participation can be summarised as follows:

1. *Incentives to motivate CHWs and build their skills, confidence and sustainability*   Incentives need to include payment of CHWs. Payments recognise the value of care work, provide validation for those involved and encourage greater participation from men and young people. Additionally there needs to be socially and medically oriented training, developing CHWs' skills and confidence to provide the care they do effectively in community settings.
2. *Incentives to build greater support for CHWs from groups internal to a community*   As mentioned above, payments for CHWs provide clear recognition of the valuable work CHWs provide and also challenges the idea of care work and women's work as having little value. Incentives also need to be responsive to what young people want to achieve out of life, and to tailor opportunities for participation accordingly.
3. *Incentives to develop greater external organisation support for CHWs*   Managers of potential support organisations external to communities, especially in public sector agencies, need to ensure that incentives support the greater involvement of their staff. These need to include the writing of community outreach and volunteer and PHC support activities into public officials' job descriptions. It also needs to be ensured that public officials receive appropriate training and the necessary authority and time to become actively involved in supporting community projects.

We hope that we have demonstrated the need to focus considerably more attention on the identification and provision of appropriate incentives for the effective participation of the three groups mentioned above: community volunteers; potential within-community support networks; and potential external support networks, particularly in the public sector. Without greater community participation, the aims of the Alma-Ata Declaration are unlikely to be realised, and the development of appropriate incentives is a vital precondition for ensuring that opportunities for such participation are optimised.

REFERENCES

Barron, P., C. Day, F. Monticelli, K. Vermaak, O. Okorafor and K. Moodley (2006), *The District Health Barometer Year 2005/06*, Durban: Health Systems Trust.
Barron, P. and J. Roma-Reardon (2008), 'Editorial – Primary Health Care in South Africa: a review of 30 years since Alma Ata', in P. Barron and J. Roma-Reardon (eds), *South African Health Review 2008*, Durban: Health Systems Trust, pp. vii–xii.

Bhattacharyya, K., P. Winch, K. LeBan and M. Tien (2001), *Community Health Worker Incentives and Disincentives*, Arlington, VA: Basic Support for Institutionalizing Child Survival Project [BASICS II] for USAID.

Campbell, C. (2003), *'Letting Them Die': Why HIV Interventions Fail*, Oxford: James Currey.

Campbell, C. (2010), 'Political will, traditional leaders and the fight against HIV/AIDS: a South African case study', *AIDS Care*, **22**(S2), 1637–43.

Campbell, C. and F. Cornish (2010), 'Development as transformative communication? Experiences from India and South Africa', HCD Working Papers, 1, London: London School of Economics and Political Science.

Campbell, C. and K. Scott (2011), 'Retreat from Alma Ata? The WHO's report on task shifting to community health workers for AIDS care in poor countries', *Global Public Health*, **6**(2), 125–38.

Campbell, C., C.A. Foulis, S. Maimane and Z. Sibiya (2005), '"I have an evil child at my house": stigma and HIV/AIDS management in a South African community', *American Journal of Public Health*, **95**(5), 808–15.

Campbell, C., Y. Nair, S. Maimane and J. Nicolson (2007), '"Dying twice": a multi-level model of the roots of AIDS stigma in two South African communities', *Journal of Health Psychology*, **12**(3), 403–16.

Campbell, C., Y. Nair, S. Maimane and Z. Sibiya (2008), 'Supporting people with AIDS and their carers in rural South Africa: possibilities and challenges', *Health and Place*, **14**(3), 507–16.

Campbell, C., Y. Nair, S. Maimane and A. Gibbs (2009a), 'Strengthening community responses to AIDS: possibilities and challenges', in P. Rohleder, L. Swartz and S. Kalichman (eds), *HIV in South Africa 25 Years on*, New York: Springer, pp. 221–36.

Campbell, C., A. Gibbs, Y. Nair and S. Maimane (2009b), 'Frustrated potential, false promises or complicated possibilities? Empowerment and participation amongst female health volunteers in South Africa', *Journal of Health Management, Special Edition on Subaltern Approaches to the Millennium Development Goals*, **11**(2), 315–36.

Campbell, C., Y. Nair, S. Maimane, Z. Sibiya and A. Gibbs (2012), 'Dissemination as intervention: building local AIDS competence through the report-back of research findings to a South African rural community', *Antipode*, **44**(3), 702–24.

Chan, M. (2008), 'Return to Alma-Ata', *Lancet*, **372**(9642), 865–6.

Chopra, M., J. Lawn, D. Sanders, P. Barron, S. Abdool Karim, D. Bradshaw, R. Jewkes, Q. Abdool Karim, A. Flisher, B. Mayosi, S. Tollman, G. Churchyard and H. Coovadia (2009), 'Achieving the Health Millennium Development Goals for South Africa: challenges and priorities', *Lancet*, **374**(9694), 1023–31.

Clarke, M., S. Dick and S. Lewin (2008), 'Community health workers in South Africa: where in this maze do we find ourselves?', *South African Medical Journal*, **98**(9), 680–81.

Cleary, S., A. Boulle, M. Castillo-Riquelme and D. McIntyre (2008), 'The burden of HIV/AIDS in the public healthcare system', *South African Journal of Economics*, **76**(S1), S3–S14.

CSDH (2008), *Closing the Gap in a Generation: Health Equity through Action on the Social Determinants of Health. Final Report of the Commission on Social Determinants of Health*, Geneva: World Health Organization.

Connelly, D., Y. Veriava, S. Roberts, J. Tsotetsi, A. Jordan, E. DeSilva, S. Rosen and M. Bachman DeSilva (2007), 'Prevalence of HIV infection and median CD4 counts among health care workers in South Africa', *South African Medical Journal*, **97**(2), 115–23.

Coovadia, H., R. Jewkes, P. Barron, D. Sanders and D. McIntyre (2009), 'The health and health system in South Africa: historical roots of current public health challenges', *Lancet*, **374**(9692), 817–34.

Gibbs, A., C. Campbell, Y. Nair and S. Maimane (2010), 'Mismatches between youth aspirations and participatory HIV/AIDS programmes', *African Journal of AIDS Research*, **9**(2), 153–63.

Lawn, J., J. Rohde, S. Rifkin, M. Were, V. Paul and M. Chopra (2008), 'Alma-Ata 30 years on: revolutionary, relevant, and time to revitalise', *Lancet*, **372**, 917–27.

Lehmann, U. (2008), 'Strengthening human resources for primary health care', in P. Barron and J. Roma-Reardon (eds), *South African Health Review 2008*, Durban: Health Systems Trust, pp. 163–78.

McCoy, D., A. Ntuli and D. Sanders (eds) (2008), *Global Health Watch 2: An Alternative World Health Report*, London and New York: Zed Books.

Nair, Y. and C. Campbell (2008), 'Building partnerships to support community-led HIV/AIDS management: a case study from rural South Africa', *African Journal of AIDS Research*, **7**(1), 45–53.

Rifkin, S. (1996), 'Paradigms lost: toward a new understanding of community participation in health programmes', *Acta Tropica*, **61**(2), 79–92.

Rosato, M., G. Laverack, L. Grabman, P. Tripathy, N. Nair, C. Mwansambo, K. Azad, J. Morrison, Z. Bhutta, H. Perry, S. Rifkin and A. Costello (2008), 'Community participation: lessons for maternal, newborn and child health', *Lancet*, **372**, 962–71.

Schaay, N. and D. Sanders (2008), 'International perspective on primary health care over the past 30 years', in P. Barron and J. Roma-Reardon (eds), *South African Health Review 2008*, Durban: Health Systems Trust, pp. 3–16.

South African Department of Health (2007), *HIV and AIDS and STI National Strategic Plan 2007–2011*, Pretoria: Department of Health.

South African Department of Health (2008), *The Birchwood National Consultative Health Forum Declaration on Primary Health Care*, Pretoria: Department of Health.

UNAIDS (2008), *Report on the Global AIDS Epidemic, 2008*, Geneva: UNAIDS.

Walker, D. and S. Jan (2005), 'How do we determine whether community health workers are cost-effective? Some core methodological issues', *Journal of Community Health*, **30**(3), 221–9.

Walt, G. (ed.) (1990), *Community Health Workers in National Programmes: Just Another Pair of Hands?* Milton Keynes: Open University Press.

WHO (1978), *Declaration of Alma-Ata, 1978*, available at www.who.int/hpr/NPH/docs/declaration_almaata.pdf (accessed 5 October 2009).

WHO (2008), *The World Health Report 2008 – Primary Health Care (Now More Than Ever)*, Geneva: WHO.

3 Socioeconomic status and access to health care: the quandary of transition economies
Heba A. Elgazzar

1. INTRODUCTION

> To sustain quality social environments with diminished resources is a difficult task. It is possible that societies with high quality social capital will be better able to adjust than will fragmented individualistic societies. Societies that have a strong, coherent sense of what is important, and a collective will, will probably be most successful.
>
> (Frank and Mustard, 1994, p. 17)

Emerging studies on income inequality point to a paradox. Despite economic progress, social inequalities such as disparities in wealth and health appear to be widening in many countries (Coburn, 2003). In the case of health, various economic barriers to accessing health care services may exist, such as a low ability to pay and a lack of access to safety nets. This chapter examines the relationship between economic status and the utilisation of health care services in middle-income countries.

Social values help to shape the debate on how health care should be organised and financed, as well as the role of the state. Where the health care system is oriented towards social solidarity, the state tends to play a more active role in ensuring that all socio-economic levels have equal access to services regardless of ability to pay. In transition economies such as middle-income countries in the Middle East, Latin America, Eastern Europe and Southeast Asia, governments are currently in the process of building institutional effectiveness, reducing corruption and strengthening overall governance. Health systems are often bimodal, where public and private systems operate in parallel and are financed through a fragmented mix of tax revenues, public and private health insurance, and out-of-pocket payments.

Households in many middle-income countries tend to rely heavily on private sources of financing to access services; on average, out-of-pocket spending tends to account for 40–50 per cent of total health care expenditure in middle-income countries (World Bank, 2011). Hence, economic status may pose a barrier to accessing health services where there exists a high reliance on ability to pay. As a result, ill health may persist among vulnerable populations, threatening welfare and furthering the cycle of economic hardship and illness. To examine the role of public policy in ensuring affordable care for citizens in transition economies, the chapter evaluates the association between economic status and health-related outcomes in various policy contexts in transition economies.

This chapter is structured as follows. The following section presents a conceptual framework for examining disparities in access to care, with particular attention given to the case of transition economies. Next, the social gradient in health and the influence of socioeconomic status on the likelihood of accessing services is examined, highlighting that the effect varies by the type of health service. Finally, policy options regarding the design of health financing systems towards alleviating disparities in middle-income countries are discussed, shedding light on the need to reconsider the role of the state in increasingly sophisticated economies.

2.   CONCEPTUAL FRAMEWORK

Demand for Health Care

Transition health systems face certain challenges that are distinct from those of low-income countries, which tend to be more resource constrained and whose disease burden is typically more heavily dominated by communicable conditions requiring population interventions. Transition economies by contrast tend to be relatively more resource rich, but their institutional governance may lack effectiveness, resulting in health service delivery that may be inefficient and inequitable in responding to the particular preferences of a growing middle class. The dual burden of both non-communicable and communicable conditions in middle-income countries renders a need for fairly sophisticated health care coordination, prevention and treatment, which the public sector struggles to achieve en masse. These conditions tend to require regular, long-term care, which can be complex (Fernández and Knapp, 2004). The prevalence of chronic health conditions also tends to be higher among the worse-off in many societies, and this group is particularly vulnerable in health systems where access depends on ability to pay (Walker, 1986; Wiener, 2004; Knapp, 2007).

Differing notions of health and its determinants have influenced the nature of health promotion, and, ultimately, the path of health systems development. The concept of health as a state of equilibrium between man and the environment, as seen through the ancient Greeks and Chinese, paves the way for examining how social conditions are associated with health. Health can be defined either through a negativist or positivist lens, with the former often dominating the discourse in middle-income countries. The negativist approach emphasises the absence of disease as the definition of health and has gained momentum with the advance of modern medicine and thus focuses on biomedical, rather than social, determinants of disease (Cockerham, 2001). As a result, health services in middle-income countries tend to be dominated by curative care with less of an emphasis placed on preventive services and the promotion of healthy social factors.

By contrast, relatively recent sociological paradigms broaden the range of influences on health, thus adopting the positivist approach, which defines health in terms of the presence of human capital and overall well-being rather than merely the absence of infirmity (World Health Organization, 1948; Labonte, 1993; Raphael, 2000). The effect of economic determinants on utilisation in middle-income countries is assessed in this chapter by applying an economic model of the demand for health care, based on the work of Grossman (1972), Anderson (1975), Wagstaff et al. (1991), Pohlmeier and Ulrich (1995), and others. While a number of theories exist regarding a vast array of determinants of health (Murray and Chen, 1993; Evans, 1994), this chapter focuses on the effect of socioeconomic status. The conceptual model is based on the behavioural model of utilization proposed by Anderson and Newman (1973), shown in Figure 3.1.

Anderson's (1975) behavioural model of utilisation characterises the choice to use

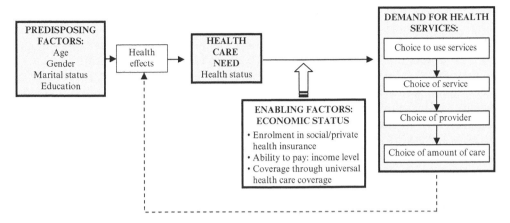

Sources: Adapted from Anderson and Newman (1973), as well as Grossman (1972); Wagstaff et al. (1991); Anderson (1995); Pohlmeier and Ulrich (1995); Marmot (2005).

Figure 3.1   *Conceptual framework for examining socioeconomic disparities in health service utilisation*

services as a function of three groups of factors, including: (a) predisposing factors, or demographic characteristics, social structure and health beliefs; (b) enabling factors, or the ability to secure resources in order to access services; and (c) medical need, which can be perceived or evaluated (Anderson, 1975; Anderson, 1995). Research has found that acute, inpatient care is typically less influenced by enabling factors than is preventive, outpatient care, which is perceived to be more discretionary (Anderson and Newman, 1973). 'Enabling factors' may be defined across societies. The nature of social safety nets is one such critical factor that may increase or reduce the role of other enabling factors. Understanding the general political-economic basis for social safety nets will help to unravel broader causes and possible policy responses to structural inequalities.

To translate Anderson's model into an empirical assessment, Grossman's (1972) model for the demand for health represents health as a matter of investment (Mushkin, 1962; Van Doorslaer, 1987). The choice to invest in health is posited within a utility-maximizing function under constraints, where an individual's total utility is a function of the utility derived from their inherited initial 'stock of health', the 'stock of health' over time, and the consumption of other commodities. In Grossman's model, the stock or amount of health at a given time *t* is subject to the amount of investment in related goods in the period immediately preceding it, such as medical care, length of time and human capital (Grossman, 1972), expressed as:

$$H_{t+1} - H_t = I_t - \delta_i H_t, \tag{3.1}$$

$$I_t = I_t (M_t, T_t; E_t) \tag{3.2}$$

where I_t is gross investment in health, δ_t is the rate of depreciation during the *t*th period, M_t is medical care, TH_t is time input, and E_t is the stock of human capital (Grossman,

1972). In effect, the demand for health is only observable through the demand for health care, given its latent properties (Culyer, 1976; Williams, 1978).

Overall, the demand for health services is a function of enabling, predisposing and medical factors that are context specific. Three fundamental principles are relevant to understanding the nature of this demand. First, the demand for health care is a derived demand for health. Second, health is an uncertain and latent variable, represented by an array of indicators. Third, the production of health is a function of health status at a given time and other inputs, such as medical care, income, education, environmental hazards and other socioeconomic determinants. The relative importance of social status, in turn, depends on the nature of the health system and the underlying welfare state, the subject of emerging empirical research.

The understanding of economic status emerges from the sociological theory of social stratification, exemplified by Weber's framework of 'lifestyle'. 'Lifestyle' (*Lebensstil*) is a function of both 'life chances' (*Lebenschancen*), or class position represented by income, norms, education and occupational category, and 'life-conduct' (*Lebensführung*), or behaviours and choices made by the individual, such as smoking habits and eating patterns (Weber, 1978). Although measures of poverty and income levels are important indicators of social deprivation, they may not indicate the extent to which access to social services is hindered in all contexts. In middle-income countries, other forms of social exclusion may be more salient, such as insurance status and educational level. As Sen (2004) states, 'income inequality' and 'economic inequality' are not necessarily the same, rendering the need to evaluate the 'impact of multiple economic and social influences on quality of life' (Sen, 2004, p. 65).

Access to Care and the Welfare State

The way that social determinants of health are addressed at a national policy level depends on underlying social values regarding social justice and the role of the state, which can be assessed using the welfare state typology described by Titmuss (1956) and Esping-Andersen (1990) (Figure 3.2). The development of a welfare state reflects a given country's history, political institutions and values, and its development trajectory is therefore path-dependent (Esping-Andersen, 2000; Klein, 2001, 2003). Notions of the welfare state in middle-income countries fall along the spectrum, ranging from the liberal or residual model as in the case of Lebanon, to the corporatist model as in Argentina and Tunisia, and finally to social-democratic variations as in Egypt, Indonesia, Morocco, and several former Soviet Union nations such as Croatia and Hungary. Many middle-income welfare systems are also witnessing shifts from a patchwork of vertical public interventions towards a systems-based approach.

The liberal welfare state represents the most conservative approach to social benefits, considered the 'liberal welfare state'. Examples from middle-income countries include Lebanon, most notably, and *de facto*, many countries in which a sizeable private market for health services, particularly for outpatient physician consultation and pharmaceuticals, has emerged catering to upper wealth groups who can afford to pay direct out-of-pocket fees. This pattern has emerged even in countries where a broader social safety net may exist in theory, but fails to provide adequate quality of care.

Many middle-income countries currently fall within the corporatist–statist cluster,

Role of:	Liberal/ residual	Conservative/ social security	Social-democratic/ statist
• Family	Limited	Significant	Limited
• Market	Significant	Limited	Limited
• State	Limited	Supplementary	Significant
Social orientation of welfare state	Individual	Kinship/family Federalist	Universal solidarity
High-income example	USA	Germany Italy France UK	Sweden
Middle-income example	Lebanon	Tunisia Argentina Egypt Indonesia	

Sources: Titmuss (1956); Esping-Andersen (1990, 2000, p. 85); Castles (2004); World Bank (2009).

Figure 3.2   Typology of welfare states

notably countries such as Argentina, Tunisia and Indonesia. A limited public fiscal capacity to fund health services directly has resulted in a reliance on social health insurance schemes and a sizeable labour market to contribute to health care financing. However, in many cases such as Tunisia, the benefits included in health insurance schemes, perverse incentives to access high-technology care and the complexity inherent in retrospective reimbursement policies have led to growing dissatisfaction among beneficiaries in these social-security-based systems. This, in turn, has propelled those who are able to pay to pursue parallel health care services in the private market by paying out of pocket.

The social-democratic model similar to the Beveridge approach has historically been the most common approach adopted, having begun to narrow in scope. Countries such as Egypt, Indonesia, Morocco, and several formal Soviet Union nations such as Croatia and Hungary had established universal public services funded largely through governmental revenues during the 1960s and 1970s. Owing to a lack of investment in public facilities, fewer and fewer incentives for providers to practise in ill-equipped structures, and increasingly liberal economic policies stimulating private investment in hospitals and clinics, many middle-income countries have been left with the burden of managing increasingly multi-tiered, fragmented and inefficient health systems.

Health Policy in Middle-income Countries

The societal perspective towards health largely defines the role of the state and that of ability to pay in mediating access to health care. Navarro and Shi (2003) show through a cross-national analysis that 'political traditions more committed to redistributive

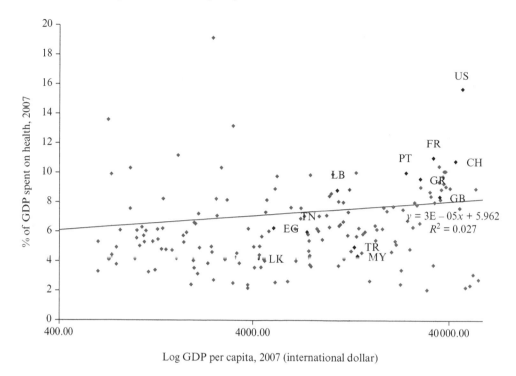

Notes: GDP = gross domestic product. EG = Egypt; CH = Switzerland; FR = France; GB = United Kingdom; GR = Greece; LB = Lebanon; LK = Sri Lanka; MY = Malaysia; PT = Portugal; TN = Tunisia; TR = Turkey; US = United States.

Source: World Bank (2011).

Figure 3.3   Total health expenditure by national income level

policies (both economic and social) . . . were generally more successful in improving the health of populations' (p. 195). Many middle-income countries in Eastern Europe, Latin America, Eastern Asia and the Middle East have been engaged in reforming their health care systems since the early 1990s, particularly in the area of equity in quality of care and health insurance coverage. A comparison of all aspects of the health systems is beyond the scope of this chapter; the main interest is the underlying state–society framework and how this influences the effect of socioeconomic factors on access to care.

Taking the case of the Middle East, there has been a recognition that social outcomes, such as education and health, have lagged behind economic development in comparison to other economies where social and economic progress have been realised at a more similar pace (Figure 3.3 and Table 3.1). Lagging social outcomes such as health indicators have been attributed in part to ill-defined state–society relationships (Turner, 1984; Issawi, 1989; Karshenas and Moghadam, 2006). That is to say, the commitment of the state towards its citizens and the trust afforded by citizens towards the state in the area of public services has been tentative at best and completely lacking at worst.

The concept of health in Middle Eastern countries, as in many middle-income coun-

Table 3.1   Health status indicators by national income level

Country	Private expenditure as % of total health expenditure	Adult literacy rate (%)	Infant mortality rate (per 1000 live births)	Health life expectancy at birth (years)	Age-standardised mortality rate for cardiovascular diseases (deaths per 100 000)
Low- and middle-income countries					
Egypt	61.6	71.4	30	59	560
Lebanon	71.7	87.0	28	60	463
Tunisia	55.7	74.3	20	62	417
Turkey	28.6	87.4	26	62	542
Sri Lanka	53.8	90.7	12	62	314
Malaysia	55.0	88.7	10	63	274
High-income countries					
Greece	57.2	96.0	4	71	258
Portugal	27.7	93.8	4	69	208
France	20.1	99.0	4	72	118
Switzerland	40.3	99.0	4	73	142
UK	12.9	99.0	5	71	182
USA	54.9	99.0	6	69	188

Note: Cardiovascular deaths shown as an indicator of the burden of non-communicable diseases in each country.

Source: World Health Organization Statistical Information System, 2008. Data are for 2002–06.

tries, has shifted from the ancient 'equilibrium' notion to one that focuses on the 'sick role' and a negativist approach (Gallagher, 2001; Adib, 2004). Preventive and primary health care, with some exceptions due to vertical or selected public health campaigns, have tended to receive relatively little governmental expenditure, with the private sector involved to varying extents.

Specialists and acute care providers have tended to dominate the provision of health services, with a tendency for citizens to bypass general practitioners and seek highly specialised services (Karshenas and Moghadam, 2006; Jabbour et al., 2006; Maziak, 2006). Family support and social arrangements also play important roles in health care in many middle-income countries, a function of both historically cultural aspects as well as the way in which public services are structured.

The performance of middle-income health systems may be more a function of how the system is governed rather than the level of public expenditure. For example, Egypt reflects a relatively solidarity-based social system and economic development has generally been state-led, with a combination of nationalisation and privatisation. By contrast, the Lebanese political system is highly fragmented, with power divided between approximately 18 different political factions. Its mercantile, *laissez-faire* economic development has continued through the civil war, leaving much of the responsibility for social support to private and non-governmental actors.

Whilst a universal system of health care provision exists for all citizens to use in many

Table 3.2   Health system comparison, Egypt and Lebanon

Parameter	Egypt	Lebanon
Overall organisation		
Degree of centralised policy making and planning by Ministry of Health	Relatively centralised	Relatively fragmented
Financing sources		
● Direct governmental revenues finance universal health system operated by Ministry of Health	National health service designed to provide most care free to all citizens	Means-tested coverage for selected treatment provided to 13% of citizens
● Social health insurance	Operates in parallel to national health service (48% of citizens enrolled)	● Social security fund covers 18% of citizens ● Other social health insurance covers 23% of citizens
● Private health insurance	Voluntary, supplementary; 1% of citizens enrolled	Voluntary, comprehensive/ supplementary; 15% of citizens enrolled
● Household out-of-pocket payments	Most households; 58.3% of total health expenditure	Most households; 58.9% of total health expenditure
Provision		
Outpatient care: % delivered through private providers	~70%	>95%
Inpatient care: % delivered through private providers	~30%	~90%
Presence of functioning gate-keeping system	Relatively weak	Negligible
Predominant provider payment mechanism:		
● Public outpatient clinics	Salary irrespective of output	Not applicable
● Private outpatient clinics	Fee for service	Fee for service or charitable
● Public inpatient hospitals	Fee for service	Fee for service
● Private inpatient hospitals	Fee for service	Fee for service

Source: Compiled by author.

middle-income countries, these systems are often underinvested and the option of last resort, as in Egypt and Lebanon. Considerable public provision is found in Egypt, although citizens prefer to go to private outpatient providers due to higher quality of care. In contrast, the vast majority of provision in Lebanon is private and dominated by hospitals. Furthermore, providers in both countries are generally paid on a fee-for-service basis, and neither health system incorporates substantive systems of performance-based payments (Table 3.2). The lack of appropriate incentive systems found in health financing schemes in middle-income health systems probably exacerbates socioeconomic disparities in access to health services.

3.   SOCIAL GRADIENT IN HEALTH AND HEALTH CARE IN TRANSITION ECONOMIES

Gaps in Household Financial Burden and Health

In many countries, direct household payments for health care can account for the single largest component of household spending after food expenditures. O'Donnell et al. (2007) demonstrated that aggregate public health expenditure tends to be concentrated among the relatively well-off in several Asian countries. These observations mirror the observation found in England at the turn of the century regarding the distribution of maternal health services. The impact of these external 'health shocks' can be catastrophic and can significantly affect the living standards of individuals.

Formal and informal out-of-pocket payments for health care may pose barriers to accessing health services. Growing out-of-pocket spending on health care has become a policy concern in middle income countries for three reasons: first, households may be pushed into poverty or into deeper poverty as a result of using catastrophic health services; second, households facing these health expenses may cut back on other essential household spending such as food and clothing; and third, households may, in fact, choose to forgo necessary health care services rather than face the steep financial consequences – creating a vicious cycle of ill health, disability and poverty. In Morocco, only 38 per cent of survey respondents reported that they were always able to receive the care they needed, as compared to 74 per cent in France; in Morocco, among those who did not use the health services they needed, 39 per cent indicated that this was due to a lack of affordability, as compared to 11 per cent in France (World Health Organization, 2004). These findings illustrate that shifting financial risk to households in health care can lower or even eliminate the chances for people to seek medical care when they need it.

Some of the most telling evidence of this impact comes from a longitudinal study in the USA showing that out-of-pocket payments can deter access and lower health status even for those with health insurance coverage (Keeler, 1992). Given relatively high resource constraints in low- and middle-income countries, out-of-pocket payments are a particular cause for concern where health-financing systems are in transition. These findings have been found for maternal and mental health services in several countries (Palmer et al., 2004; Ensor and Ronoh, 2005; Knapp et al., 2006). Evidence from Egypt (Rannan-Eliya et al., 1999; Elgazzar, 2009), Jordan (Ekman, 2007), Iran (Hosseinpour et al., 2005), Lebanon (Elgazzar, 2009) and other countries suggests that socioeconomic inequities are apparent in terms of maternal and child health status, many non-communicable chronic conditions, and self-assessed health and pain levels.

Risk-pooling schemes such as public and private health insurance tend to reduce the amount of out-of-pocket expenditure in some cases, particularly pharmaceutical expenditure (Kanavos and Gemmill, 2004). Several studies have shown that out-of-pocket payments for health care can aggravate poverty levels in developing countries, as observed throughout Asian countries (Grogan, 1995; O'Donnell et al., 2007; Lu et al., 2007; van Doorslaer et al., 2007). Although the effect is more prominent in low-income countries than in middle-income countries, out-of-pocket payments coupled with poor-quality health services contribute to ever-growing social rifts regarding ability to pay for and to access health services.

Gaps in Health Service Utilisation

Disparities in health care use are more apparent in the chances of using outpatient services, such as physician consultations, than in inpatient services, such as overnight hospital admissions. This has been observed in low- and middle-income countries such as Malaysia, Egypt and Lebanon, as well as several high-income countries such as the UK and other OECD countries (van Doorslaer et al., 2004; Morris et al., 2005; van Doorslaer et al., 2008; Elgazzar, 2009).

In Egypt and Lebanon, the effect of income and insurance is larger on the probability of using most outpatient services, including hospital outpatient care, than their effect on the use of inpatient care (Elgazzar, 2009). This is consistent with most of the literature, which shows that income and insurance influence the use of preventive and outpatient services to a greater extent than that of acute, urgent services (Anderson and Benham, 1970; Phelps, 1975; Ware et al., 1986; van Doorslaer, 1987; Noro et al., 1999; van Doorslaer et al., 2004).

In addition, health care use has been found to be more closely associated with insurance than with income *per se*, particularly in Lebanon. The effect of insurance on the likelihood of accessing health services is generally larger than the effect of income after adjusting for endogeneity to the extent possible. Insurance also tends to play a greater role in Lebanon than in Egypt for most health services, notably for physician, pharmacy and hospital outpatient care. The findings are consistent with those from other countries, which indicate that people are more likely to use health care in systems that are not heavily based on ability to pay (Newhouse, 1993; van Doorslaer et al., 2004; van Doorslaer et al., 2006). It also supports the notion that insurance is more beneficial to the worse off (Wagstaff and van Doorslaer, 2001; Jowett et al., 2003).

Further, the relationship between economic status and utilisation differs between the probability and the intensity of care. In Lebanon, income and insurance influenced the *probability* of care, but not necessarily the *number* of visits. The Lebanese case is an example of a market-based financing system. The few who can afford to contact the system do so; among those individuals, *intensity* is largely determined by health need and providers' choices. This pattern is similar to that found in other market-based systems (Anderson and Newman, 1973; Pohlmeier and Ulrich, 1995; Santos Silva and Windmeijer, 2001).

4.   POLICY IMPLICATIONS

The role of economic status in access to health care depends on factors that often receive relatively little policy attention in middle-income, transition economies. These factors include: (i) varying conceptual definitions of health and the health system; (ii) the role of the state in health financing and provider incentives; and (iii) the relative impact of other social factors on the demand for health care services. Comprehensive social safety nets for health care typically arise from a social orientation towards health and health care. Yet many middle-income countries in Latin America, Eastern Europe, the Middle East and parts of Asia have historically viewed health through a disease-oriented lens, resulting in health systems that typically fall short of meeting the health needs of the most vulnerable populations. Three key policy implications regarding health systems development emerge based on the nature of socioeconomic health disparities in middle-income countries.

First, the role of state-funded, comprehensive social safety nets for health care may partially explain why the effects of income and insurance are relatively smaller in solidarity-oriented systems than in privately oriented systems, particularly for outpatient care. Where social safety nets are relatively more comprehensive, people may be more encouraged to seek care when needed regardless of ability to pay or enrolment in health insurance schemes other than the national health service system. Although certain types of health care financing may not alleviate income inequality *per se*, universal social safety nets, for example, provide a means of alleviating health care inequality for those who are otherwise unequal based on income. At the same time, a number of other factors may have explained the difference in the effects of income and insurance, such as differences between countries regarding the quality of service delivery; the nature and distribution of the supply of health services and providers; and social beliefs about curative versus preventive care.

Second, the utilisation of health care among the worst-off citizens should be addressed in order to improve overall equality in health care. Research has found that the degree of inequity in health care was driven by patterns among the poorest quintiles in many societies, such as in Egypt and Lebanon (Jurjus, 1995; Ellis et al., 1994; Rannan-Eliya et al., 1999; Nandakumar et al., 2000; Elgazzar, 2009), as well as high-income countries (Deaton, 2002; Muennig et al., 2005; Ross et al., 2006; Hernández-Quevedo et al., 2006).

Therefore health insurance schemes and service delivery systems should prioritise the needs of those at the lowest ends of the income ladder. Eligibility criteria for risk-pooling schemes are central. Lower-income groups tend to face a higher burden of out-of-pocket payments. They are more likely to be pushed further into poverty as a result of using health care. Yet insurance coverage tends to be more concentrated among the well-off, which only exacerbates inequity.

Although social values play a part in shaping criteria, the most vulnerable should at the very least be relieved of economic burdens associated with care. Because the most vulnerable pay for health care does not mean that they can 'afford' the costs; costs extend beyond financial consequences (Russell, 1996). They include opportunity costs such as forgoing necessities, selling assets, reshuffling family labour arrangements and delaying other health care needs. These consequences have been observed in many societies (Russell, 1996; Segall et al., 2002; Russell, 2005). This evidence shows that 'affordability', 'ability to pay' and 'willingness to pay' are not synonymous. Providing protection from unforeseen health and economic consequences should reduce the likelihood that people delay necessary care, which leads to a vicious cycle of ill health and poverty.

Finally, the nature of health insurance coverage influences the utilisation of services, particularly in health systems where the overall financing scheme is highly fragmented. Demand- and supply-side incentives built into health insurance systems for the use of outpatient care in particular should be considered carefully in policy setting. This careful consideration of incentives equally applies to other forms of financing, such as universal, public provision. Although comparisons of aggregate expenditures may suggest that the amount of public expenditure is similar between countries, the nature of expenditure is often more important (Castles, 2004).

For example, economic inequity may persist despite the existence of a universal social safety net for health care as represented by a national health service. This pattern leads to questions regarding whether the concentration of public resources on hospital care and in relatively well-off areas in many middle-income countries exacerbates inequity. This highlights that it is not just sufficient for the state to *spend*. It is equally, if not more, important to *spend appropriately*.

Overall, economic equity in the use of health services, particularly outpatient care, tends to be greater in health systems in which social safety nets are comprehensive, and this pattern appears to transcend a country's economic level. Inequity has been attributed to several factors, such as the distribution of supply and fees charged at the point of service. The evidence reviewed in this chapter suggests that health insurance and risk-pooling schemes in middle-income countries that are based on ability to pay tend to increase financial barriers to accessing health care. Therefore enabling factors such as income level and social or private health insurance coverage become more important in systems where social safety nets do not exist or fail to provide adequate coverage for health care. Middle-income countries that face challenges in terms of equity and financial sustainability of health financing, such as the case of the Middle East, would benefit from instituting comprehensive and effective systems of universal risk pooling based on a more prospective, socially oriented framework for health care. Addressing the fragmented nature of policy making will prove invaluable to overcoming the quandary of socioeconomic disparities despite economic growth in middle-income economies.

REFERENCES

Adib, S.M. (2004), 'From the biomedical model to the Islamic alternative: a brief overview of medical practices in the contemporary Arab world', *Social Science and Medicine*, **58**, 697–702.

Anderson, R.M. (1975), 'Introduction', in R.M. Anderson, J. Kravits and O.W. Anderson (eds), *Equity in Health Services*, Boston, MA: Ballinger Publishing Company, pp. 3–8.

Anderson, R.M. (1995), 'Revisiting the behavioural model and access to medical care: does it matter?', *Journal of Health and Social Behaviour*, **36**(March), 1–10.

Anderson, R.M. and L. Benham (1970), 'Factors affecting the relationship between family income and medical care consumption', in Herbert E. Klarman (ed.), *Empirical Studies in Health Economics*, Baltimore, MD: Johns Hopkins University Press, pp. 73–95.

Anderson, R.M. and J.F. Newman (1973), 'Societal and individual determinants of medical care utilisation in the United States', *The Milbank Memorial Fund Quarterly. Health and Society*, **51**(1), 95–124.

Castles, Francis G. (2004), *The Future of the Welfare State*, Oxford: Oxford University Press.

Coburn, D. (2003), 'Income inequality, social cohesion, and the health status of populations', in R. Hofrichter (ed.), *Health and Social Justice: Politics, Ideology, and Inequity in the Distribution of Disease*, San Francisco, CA: Jossey-Bass, pp. 335–55.

Cockerham, W.C. (2001), 'Medical sociology and sociological theory', in W.C. Cockerham (ed.), *The Blackwell Companion to Medical Sociology*, Malden, MA: Blackwell Publishers, pp. 3–22.

Culyer, A.J. (1976), *Need and the National Health Service*, London: Martin Robertson.

Deaton, A. (2002), 'Policy implications of the gradient of health and wealth. An economist asks, would redistributing income improve population health?', *Health Affairs*, **21**(2), 13–30.

Ekman, B. (2007), 'The impact of health insurance on outpatient utilization and expenditure: evidence from one middle-income country using national household survey data', *Health Research Policy and Systems*, **5**(6).

Elgazzar, H. (2009), 'Income and the use of health care: an empirical study of Egypt and Lebanon', *Health Economics, Policy and Law*, **4**(4), 445–78.

Ellis, R.P., D.K. McInnes and E.H. Stephenson (1994), 'Inpatient and outpatient health care demand in Cairo, Egypt', *Health Economics*, **3**(3), 183–200.

Ensor, T. and J. Ronoh (2005), 'Effective financing of maternal health services: a review of the literature', *Health Policy*, **75**, 49–58.

Esping-Andersen, G. (1990), *The Three Worlds of Welfare Capitalism*, Cambridge: Polity Press.

Esping-Andersen, G. (2000), *Social Foundations of Postindustrial Economies*, Oxford: Oxford University Press.

Evans, R.G. (1994), 'Introduction', in R.G. Evans, M.L. Barer and T.R. Marmor (eds), *Why Are Some People Healthy and Others Not?*, Berlin: Walter de Gruyter, pp. 3–26.

Fernández, J.-L. and M. Knapp (2004), 'Production relations in social care', in M. Knapp, D. Challis, J.-L. Fernandez and A. Netten (eds), *Long-Term Care: Matching Resources and Needs*, Aldershot, UK: Ashgate Publishing, pp. 171–82.

Frank, J.W. and J.F. Mustard (1994), 'The determinants of health from a historical perspective', *Dædalus*, **123**(4), 1–19.

Gallagher, E. (2001), 'Health, health care, and medical education in the Arab world', in W.C. Cockerham (ed.), *The Blackwell Companion to Medical Sociology*, Malden, MA: Blackwell Publishers, pp. 393–409.

Grogan, C.M. (1995), 'Urban economic reform and access to health care coverage in the People's Republic of China', *Social Science and Medicine*, **41**(8), 1073–84.

Grossman, M. (1972), 'The demand for health: a theoretical and empirical investigation', National Bureau of Economic Research Occasional Paper No. 119, New York: National Bureau of Economic Research.

Hernández-Quevedo, C., A.M. Jones, Á. López-Nicolás and R. Rice (2006), 'Socioeconomic inequalities in health: a comparative analysis using the European Community Household Panel', *Social Science and Medicine*, **63**, 1246–61.

Hosseinpour, A.R., K. Mohammad, R. Majdzadeh, M. Naghavi, F. Abolhassani, A. Sousa, N. Speybroeck, H.R. Jamshidi and J. Vega (2005), 'Socioeconomic inequality in infant mortality in Iran and across its provinces', *Bulletin of the World Health Organization*, **83**, 837–44.

Issawi, C. (1989), 'The Middle East in the world context: a historical view', in Georges Sabagh (ed.), *The Modern Economic and Social History of the Middle East in its World Context*, Cambridge: Cambridge University Press, pp. 3–28.

Jabbour, S., A. El-Zein, I. Nuwayhid and R. Giacaman (2006), 'Can action on health achieve political and social reform?', *British Medical Journal*, **333**(7573), 837–9.

Jowett, M., P. Contoyannis and N.D. Vinh (2003), 'The impact of public voluntary health insurance on private health expenditures in Vietnam', *Social Science and Medicine*, **56**, 333–42.

Jurjus, A.R. (1995), 'Health financing in Lebanon: cost and insurance coverage', Beirut: Ministry of Public Health.

Kanavos, P. and M. Gemmill (2004), 'Senior citizens and the burden of prescription drug outlays: what lessons for the Medicare Prescription Drug Benefit?', *Applied Health Economics and Health Policy*, **3**(4), 217–27.

Karshenas, M. and V.M. Moghadam (2006), 'Social policy in the Middle East: introduction and overview', in M. Karshenas and V.M. Moghadam (eds), *Social Policy in the Middle East: Economic, Political, and Gender Dynamics*, New York: Palgrave Macmillan and United Nations Research Institute for Social Development, pp. 1–30.

Keeler, E.B. (1992), 'Effects of cost sharing on use of medical care and health', *Journal of Medical Practice Management*, **8**, 317–21.

Klein, R. (2001), *The New Politics of the NHS*, 4th edn, Harlow, UK: Prentice-Hall.

Klein, R. (2003), 'Lessons for (and from) America', *American Journal of Public Health*, **93**(1), 61–3.

Knapp, M. (2007), 'Economic outcomes and levers: impacts for individuals and society', *International Psychogeriatrics*, **19**(3), 483–95.

Knapp, M., M. Funk, C. Curran, M. Prince, M. Grigg and D. McDaid (2006), 'Economic barriers to better mental health practice and policy', *Health Policy and Planning*, **21**(3), 157–70.

Labonte, R. (1993), *Health Promotion and Empowerment: Practice Frameworks*, Toronto: Centre for Health Promotion and ParcipAction, available from http://www.utoronto.ca/chp.

Lu, J.F., G.M. Leung, S. Kwon, K.Y. Tin, E. van Doorslaer and O. O'Donnell (2007), 'Horizontal equity in health care utilization evidence from three high-income Asian economies', *Social Science and Medicine*, **64**(1), 199–212.

Marmot, M. (2005), 'Social determinants of health inequalities', *Lancet*, **365**(9464), 1099–104.

Maziak, W. (2006), 'Health in the Middle East', *British Medical Journal*, **333**(7573), 815–16.

Morris, S., M. Sutton and H. Gravelle (2005), 'Inequity and inequality in the use of health care in England: an empirical investigation', *Social Science and Medicine*, **60**, 1251–66.

Muennig, P., P. Franks, E. Haomiao, E. Lubetkin and M. Gold (2005), 'The income-associated burden of disease in the United States', *Social Science and Medicine*, **61**, 2018–26.

Murray, C.J.L. and L.C. Chen (1993), 'In search of a contemporary theory for understanding mortality change', *Social Science and Medicine*, **36**(2), 143–55.

Mushkin, S.J. (1962), 'Health as an investment', *Journal of Political Economy*, **70**(5, Part 2: Investment in Human Beings), 129–57.

Nandakumar, A.K., M. Chawla and M. Khan (2000), 'Utilization of outpatient care in Egypt and its implications for the role of government in health care provision', *World Development*, **28**(1), 187–96.

Navarro, V. and L. Shi (2003), 'The political context of social inequalities and health', in Richard Hofrichter (ed.), *Health and Social Justice: Politics, Ideology, and Inequity in the Distribution of Disease*, San Francisco, CA: Jossey-Bass, pp. 195–216.

Newhouse, J.P. (1993), *Free For All? Lessons from the RAND Health Insurance Experiment*, Cambridge, MA: Harvard University Press.

Noro, A.M., U.T. Hakkinen and O.J. Laitinen (1999), 'Determinants of health service use and expenditure among the elderly Finnish population', *European Journal of Public Health*, **9**(3), 174–80.

O'Donnell, O., E. van Doorslaer, R. Rannan-Eliya et al. (2007), 'The incidence of public spending on health care: comparative evidence from Asia', *World Bank Economic Review*, **21**(1), 93–123.

Palmer, N., D.H. Mueller, L. Gilson, A. Mills and A. Haines (2004), 'Health financing to promote access in low-income settings – how much do we know?', *Lancet*, **364**(9442), 1365–70.

Phelps, C.E. (1975), 'Effects of insurance on demand for medical care', in R. Anderson, J. Kravits and W. Anderson (eds), *Equity in Health Services: Empirical Analyses in Social Policy*, Cambridge: Ballinger Publishing Co., pp. 105–29.

Pohlmeier, W. and V. Ulrich (1995), 'An econometric model of the two-part decision-making process in the demand for health care', *The Journal of Human Resources*, **30**(2), 339–61.

Rannan-Eliya, R., C. Blanco-Vidal and A.K. Nandakumar (1999), 'The distribution of health care resources in Egypt. Implications for equity: an analysis using a national health accounts framework', Report No. 81, Boston, MA: Harvard School of Public Health.

Raphael, D. (2000), 'Health inequities in the United States: prospects and solutions', *Journal of Public Health Policy*, **21**(4), 394–427.

Ross, J.S., E.H. Bradley and S.H. Busch (2006), 'Use of health care services by lower-income and higher-income uninsured adults', *Journal of the American Medical Association*, **295**(17), 2027–36.

Russell, S. (1996), 'Ability to pay for health care: concepts and evidence', *Health Policy and Planning*, **11**(3), 219–37.

Russell, S. (2005), 'Illuminating cases: understanding the economic burden of illness through case study household research', *Health Policy and Planning*, **20**(5), 277–89.

Santos Silva, J.M.C. and F. Windmeijer (2001), 'Two-part multiple spell models for health care demand', *Journal of Econometrics*, **104**, 67–89.

Segall, M., G. Tipping, H. Lucas, T.V. Dung, N.T. Tam, D.X. Vinh and D.L. Huong (2002), 'Economic transition should come with a health warning: the case of Vietnam', *Journal of Epidemiology and Community Health*, **56**, 497–505.

Sen, A. (2004), 'From income inequality to economic inequality', in C.M. Henry (ed.), *Race, Poverty and Domestic Policy*, New Haven, CT and London: Yale University Press, pp. 59–82.

Titmuss, R.M. (1956), *The Social Division of Welfare: Some Reflections on the Search for Equity*, reprinted in R.E. Goodin and D. Mitchell (eds) (2000), *The Foundations of the Welfare State, Volume I*, Cheltenham, UK and Northampton, MA, USA: Edward Elgar Publishing Limited, pp. 146–67.

Turner, Bryan S. (1984), *Capitalism and Class in the Middle East: Theories of Social Change and Economic Development*, London: Heinemann.

van Doorslaer, E.K. (1987), *Health, Knowledge and the Demand for Medical Care*, Assen: Van Gorcum.

van Doorslaer, E., P. Clarke, E. Savage and J. Hall (2008), 'Horizontal inequities in Australia's mixed public/private health care system', *Health Policy*, **86**, 97–108.

van Doorslaer, E., C. Masseria and the OECD Health Equity Research Group Members (2004), 'Income-related inequality in the use of medical care in 21 OECD countries', OECD Health Working Paper No. 14, Paris: OECD.

van Doorslaer, E., O. O'Donnell, R.P. Rannan-Eliya, A. Somanathan, S.R. Adhikari, C.C. Garg, D. Harbianto, A.N. Herrin, M.N. Huq, S. Ibragimova, A. Karan, T.J. Lee, G.M. Leung, J.F. Lu, C.W. Ng, B.R. Pande, R. Racelis, S. Tao, K. Tin, K. Tisayaticom, L. Trisnantoro, C. Vasavid and Y. Zhao (2007), 'Catastrophic payments for health care in Asia', *Health Economics*, **16**(11), 1159–84.

van Doorslaer, E., O. O'Donnell, R.P. Rannan-Eliya, A. Somanathan, S.R. Adhikari, C.C. Garg, D. Harbianto, A.N. Herrin, M.N. Huq, S. Ibragimova, A. Karan, C.W. Ng, B.R. Pande, R. Racelis, S. Tao, K. Tin, K. Tisayaticom, L. Trisnantoro, C. Vasavid and Y. Zhao (2006), 'Effect of payments for health care on poverty estimates in 11 countries in Asia: an analysis of household survey data', *Lancet*, **368**(9544), 1357–64.

Wagstaff, A., P. Paci and E. van Doorslaer (1991), 'On the measurement of inequalities in health', *Social Science and Medicine*, **33**(5), 545–57.

Wagstaff, A. and E. van Doorslaer (2001), 'Paying for health care: quantifying fairness, catastrophe, and impoverishment, with applications to Vietnam, 1993–98', Policy Research Working Paper No. 2715, Washington, DC: The World Bank.

Walker, G.K. (1986), 'Reforming Medicare: the limited framework of political discourse on equity and economy', *Social Science and Medicine*, **23**(12), 1237–50.

Ware, J.E., W.H. Rogers, A.R. Davies, G.A. Goldberg, R.H. Brook, E.B. Keeler, C.D. Sherbourne, P. Camp and J.P. Newhouse (1986), 'Comparison of health outcomes at a health maintenance organisation with those of fee-for-service care', *Lancet*, **327**(8488), 1017–22.

Weber, Max (1978), 'Class and status', in G. Roth and C. Wittich (eds), *Economy and Society: An Outline of Interpretive Sociology, Volume 2*, Berkeley, CA: University of California Press, pp. 926–49.

Wiener, J. (2004), 'Home and community-based services in the United States', in M. Knapp, D. Challis, J.-L. Fernández and A. Netten (eds), *Long-Term Care: Matching Resources and Needs*, Aldershot: Ashgate Publishing, pp. 83–100.

Williams, A. (1978), 'Need – an economic exegesis', in A.J. Culyer (ed.) (1991), *The Economics of Health, Volume I*, Aldershot, UK and Brookfield, US: Edward Elgar Publishing, pp. 259–72.

World Bank (2009), 'Health financing in Indonesia: a reform road map', Washington, DC: The World Bank Group.

World Bank (2011), World Development Indicators, Washington, DC: The World Bank, available from http://www.worldbank.org, accessed 6 March 2011.

World Health Organization (1948), 'World Health Organization Constitution', in *Basic Documents*, Geneva: World Health Organization.

World Health Organization (2004), *World Health Survey*, Geneva: World Health Organization.

4 Quality of ambulatory care: hospitalisations for ambulatory care sensitive conditions
Lucia Kossarova

1. INTRODUCTION

Performance measurement in the different areas of health care has become increasingly important in recent decades. Primary care and the hospital sector have been addressed extensively in the literature (Lester and Roland, 2009; McKee and Healy, 2002). With the increasing burden of chronic diseases, there has also been growing interest in measuring the performance of chronic care (McKee et al., 2009) where indicators may capture the care patients receive at both the ambulatory and hospital level for the selected chronic conditions. Less attention has been given to measuring the performance of ambulatory or outpatient care. This chapter looks at how hospitalisations for ambulatory care sensitive conditions (ACSCs) can be used as a performance indicator of the quality of ambulatory care.

Measuring the performance of ambulatory care[1] is important for several reasons. First, health care is generally more expensive to provide in inpatient than outpatient settings, and potential savings can be made from reduced hospital admissions (Kovner and Knickman, 2008); the hospital sector usually absorbs as much as 50 per cent of national expenditure on the health care system (Rechel et al., 2009). Besides the cost of hospital care, a hospital admission is likely to cause disruptions in the patient's life, as well as in his or her family's (Rechel et al., 2009). Also, repeated hospitalisations may lead to the overall deterioration of the patient's condition (Chu et al., 2004). Therefore quality ambulatory care and reduced hospital admissions are not only a potential cost-reduction strategy but also an obligation towards the patients by those who design and regulate the health care system.

While some hospitalisations may be necessary, often patients are hospitalised for so-called 'ambulatory care sensitive conditions' such as asthma or urinary infection which could be treated with timely and effective ambulatory care. It is these types of avoidable or unnecessary hospitalisations that can be used as an indicator of the quality of outpatient care. The purpose of this chapter is to review the use of hospitalisations for ambulatory care sensitive conditions (ACSHs) as a measure of performance of *ambulatory care*. The chapter begins by defining ambulatory care. Then the concepts important for defining quality and measuring performance in general, and more specifically to ambulatory care, are presented. Third, the chapter reviews the literature on ACSHs and the factors that help to explain hospitalisations for these conditions. Finally, the chapter concludes with policy and future research recommendations.

Ambulatory care can be defined as all the services provided on an outpatient basis, requiring no overnight hospital stay, including (i) primary care, (ii) emergency care and (iii) ambulatory specialty care as well as diagnostics services, provided by a range of health care professionals (Kovner and Knickman, 2008). In this chapter, 'ambulatory' and 'outpatient' care will be used interchangeably. *Primary care* can have a range of meanings, including care provided by general practitioners, family physicians, nurse practitioners, specialists or others, depending on the specific country (Lester and Roland, 2009). Lester and Roland (2009) described primary care in terms of its functions with a number of critical elements, including: (i) first contact accessible services where demands are clarified and information, reassurance or advice are given or diagnosis made; (ii) provision of comprehensive services to meet the needs of their patients, focusing on generalism rather than specialism; (iii) provision of patient-centred rather than disease-centred care; (iv) provision of longitudinal relationship between individual patient and their health care provider; (v) coordination of care for individual patients; (vi) integration of biomedical, psychological and social dimensions of the patient's problem; and (vii) a focus on health promotion and disease prevention as well as management of established health problems.

Specialty care is care given by physicians who have received additional training in a specific area of expertise, for example cardiologists, endocrinologists and so on. Finally, *emergency care*, while designed to care for the acutely ill or injured patient, serves also as a major source of walk-in services for less sick patients because it is more convenient. While emergency services could be less costly, there is broad consensus that it is an inappropriate place to obtain primary care because some elements of care, for example continuity, receive little or no attention; at the same time these types of visits, while not equivalent to hospitalisations, may also suggest weaknesses of primary care in preventing exacerbations of number of chronic conditions, for example asthma, diabetes, and acute conditions, e.g. influenza or common types of pneumonia (Kovner and Knickman, 2008).

2.   MEASURING THE QUALITY OF AMBULATORY CARE

Measuring performance is particularly important in health care because it is people's health or life that is at stake and it is vital to know whether steps are being taken towards avoiding unnecessary illness or death. In general, performance measurement seeks to monitor, evaluate and communicate the extent to which various aspects of the health system are meeting key objectives (Smith et al., 2009). These key objectives can be general health systems goals or components of quality of care.

One of the pioneers in the area of quality of care, Avedis Donabedian, wrote in his last book that 'some believe quality in health care is too abstract and nebulous a concept to be precisely defined or objectively measured' (Donabedian, 2003, p. xxxi). Yet he correctly stated that if quality was so difficult to define and measure, it would be difficult to 'set it apart as a goal an individual or an organization can aspire to' (ibid., p. xxxii). Definitions of quality may differ in the breadth and focus, or the dimensions that define it (Legido-Quigley et al., 2008) but they may all be suitable depending on the level of the system at which they are to be used and the nature and scope of the responsibilities of the person who is defining them (Donabedian, 1988). It is also essential to distinguish between clinical quality and quality of care in more general terms. The definition below addresses quality of care in general terms.

Main goals of health systems

1. Health (improvement) – absolute level and equity
2. Fair financial contribution – equity
3. Responsiveness – absolute level and equity

Dimensions of quality

Effectiveness, efficiency, access, safety, equity, appropriateness, timeliness, acceptability, satisfaction, continuity, choice, efficacy etc.

Source: Based on World Health Organization (2000) and Legido-Quigley et al. (2008).

Figure 4.1   Goals of health systems and dimensions of quality

Legido-Quigley and colleagues (2008) reviewed a number of 'quality of care' definitions. For the purposes of this chapter the 'quality of care' definition of the Institute of Medicine (Institute of Medicine, 1990, p. 4) will be used, defining quality as 'the degree to which health services for individuals and populations increase the likelihood of desired health outcomes and are consistent with current professional knowledge'. This definition 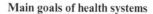 of quality can be made more specific by understanding the different dimensions of quality. Several different dimensions have been identified in earlier publications, but it has been noted that these are 'neither comprehensive nor mutually exclusive' (Legido-Quigley et al., 2008, p. 4). These dimensions include effectiveness, efficiency, access, safety and others that are relevant when evaluating the different areas or levels of a health system but alone are not sufficient to capture the quality of the entire health care system. These dimensions of quality are also sometimes referred to as 'health system goals'.

The World Health Organization report (2000) identified three principal goals of any health system: (i) to improve the health of citizens; (ii) to respond to the needs of the individuals; and (iii) to provide financial protection. In achieving these goals, it is not only the absolute level that is important but also an equitable distribution across the population groups. These three goals correspond to nearly all the dimensions of quality of care as summarized by Legido-Quigley and colleagues (Figure 4.1). For example, the dimensions of choice, acceptability and satisfaction all reflect the responsiveness of a health care system. Depending on the stakeholder interested (e.g. purchasing organization, provider, policy makers etc.) or the level at which performance is being measured (e.g. single provider, provider organization, regional, national level), different dimensions or health system goals receive priority and different indicators are used to measure how the system is performing.

Various indicators have been proposed to measure these different dimensions of quality (Smith et al., 2009). Most of the process and outcome indicators (McGlynn, 2009; McGlynn et al., 2003; McKee et al., 2009; McKee and Healy, 2002; Nolte and McKee, 2008) used to measure performance capture selected levels of care (e.g. primary, specialty, chronic) but not the performance of ambulatory care in general. For example, a process indicator for diabetes such as 'patients with diabetes should have an annual eye and visual exam' or outcome indicator 'the percentage of patients with diabetes in whom the last blood pressure was 145/85 mgHg or less' only capture care provided at primary care level. On the other hand, indicators such as 'women who have a hysterectomy for post-menopausal bleeding should have been offered a biopsy of the endometrium within six months prior to the procedure' or 'rate of diabetes related blindness or amputation' only measure specialist outpatient care. The advantage of the indicator of ACSHs is that it captures the performance of all the care provided at the outpatient level. It is an indicator of weaknesses in the performance of the ambulatory care sector, including primary, specialist, chronic, acute as well as diagnostic care. At the same time, it is an indicator that captures a range of quality of care dimensions such as access to, effectiveness, equity, appropriateness and efficacy of ambulatory care.

3. HOSPITALISATIONS FOR AMBULATORY CARE SENSITIVE CONDITIONS

Several definitions of ACSCs have been put forward since the concept originated. We will not review all of them in this chapter but will highlight the need for having clear definitions when using the indicator to measure health system performance. One of the first ones is by Billings and colleagues (1993), who defined ACSCs as 'conditions for which timely and effective ambulatory care can help reduce the risks of hospitalisation by preventing the onset of an illness or condition, controlling an acute episodic illness or condition, or managing a chronic disease or condition'. While this definition refers to the performance of ambulatory care, Billings and colleagues (1993) stressed that both 'access to ambulatory care and the performance of outpatient care delivery system may have a substantial effect on admission rates'. In addition, other factors, including environmental, personal, access barriers, the organization and mix of available outpatient resources and others need to be considered. The Institute of Medicine (Millman, 1993), building on the work by Billings, referred to ACSCs as 'avoidable hospitalisations' that 'might not have occurred had the patient received effective, timely, and continuous outpatient (ambulatory) medical care for certain chronic disease conditions'. In this context, ACSHs should not be considered simply as a utilisation measure but as a costly adverse event that can be avoided if patients have timely access to effective ambulatory care (Millman, 1993).

The Agency for Healthcare Research and Quality (AHRQ) in the USA has been using a set of ACSCs as its Prevention Quality Indicators. Their definition of ACSCs refers to the importance of 'adequate primary care' (Agency for Healthcare Research and Quality, 2001) as well as 'good outpatient care that can potentially prevent need for hospitalisation, or of which early intervention can prevent complications or more severe disease' (Agency for Healthcare Research and Quality, 2004). Other researchers focus on ACSHs as an indicator of quality and access to primary health care (Ansari, 2007a) and there are many other, all somewhat similar, definitions in circulation.

The above definitions of ACSCs refer to the importance of *outpatient, ambulatory* as well as *primary care* for preventing unnecessary hospitalisations. It is possible that researchers use different terms but refer to the same elements of care or may indeed be measuring different things. Therefore, it is important to be clear which aspects of care are being measured with ACSCs especially as someone's chances of being hospitalised may depend on factors that are not only in the responsibility of primary care providers but also a consequence of the care provided by other outpatient specialists and health care staff, as well as appropriate coordination across the different levels of care, continuity, patient management and others. In addition, ACSHs may be measuring the contribution of non-health system factors, which will be addressed later in the chapter.

This indicator is conceptually related to and has been developed on the basis of an indicator of population health – 'avoidable' mortality (Millman, 1993). 'Avoidable' mortality can be defined as the deaths from certain causes that should not occur in the presence of timely and effective health care (Holland, 1988; Nolte and McKee, 2004; Rutstein et al., 1976). It is an indicator that is a marker for population health while at the same time encompassing the quality of the entire health system. Both 'avoidable' mortality and hospitalisations for ACSCs are meant to be used as 'screening tools' for potential problems in the health system to be further investigated – in other words, to provide a 'snapshot' on the quality of the health system overall, or ambulatory care more specifically.

The first list of ACSCs was developed in the early 1990s in the USA by Weissman (Weissman et al., 1992) with 12 conditions and Billings (Billings et al., 1993) with 28 conditions when the Institute of Medicine suggested that ACSHs be used as a measure of access problems and deficiencies in outpatient management (Millman, 1993). In general, ACSCs have been identified through consensus processes with panels of clinicians, using various methodologies and decision criteria (Ansari, 2007a). ACSCs can be classified into three broad categories as follows:

- *Vaccine-preventable* ACSCs where the vaccine prevents the occurrence of the condition (not actually the hospitalisation) and thus the incidence of preventable diseases (e.g. measles, rubella etc.)
- *Acute* ACSCs for which timely and appropriate care reduces morbidity and pain (e.g. dehydration/gastroenteritis, perforated ulcer, pelvic inflammatory disease, kidney infection etc.)
- *Chronic* ACSCs where appropriate outpatient care reduces the effect of particular chronic disease and prolongs life (e.g. asthma, hypertension, angina, congestive heart failure, diabetes etc.)

Many countries, including Canada, the USA, the UK, Italy, Spain and Australia, have already developed their country-specific lists and have been monitoring ACSHs during the last decade (Ansari et al., 2006; Billings et al., 1996; Caminal et al., 2004; CIFHI, 2008; Giuffrida et al., 1999; Magan et al., 2008; Rizza et al., 2007). While countries differ in how the indicator is applied and the lists of conditions and ICD codes being monitored, the fact that easily accessible and cheap administrative data may be used makes this indicator attractive to health policy and decision makers alike. However, it is important to acknowledge any methodological differences, especially when making comparisons over time or across countries.

Hospitalisations for *individual* ambulatory care sensitive conditions (e.g. asthma or gastroenteritis only) have been carefully evaluated and proposed as area-level indicators by the Agency for Healthcare Research and Quality (AHRQ) in the USA as part of the Healthcare Cost and Utilization Project, an ongoing Federal State–private sector collaboration to build uniform databases from administrative hospital based data (AHRQ, 2001). The AHRQ evaluated the validity of admissions for all the ambulatory care sensitive conditions together[2] along the following dimensions: face validity, precision, minimum bias, construct validity, fosters true quality improvement, and prior use and application. Given the limitations of the measure, the Agency recommended that ACSHs be used alongside other quality indicators as a 'quality screen' that can provide initial information about a potential problem in the health system that should be analysed in more depth (AHRQ, 2001, 2004).

It is difficult to establish the appropriate rate of hospitalisations for ACSCs, but a rate that is too high may indicate poor access to, underuse or inappropriate outpatient care or low threshold for admissions by the admitting physician. Overall, it is important to explore the causes of variations in admissions rates where the best benchmark would be comparisons with national, regional or peer group means (AHRQ, 2001). Wennberg and colleagues (Wennberg, 1999, 2004; Wennberg et al., 2004) have extensively studied variations in health care utilisation and expenditures in the USA and shown the importance of understanding the factors that explain such variations – in particular, how the care provided for the same condition differs across regions. For example, if high rates persist in some regions over time, there may be some systematic differences in access to and appropriateness of the treatment, or other factors.

Many of the ACSCs have clinical practice guidelines, and studies have shown that better outpatient care can reduce patient complication rates of existing disease, including the complications leading to hospital admissions. Empirically, most of the hospital admission rates for ACSCs are correlated, suggesting that common underlying factors influence many of the rates (AHRQ, 2007). However, exploring concrete aspects of clinical quality of care and how these are linked to hospitalisation levels requires a condition-specific analysis. Yet studies that look at sets of ACSCs have not been able to include clinical quality of care variables such as appropriate treatment.

Preventable hospitalisations have primarily been proposed as a single outcome-based measure of *access*, after acknowledging that evaluating all the different dimensions of access (availability, accessibility, affordability etc.) is often not feasible (Ansari, 2007b). In fact, most of the available literature focuses on ACSH rates as a measure of access to health care where different factors, predominantly socioeconomic, are used as a proxy for access to health care; an inverse relationship with ACSH rates suggests reduced access. In addition, the relationship of other variables (e.g. lifestyle factors, prevalence, environment etc.) and ACSHs have also been explored. The large amount of non-health system factors that have a relationship with ACSH rates may suggest that the reporting of ACSHs figures is not likely to foster change in the quality of services provided. However, if all the different factors are appropriately accounted for, changes in ACSH rates are likely to at least indicate areas of weakness in the health system and provide the initial motivation for further enquiries and potential for improvement.

4.   FACTORS ASSOCIATED WITH ACSHS

A systematic review[3] has been carried out to bring together the existing body of evidence on the factors that explain ACSHs. Such evidence should enable the better application of this indicator to the measurement of performance of ambulatory care. As a result, any subsequent policy changes and improvements in access and quality of care should not only save costs but also avoid unnecessary hospital stays for patients.

In the process of carrying out the initial literature search for the systematic review in the Medline and Embase databases, a comprehensive literature review[4] (Ansari, 2007a) has been identified. The Ansari review covers evidence from 1970 until August 2005; it explores the validity of ACSC admissions as proxy indicators for access to primary health care, and summarises all the different factors associated with ACSHs rates across geographic areas and population groups. The author of the review grouped the evidence along several areas:

- Demographics (age, race, gender)
- Socioeconomic status
- Rurality
- Health system factors (primary care physician supply, regular source of care, self-rated access to care, presence of subsidised primary care, inpatient bed supply, clinical threshold for admission/physician practice style)
- Prevalence
- Lifestyle factors
- Environment
- Adherence to medication
- Severity of illness
- Propensity to seek care

Ansari concluded that ACSC admissions are valid proxy indicators of access to primary health care. ACSHs result from a number of key reasons, including insufficiency and maldistribution of primary health care resources, evidence of the existence of barriers to accessing primary care services (e.g. socioeconomic), problems with continuity of care and inefficient use of resources (e.g. may occur if the patient finds it easier or cheaper to go directly to the hospital instead of getting care in an ambulatory setting) (Ansari, 2007a). Overall, this review revealed that socioeconomic factors seem to be the most important predictors of ACSHs. While some factors are addressed much more extensively (e.g. supply of physicians), others such as lifestyle, prevalence, adherence to medication and, in more general terms, utilisation and clinical quality of care that patients receive are covered to a more limited extent.

We have systematically updated the Ansari review to encompass new evidence from 2005 until March 2009 to see whether the effects of any additional factors that influence ACSHs have since been identified. The results from the Ansari review as well as the systematic review can be summarised in light of a conceptual framework adapted from models for access to care, in particular earlier behavioural models (Andersen, 1995; Andersen et al., 1983), supply–demand models (Basu et al., 2004), Chang's model (Chang et al., 2008) and the World Bank's health outcome model.[5] This framework does

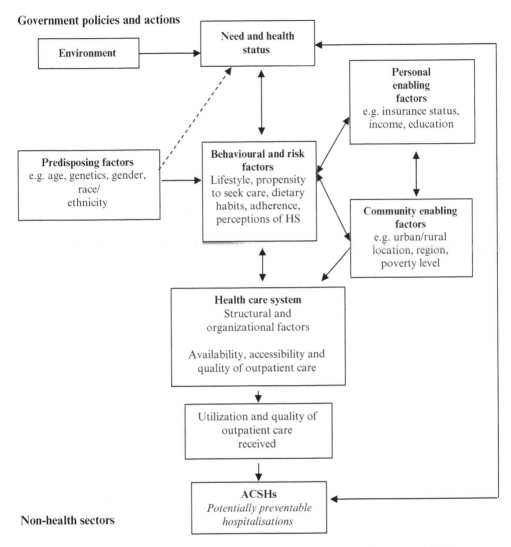

Source: Adjusted and based on Chang et al. (2008); Andersen et al. (1983, 1995); Basu et al. (2004); Klugman (2002).

Figure 4.2   Conceptual framework for ACSHs

not, however, only focus on ACSHs as a measure of access since other variables not associated with access may have an effect on preventable hospitalisations. Figure 4.2 summarises the conceptual framework that has been applied when reviewing the literature and shows which factors are likely to influence ACSHs, and how.

Any individual begins with the onset of a certain condition (need) that is influenced by the environment, behavioural and risk factors, as well as the person's predisposing factors such as genetic characteristics, age, gender or ethnicity. Then there are the behavioural and risk factors, which include the person's lifestyle (e.g. exercise, eating and smoking habits), attitude towards taking medication and propensity to seek care. These are influenced both by predisposing as well as enabling personal factors (e.g. insurance status, income) and enabling community factors (e.g. community poverty level); both provide the 'means' to utilise services (Chang et al., 2008). Depending on the person's perception of the health care system, its availability, quality and accessibility, individuals utilise health care. Finally, the number of times the person comes into contact with the outpatient health system (primary and/or specialist care), as well as the quality of care he or she receives, determine ACSH rates.

Therefore, while ACSH rates may be used as a measure of access to effective out-patient care, it is important to take into account all the different factors that may confound this relationship, to the extent that this is possible. Some of these variables (e.g. age, gender, ethnicity) may capture differences in preferences for and utilisation of outpatient treatment, or quality of treatment offered by providers and not just biological predispositions. For example, ethnicity may not be an important factor after additional variables such as patient attributes, lifestyle, level of poverty and others are included. Therefore, instead of risk adjustment, which may hide important gender or ethnic differences, these may be better accounted for through a stratified analysis where the results are examined separately – that is, for women and men, different ethnic groups and so on.

In addition, some variables in the framework, for example genetics, may not only explain access to care, but, through the concept of health need, may have a direct relationship to ACSHs (see dashed line in Figure 4.2). These are hospitalisations that are not preventable but need to be accounted for.

Fourteen new studies have been included and analysed as part of the systematic review. Information on key aspects that are relevant for analysis has been extracted and can be found in Appendix Table 4A.1. The findings of the reviewed studies are summarised in Table 4.1. The table highlights the variables of interest[6] that have been selected on the basis of the factors identified in the Ansari review. We have also identified new determinants of ACSHs.

The literature search yielded highly heterogeneous studies that may partially be explained by the search strategy, which did not focus only on certain variables of interest. A broad search may be more informative and useful for researchers or policy makers who are interested in the general application and use of the ACSH indicator. This is also suggested by the way the Ansari review was carried out; it did not include an in-depth comparison of the studies but instead focused on their results.

Overall, the variety of settings and chosen variables of interest, differences in ACSCs lists used, the target population, number and type of confounders, study designs, methods and data sources made it difficult to compare and assess the quality of studies. Therefore it was difficult to draw sound conclusions about the overall effects and strengths of associations of the different factors and ACSHs. However, despite these limitations, this systematic review, together with the Ansari review, provides interesting findings for future research and policy application of the ACSHs indicator.

Most of the studies did not apply a conceptual framework in their analysis, which may have influenced the overall quality and results. As in earlier research, these studies again focused on demographic, socioeconomic and a few health system factors. Also, the factors assessed were those that are generally easier to assess and measure. While this may not be a problem as such, it may lead to incomplete conclusions about ACSHs

Table 4.1   Summary of results

Study	1	2	3	4	5	6	7	8	9	10	11	12	13	14	Association with ACSHs
Demographics															
Age					X										YES
Gender			X												YES
Race	X						X						X		MIXED
Socioeconomic status															
Insurance status	X	X		X					X			X			YES
Poverty among elderly											X				YES
Managed care penetration											X				YES
Availability of supplemental coverage											X				YES
Rurality															
Urban sprawl											X				YES
Health system factors															
Self-rate access						X									YES
Continuity of care/ regular source of care								X						X	YES
Presence of rural clinic										X					YES
Physician supply (providers other than GPs)											X				YES
Physician visits											X				YES
Prevalence, lifestyle factors, environment, adherence to medication, propensity to seek care, severity of illness															

as a performance indicator for the quality of ambulatory care. When the studies were reviewed using our conceptual framework, the literature predominantly deals with predisposing factors, personal enabling factors and health system factors and how these explain ACSH rates, while other factors are not addressed.

Besides one study that included physician visits, no new evidence has been identified that would consider health services utilisation (intensity of care) and clinical quality of care variables, such as appropriate drug treatment for a specific condition[7] or adherence to the prescribed treatment. Yet it is important to acknowledge that including these types of variables may only be possible if ACSCs are monitored individually at the patient level. This has been done in condition-specific studies, for example diabetes or asthma, where it has been established that hospitalisations for these conditions can be controlled with appropriate care. Also, none of the studies looked at the relationship between all the key factors together – predisposing (e.g. age, gender), enabling (e.g. income, insurance), behaviour and risk (e.g. adherence, smoking), utilisation (e.g. primary and specialist visits) and quality of care (e.g. type of drug treatment) – and ACSHs. Finally, the indicator of ACSHs continued to be applied mainly in the USA, as well as Canada, Australia and Spain, but not in new country contexts.

5.   CONCLUSIONS AND RECOMMENDATIONS

This chapter highlighted how hospitalisations for ACSCs may be a suitable performance indicator of the quality of ambulatory care. The systematic literature review revealed that further research is required to better understand the association of new factors with ACSHs besides those that have been more commonly researched. Also, it would be significant if future reviews of evidence carried out a more in-depth analysis of the study designs, methods, data sources and ASCSs lists used in order to provide better-quality evidence to policy makers. This chapter did not review the condition-specific literature (e.g. diabetes, asthma and hypertension) that may have identified a range of additional factors, especially clinical, associated with preventable hospitalisations. These may include, for example, appropriateness of clinical care according to evidence-based guidelines, adherence or others.

In order to make the ACSHs useful for policy makers at the country level, it is important that future studies focus on factors that are specific to the country's health system context, particularly in countries where, to date, little or no research has been carried out. For example, in systems of social health insurance where entire populations are covered, exploring the association of insurance status with hospitalisations may not be relevant. Instead, coordination of care or adherence and their association with preventable hospitalisations may need to be measured. In addition, it may be important to understand the hospital payment scheme, which may influence the admission threshold and patient management of the admitting physicians.

Ansari (2007a) suggested that ACSHs be used by policy makers as an information and evaluation tool for continuous monitoring of health services or as an outcome indicator for small area analysis where communities or regions with problems accessing primary care can be identified. However, the indicator not only reveals problems in accessing primary health care but also problems with the quality of the entire ambulatory care level of the health system. Large variations in ACSHs should serve as the warning flag, requiring more in-depth investigations of factors associated with such preventable hospitalisations and careful consideration of future actions. Better understanding of country-specific determinants of ACSHs will allow policy makers and managers in the countries to take the necessary quality improvement actions at the different levels of ambulatory care. These may be actions focused on improving access to primary care, specialist care or diagnostic services, coordination of care across these providers as well as improvement of clinical quality and appropriateness of care provided. Finally, non-health system determinants of preventable hospitalisations as highlighted in the conceptual framework (e.g. behavioural and risk factors) should also be considered.

ACSHs can rely on easily accessible administrative or billing data available from purchasing organisations or discharge data from hospitals, which makes this indicator more appealing to policy makers and managers. Analysing patient-level panel data allows for the examination of the factors influencing ACSHs over an extended period of time. While most administrative and billing databases may lack clinical information about the patient (e.g. severity of the disease at presentation, behavioural risk factors), basic demographic data, information about physician contacts and services provided (e.g. types of drugs prescribed, diagnostic tests carried out etc.) may reveal a wealth of information about the quality of care provided to patients. If necessary, additional databases and surveys (e.g. censuses) may be used to supplement the missing information.

NOTES

1. In this chapter ambulatory care and outpatient care are used interchangeably.
2. Most evidence applies to sets of conditions. The indicators included are: perforated appendix; diabetes short-term complication; diabetes long-term complication; chronic obstructive pulmonary disease; hypertension; congestive heart failure; low birth weight; dehydration; bacterial pneumonia; urinary tract infection; angina without procedure; uncontrolled diabetes; adult asthma; and rate of lower-extremity amputation among patients with diabetes.
3. Detailed methodology of the systematic review can be requested from the author.
4. From here onwards this literature review may be referred to as 'Ansari review' only.
5. The World Bank, www.worldbank.org.
6. Variables controlled for/confounding variables are not included.
7. Literature on determinants of hospitalisations for individual conditions has not been reviewed.

REFERENCES

Agency for Healthcare Research and Quality (2001), *Refinement of the HCUP Quality Indicators*, Rockville, MD: US Department of Health and Human Services.
Agency for Healthcare Research and Quality (2004), *AHRQ Quality Indicators – Guide to Prevention Quality Indicators: Hospital Admission for Ambulatory Care Sensitive Conditions*, Revision 4, Rockville, MD: US Department of Health and Human Services.
Agency for Healthcare Research and Quality (2007), *Guide to Prevention Quality Indicators: Hospital Admission for Ambulatory Care Sensitive Conditions*, Rockville, MD: US Department of Health and Human Services.
Andersen, R.M. (1995), 'Revisiting the behavioral model and access to medical care: does it matter?', *Journal of Health and Social Behavior*, **36**(3), 1–10.
Andersen, R.M., McCutcheon, A., Aday, L.A., Chiiu, G.Y. and Bell, R. (1983), 'Exploring dimensions of access to medical care', *Health Services Research*, **18**(1), 49–74.
Ansari, Z. (2007a), 'The concept and usefulness of ambulatory care sensitive conditions as indicators of quality and access to primary health care', *Australian Journal of Primary Health*, **13**(3), 91–110.
Ansari, Z. (2007b), 'A review of literature on access to primary health care', *Australian Journal of Primary Health*, **13**(2), 80–95.
Ansari, Z., Laditka, J.N. and Laditka, S.B. (2006), 'Access to health care and hospitalization for ambulatory care sensitive conditions', *Medical Care Research and Review*, **63**(6), 719–41.
Basu, J., Friedman, B. and Burstin, H. (2004), 'Managed care and preventable hospitalization among Medicaid adults', *Health Services Research*, **39**(3), 489–510.
Billings, J., Anderson, G.M. and Newman, L.S. (1996), 'Recent findings on preventable hospitalizations', *Health Affairs*, **15**(3), 239–49.
Billings, J., Zeitel, L., Lukomnik, J., Carey, T.S., Blank, A.E. and Newman, L. (1993), 'Impact of socioeconomic status on hospital use in New York City', *Health Affairs*, **12**, 162–73.
Bindman, A.B., Chattopadhyay, A. and Auerback, G.M. (2008), 'Interruptions in Medicaid coverage and risk for hospitalization for ambulatory care-sensitive conditions', *Annals of Internal Medicine*, **149**(12), 854–60.

Bindman, A.B., Chattopadhyay, A., Osmond, D.H., Huen, W. and Bacchetti, P. (2005), 'The impact of Medicaid managed care on hospitalizations for ambulatory care sensitive conditions', *Health Services Research*, **40**(1), 19–38.

Caminal, J., Starfield, B., Sanchez, E., Casanova, C. and Morales, M. (2004), 'The role of primary care in preventing ambulatory care sensitive conditions', *European Journal of Public Health*, **14**(3), 246–51.

Carter, M.W., Datti, B. and Winters, J.M. (2006), 'ED visits by older adults for ambulatory care-sensitive and supply-sensitive conditions', *American Journal of Emergency Medicine*, **24**(4), 428–34.

Chang, C.F., Mirvis, D.M. and Waters, T.M. (2008), 'The effects of race and insurance on potentially avoidable hospitalizations in Tennessee', *Medical Care Research and Review*, **65**(5), 596–616.

Chu, C.M., Chan, V.L., Lin, A.W.N., Wong, I.W.Y., Leung, W.S. and Lai, C.K.W. (2004), 'Readmission rates and life threatening events in COPD survivors treated with non-invasive ventilation for acute hypercapnic respiratory failure', *Thorax*, **59**(12), 1020–25.

CIFHI (2008), *Health indicators*, Ottawa: Canadian Institute for Health Information.

Donabedian, A. (1988), 'The quality of care. How can it be assessed?', *Journal of the American Medical Association*, **260**(12), 1743–48.

Donabedian, A. (2003), *An Introduction to Quality Assurance in Health Care*, New York: Oxford University Press.

Falik, M., Needleman, J., Herbert, R., Wells, B., Politzer, R. and Benedict, M.B. (2006), 'Comparative effectiveness of health centers as regular source of care: application of sentinel ACSC events as performance measures', *The Journal of Ambulatory Care Management*, **29**(1), 24–35.

Giuffrida, A., Gravelle, H. and Roland, M. (1999), 'Measuring quality of care with routine data: avoiding confusion between performance indicators and health outcomes', *British Medical Journal*, **319**(7202), 94–8.

Holland, W. (ed.) (1988), *European Community Atlas of 'Avoidable Death'*, Commission of the European Communities Health Services Research Series No. 3, Oxford: Oxford University Press.

Howard, D.L., Hakeem, F.B., Njue, C., Carey, T. and Jallah, Y. (2007), 'Racially disproportionate admission rates for ambulatory care sensitive conditions in North Carolina', *Public Health Reports*, **122**(3), 362–72.

Institute of Medicine (1990), *Medicare: A Strategy for Quality Assurance*, Vol. 1, Washington, DC: National Academy Press.

Klugman, J. (2002), *A Sourcebook for Poverty Reduction Strategies: Volume 2, Macroeconomic and Sectoral Approaches*, Washington, DC: World Bank.

Kovner, A.R. and Knickman, J.R. (2008), *Jonas and Kovner's Health Care Delivery in the United States*, 9th edn, New York: Springer.

Ladltka, J.N. and Ladltka, S.B. (2006), 'Race, ethnicity and hospitalization for six chronic ambulatory care sensitive conditions in the USA', *Ethnicity and Health*, **11**, 247–63.

Legido-Quigley, H., McKee, M., Nolte, E. and Glinos, I. (2008), *Assuring the Quality of Health Care in the European Union*, Copenhagen: European Observatory on Health Systems and Policies.

Lester, H. and Roland, M. (2009), 'Performance measurement in primary care', in P.C. Smith, E. Mossialos, I. Papanicolas and S. Leatherman (eds), *Performance Measurement for Health System Improvement: Experiences, Challenges and Prospects*, Cambridge: Cambridge University Press, pp. 371–405.

Magan, P., Otero, A., Alberquilla, A. and Ribera, J.M. (2008), 'Geographic variations in avoidable hospitalizations in the elderly, in a health system with universal coverage', *BMC Health Services Research*, **8**, 48–52.

McCall, N., Harlow, J. and Dayhoof, D. (2001), 'Rates of hospitalization for ambulatory care sensitive conditions in the Medicare+Choice population', *Health Care Financial Review*, **22**, 127–45.

McGlynn, E.A. (2009), 'Measuring clinical quality and appropriateness', in P.C. Smith, E. Mossialos, I. Papanicolas and S. Leatherman (eds), *Performance Measurement for Health System Improvement: Experiences, Challenges and Prospects*, Cambridge: Cambridge University Press, pp. 87–113.

McGlynn, E.A., Asch, S.M., Adams, J., Keesey, J., Hicks, J., DeCristofaro, A. et al. (2003), 'The quality of health care delivered to adults in the United States', *The New England Journal of Medicine*, **348**(26), 2635–45.

McKee, M., Bain, C. and Nolte, E. (2009), 'Chronic care', in P.C. Smith, E. Mossialos, I. Papanicolas and S. Leatherman (eds), *Performance Measurement for Health System Improvement: Experiences, Challenges and Prospects*, Cambridge: Cambridge University Press, pp. 406–25.

McKee, M. and Healy, J. (eds) (2002), *Hospitals in a Changing Europe*, European Observatory on Health Care Systems Series, Maidenhead: Open University Press.

Menec, V.H., Sirski, M., Attawar, D. and Katz, A. (2006), 'Does continuity of care with a family physician reduce hospitalizations among older adults?', *Journal of Health Services Research and Policy*, **11**(4), 196–201.

Millman, M. (1993), *Access to Health Care in America*, Washington, DC: Institute of Medicine, National Academy Press.

Mobley, L.R., Root, E., Anselin, L., Lozano-Gracia, N. and Koschinsky, J. (2006), 'Spatial analysis of elderly access to primary care services', *International Journal of Health Geographics*, **5**, Article Number 19.

Nolte, E. and McKee, M. (2004), *Does Health Care Save Lives? Avoidable Mortality Revisited*, London: The Nuffield Trust.

Nolte, E. and McKee, M. (eds) (2008), *Caring for People with Chronic Conditions: A Health System Perspective*, Maidenhead: Open University Press.

Rechel, B., Wright, S., Edwards, N., Dowdeswell, B. and McKee, M. (eds) (2009), *Investing in Hospitals of the Future*, Copenhagen: World Health Organization, on behalf of the European Observatory on Health Systems and Policies.

Rizza, P., Bianco, A., Pavia, M. and Angelillo, I. (2007), 'Preventable hospitalization and access to primary health care in an area of Southern Italy', *BMC Health Services Research*, 7(1), 134.

Rutstein, D.D., Berenberg, W., Chalmers, T.C., Child, C.G., Fishman, A.P. and Perrin, E.B. (1976), 'Measuring the quality of medical care. A clinical method', *New England Journal of Medicine*, 294(11), 582–8.

Saha, S., Solotaroff, R., Oster, A. and Bindman, A.B. (2007), 'Are preventable hospitalizations sensitive to changes in access to primary care? The case of the Oregon Health Plan', *Medical Care*, 45(8), 712–19.

Smith, P.C., Mossialos, E., Papanicolas, I. and Leatherman, S. (2009), *Performance Measurement for Health System Improvement: Experiences, Challenges and Prospects*, Cambridge: Cambridge University Press.

Weissman, J.S., Gatsonis, C. and Epstein, A.M. (1992), 'Rates of avoidable hospitalization by insurance status in Massachusetts and Maryland', *Journal of the American Medical Association*, 268(17), 2388–94.

Wennberg, J.E. (1999), 'Understanding geographic variations in health care delivery', *New England Journal of Medicine*, 340(1), 52–3.

Wennberg, J.E. (2004), 'Practice variations and health care reform: connecting the dots', *Health Affairs (Millwood), Suppl. Web Exclusives*, VAR140-144.

Wennberg, J.E., Fisher, E.S., Stukel, T.A. and Sharp, S.M. (2004), 'Use of Medicare claims data to monitor provider-specific performance among patients with severe chronic illness', *Health Affairs (Millwood), Suppl. Web Exclusives*, VAR5-18.

World Health Organization (2000), *The World Health Report 2000: Health Systems: Improving Performance*, Geneva: World Health Organization.

Zeng, F., O'Leary, J.F., Sloss, E.M., Lopez, M.S., Dhanani, N. and Melnick, G. (2006), 'The effect of medicare health maintenance organizations on hospitalization rates for ambulatory care-sensitive conditions', *Medical Care*, 44(10), 900–907.

Zhang, W., Mueller, K.J., Chen, L.-W. and Conway, K. (2006), 'The role of rural health clinics in hospitalization due to ambulatory care sensitive conditions: a study in Nebraska', *Journal of Rural Health*, 22(3), 220–23.

APPENDIX

Table 4A.1 Summary of included studies

Study	Setting	Participants	Dependent variable and Factors of interest	Confounders	Conditions included	Result/Effect	Data source/ Methods	Limitations of study acknowledged by original author(s)
1. Chang et al. (2008)	USA, Tennessee 2002–04	<1 18+	Unadjusted overall ACSHs rates; Unadjusted chronic ACSHs rates; Unadjusted acute ACSHs rates; **Variables of interest:** Race; Insurance coverage	Age; Ethnicity; Gender; County poverty levels; Urban/rural; Region of state; Charlson Index (health status); No of hospital beds; PCP/population unit	AHRQ (2007); 14 ACSCs	Hospitalised black patients more likely than white experienced chronic ACSHs; For acute conditions the risk was lower for black patients after controlling for covariates; Insurance a strong predictor of risk of hospitalisations; Hospitalised uninsured black patients faced highest relative risk for ACSHs	Hospital discharge records; Areas resource file; Unit of analysis: individual patient; Logistic regression	Age, gender, Charlson Comorbidity Index may not fully account for underlying health care needs. Thus race and insurance variables may have picked up the effects of unobserved differences in health needs; Repeated admission of minority individuals; Race and insurance may be

| 2. Bindman et al. (2008) | USA 1998–2002 | California Medicaid population. Population covered: 4 735 797. Adults aged 18–64 with a minimum of 1 month coverage between 1998 and 2002 | Time to ACSHs. **Variable of interest:** Medicaid interruption | Demographic characteristics: age, sex, race/ethnicity. Medicaid aid category (estimate for health status). Medicaid health care delivery model. Other form of insurance. Elixhauser comorbid condition | AHRQ (2001) list | Interruption in Medicaid insurance coverage associated with higher risk for ACSH. Beneficiaries who were older, black or Hispanic were eligible for Medicaid through Supplemental Security Program or aid categories other than TANF, or were receiving services through managed care had higher risk of ACSHs. Racial disparities exist also among those with similar insurance type compared to white uninsured | Hospital patient discharge data linked to Medicaid eligibility file. Retrospective cohort study. Life-table technique + Cox proportional model | Lack of information about why interruptions occurred and whether beneficiaries changed to another insurance coverage. Additional confounding possible due to patients' health status or other unmeasured factors. No information on the use of ambulatory care services. correlated – stratification carried out |

Table 4A.1 (continued)

Study	Setting	Participants	Dependent variable and Factors of interest	Confounders	Conditions included	Result/Effect	Data source/ Methods	Limitations of study acknowledged by original author(s)
3. Magan et al. (2008)	Spain (universal coverage) 2001–03 34 health districts of Community of Madrid (CM)	65+ Population covered: 5 372 433	Age and sex ACSH rates combined for the 3 years Only ACSHs in public hospitals (71% of all hospital-isations in CM) **Variable of interest:** Gender	None	List of conditions validated for Spain Acute Chronic Vaccine preventable	ACSH rates higher for men than women in all age groups Considerable variation across the 34 districts	Hospital discharge data including adminis-trative and clinical data Cross-sectional, ecologic study	ACSH used as an indirect measure of access to and receipt of care Based on secondary data – limitations with regard to validity of principal diagnosis at discharge and completeness of variables Study only in public hospitals Not possible to eliminate readmission because not all patients

66

Study	Country / Years	Outcome measures	Variables	Methods	Results	Limitations
						could be identified across the three databases
						Associations at the aggregate level in this study do not necessarily apply to individual level
						List of conditions validated for Spain but not for population of 65 and older
						Lack of control for confounders (no. of doctors, income etc.)
4. Saha et al. (2007)	USA 1990–93 1995–2000	Age- and sex-adjusted ACSH rates **Variable of interest:** Payer (insurance)	Age Sex Marker conditions Time Comorbidities	Discharge database Retrospective time-series analysis Logistic regression	ACSH rates increased with increased insurance coverage likely due to increased access to inpatient care	Data sources may have biased the results (dynamic nature of insurance status hard to account for)

Table 4A.1 (continued)

Study	Setting	Participants	Dependent variable and Factors of interest	Confounders	Conditions included	Result/Effect	Data source/ Methods	Limitations of study acknowledged by original author(s)
5. Carter et al. (2006)	USA 2000–2002	65+	ACSH rates **Variable of interest:** Age	Sex Race Nursing home Urgent visit Location of ED	Based on Millman (1993)	ACSH rates increase with age over 85, for those from nursing residency and urgent status; ACSH rates decrease for non-white older adults. However, older adults account disproportionately for ED visits	Ambulatory care survey Logistic regression	Adjustments for non-response bias Case-mix not adjusted for Sample includes only those actually visiting ED
6. Ansari et al. (2006)	Australia (Victoria) 1999–2000 32 geographically defined primary care partnerships	18+	Age- and sex-standardized ACSH rates **Variable of interest:** Self-rated access	Access and health factors: disease burden prevalence propensity to seek care; primary physician supply per 1000, urban/ rural	Combination of Millman (1993) and AHRQ (2001) Acute Chronic Vaccine preventable	Higher ACSH rates in areas with perceived problems accessing medical care, after controlling for prevalence, disease burden, propensity	Hospital discharge data for all public and private acute care hospitals Victorian Population Health Survey	

		accessibility/ remoteness index		to seek care and physician supply	OLS	
		Social determinants: income, employment, education		Rural residence may be a greater risk factor for ACSH than poor self-rated access		
		Behavioural risk factors: smoking, vegetable consumption, alcohol, physical activity		Positive association with ACSH: low income; low education; smoking; low physician supply		
7. Laditka and Laditka (2006)	USA 1997	19–64 65+	ACSHs rates **Variables of interest:** Race Ethnicity	Disease prevalence Unmeasured hospital effects (physician supply, treatment preferences and patients' preferences etc.)	Six conditions separately: angina; asthma; COPD; CHF; hypertension; diabetes	ACSH rates for almost all conditions were higher for African Americans and Hispanics than for non-Hispanics, in both age groups and both males and females	Hospital discharge data Survey for prevalence Census for population estimates	Prevalence information relies on self-reporting Results may not be representative because states choose to participate in the Nationwide Inpatient Sample

Table 4A.1 (continued)

Study	Setting	Participants	Dependent variable and Factors of interest	Confounders	Conditions included	Result/Effect	Data source/Methods	Limitations of study acknowledged by original author(s)
8. Menec et al. (2006)	Canada 1990–91 1996–97	Province of Manitoba 67+	ACSH rates **Variable of interest:** Continuity of care	Demographics: age; gender; marital status; education; mobility Self-reported, health-related measures: self-rated health; mortality index; functional status; cognitive impairment	Billings (1993)	High continuity of care associated with reduced odds of ACSHs	Survey data from representative sample Administrative data with complete physician visits and hospitalisations Logistic regression	Limitations of study acknowledged by original author(s)
9. Zeng et al. (2006)	USA Jan.–Dec. 1996	65+ (other exclusions specified in the study) 2% stratified random sample from 4 California counties with largest Medicare	Probability of joining HMO Probability of ACSH Inpatient days for ACSCs **Variable of interest:** Medicare Health Maintenance	Selection Age, gender, eligibility for Medicaid, disability, death during study period, county of residence	15 ACSCs relevant to the elderly McCall et al. (2001)	Medicare HMO enrolees have lower ACHSs rates and fewer total inpatient days for 15 ACSCs than Medicare FFS beneficiaries. Selection of healthier beneficiaries	Medicare enrolment data Hospital discharge data Discrete factor selection model	Computational complexity of discrete factor model can lead to unreliable estimates Limited generalisability No access to

70

Author	Country Year	Sample	Variables	ACSC definition	Measures	Findings	Limitations
		enrolment = 10448 HMO 11803 FFS enrolees	Organization (HMO) enrolment			into HMOs does not completely explain their lower ACSHs	quality of care information (e.g. timing of admission, care received inpatient/ outpatient)
10. Zhang et al. (2006)	USA 1999–2001	Patients from 28 rural Nebraska counties designated as health professional shortage areas (HPSAs) Age groups: 0–17 18–64 65+	ACSH rates **Variable of interest:** Presence of rural clinic Individual characteristics: age; gender County-level contextual factors: % persons in poverty, % persons aged 65+, income per capita, hospital beds per capita, % persons 25+ with college education	Millman (1993) Chronic Acute	Hospital discharge data Area resource file Multilevel logistic regression	Elderly patients residing in rural Nebraska HPSAs with at least one rural health clinic were significantly less likely to have ACSHs due to chronic condition	Lack of data on individual rural health clinic visits for specific ACSCs Not all discharges may be reported Inaccurate diagnoses due to nature of administrative databases ACSHs should be used with other measures because some ACSHs may be due to non-primary care factors

Table 4A.1 (continued)

Study	Setting	Participants	Dependent variable and Factors of interest	Confounders	Conditions included	Result/Effect	Data source/ Methods	Limitations of study acknowledged by original author(s)
11. Mobley et al. (2006)	USA 1998–2000	FFS Medicare population 65+	ACSH rates **Variables of interest:** Physician supply Physician visits Poverty among elderly Managed care penetration Availability of supplemental coverage Urban sprawl	Disease severity Demographics Demand factors: % elderly in poverty; % total population in poverty; relative isolation of elderly Supply factors: availability and mix of physician specialties; non-physician clinicians Intervening factors: travel time; managed care prevalence; Medicare HMO, private sector HMO	11 ACSCs	Elderly living in impoverished rural areas or in sprawling suburban places are equally likely to be admitted for ACSCs While greater availability of physicians does not matter, greater prevalence of non-physician clinicians and international medical graduated, relative to US medical graduates, reduces ACSHs, especially in poor rural areas	Medicare FS beneficiary data Demographic census data Facilities and utilisation data Practitioner data Market conditions data Ecological model of spatial interaction	

| 12. Bindman et al. (2005) | USA | 1994-99 | California temporary assistance to needy families eligible Medicaid beneficiaries <65 | Average monthly ACSH rates

Variables of interest: Medicaid voluntary managed, mandatory managed and FFS care | and PPO penetration and changes in these over time; insurance industry concentration/ prevalence of employer-sponsored retirement plan; private insurance market's concentration, prevalence of employer-sponsored retirement insurance; average price of a standard MediGap plan in the area

Admission month
Admission year
Age
Sex
Race/ethnicity
County of residence | Institute of Medicine (1990) and Billings (1993) List

Control condition: average monthly appendicitis rate | Medicare managed care compared to FFS care is associated with a large reduction in ACSH rates with a greater effect for minority groups | Cross-sectional comparison

Discharge data
Eligibility file |

Table 4.1 (continued)

Study	Setting	Participants	Dependent variable and Factors of interest	Confounders	Conditions included	Result/Effect	Data source/Methods	Limitations of study acknowledged by original author(s)
						Appendicitis hospitalisation rates were not significantly different across the 3 groups		
13. Howard et al. (2007)	USA 1999–2002	Medicare population Aged 65+	ACS admission rates **Variables of interest:** Race Year	Gender	Based on Billings (1993) Bacterial pneumonia, CHF, diabetes, COPD, dehydration, UTI, angina, asthma Control conditions: appendicitis w/ appendectomy, fracture of hip/femur, gastrointestinal obstruction	Admissions for ACS conditions between African American and white patients differ but it is unclear why	Discharge data Census data Descriptive statistics	Focus on people aged 65 and older No control for income and other social and economic factors Study measures hospitalisation for a population with greater prevalence of an ACS condition along with

74

						an equivalent risk of hospitalisation per person – therefore the rate of hospitalisation will appear greater for that ethnic group
14. Falik et al. (2006)	USA	1.6 million Medicaid beneficiaries	ACS hospitalisations ACS emergency visits **Variables of interest:** Regular source of care (community health centres vs other Medicaid providers)	Insurance, scope of benefits, socioeconomic status, community resources, health status and comorbidity, demographics	19 ACSCs based on earlier studies	The community health centres compared with the other Medicaid providers experienced one-third fewer sentinel ACS events	Retrospective analysis of claims data Logistic regression

PART II

SUPPLY AND HEALTH CARE MARKETS

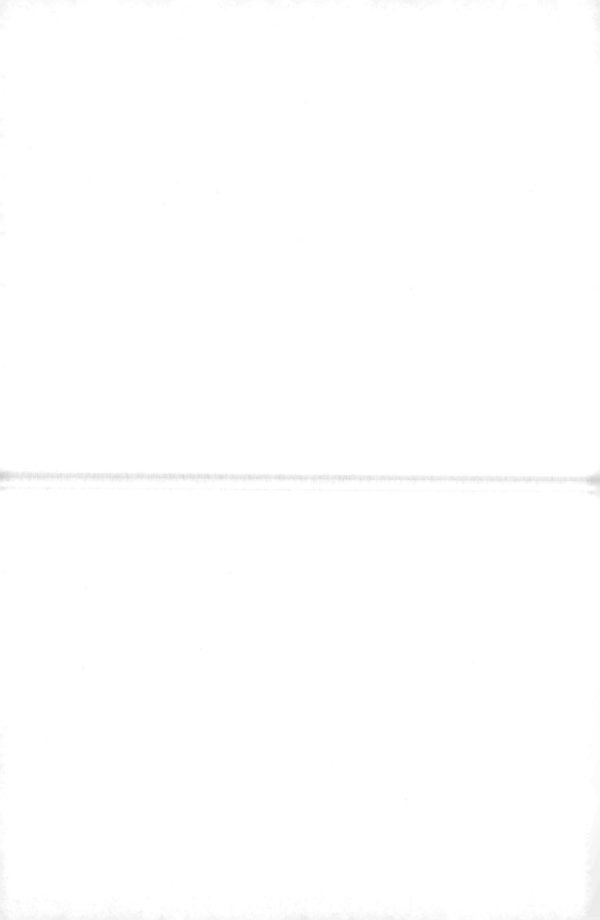

5   Choice in health care: drivers and consequences
Valentina Zigante, Joan Costa-Font and Zack Cooper

1.   INTRODUCTION

Choice and competition policies, and particularly the expansion of user choice, are increasingly promoted instruments in public health care systems. The policies are viewed as the modern answer to the tension that is inherent to health care: how to ensure equity while maintaining efficiency, and at the same time constrain costs (Bevan et al., 2010). Choice and competition, in quasi-market or managed competition structures of health care provision, are argued to constrain costs, improve equity in the provision of health care, but also to improve the *responsiveness* of health care systems (Le Grand, 2007). These visualised improvements respond to the contemporary challenges of health care systems: cost containment; inequalities in the access to health care; and a perception that health care systems are unresponsive to patients (Schoen et al., 2005). These developments in the health care sector further correspond to a more general lack of public participation in decision making, particularly in regard to public services, where consumerism has become a common answer.

The motivations found in the literature for increasing user choice and competition in the health care sector can be attributed to two broad categories, which we in this chapter discuss in terms of *extrinsic values* and *intrinsic values* of choice (following Dowding and John, 2009). The *intrinsic* value of choice, in and of itself, is in essence the value attributed to the act of choosing. This would imply that choice is valued above and beyond instrumental welfare gains and that by allowing or increasing choice, patients' preferences for health care are more likely to be satisfied, and individual autonomy and control is enhanced (Dowding and John, 2009). Further, the *extrinsic* or instrumental values, rendering improved outcomes, are based on 'micro-efficiency' arguments, whereby more choice is assumed to lead to more competition, which, in line with economic theory, will catalyse efficiency improvements. The choice of provider, and the incentives for providers to attract users, is argued to bring financial incentives for providers to improve their performance and quality of service.

Choice and competition policies have been implemented in the provision as well as in the financing of health care in countries across Europe, albeit the extent of available choice varies, along with the degree of competition (Kreisz and Gericke, 2010). This brings differences in incentive structures, depending on whether and to what extent competition is allowed, in conjunction with user choice. Choice and competition reforms in England have been widely debated; central themes of the last decade have been expanding choice, diversifying supply and introducing hospital competition into the state-funded National Health Service (NHS). The English reforms have served as inspiration for other European countries such as Spain and Italy (Cabiedes and Guilleen, 2001). In many countries, for example Germany, the Netherlands and France, choice has been a traditional aspect of the provision of health care, but these countries have also introduced policies and institutional reforms to increase competition as well as choice in their health systems.

Regardless of the motivations, and the degree of marketisation and privatisation, expanding choice in health care remains politically controversial. This is especially the case in countries where the status quo is a heavily integrated, centralised and hierarchical health system. Allowing choice is often perceived as the state losing control of the system, and competition is viewed as a first step towards privatisation. Further, critics often express concerns that choice will harm the equity of access to care and the quality of publicly provided care. However, contrary to popular belief, choice policies are not a natural fit – neither in liberal right-leaning political parties nor in the traditional left, and the policies have been key aspects of reform of health care policy in many European countries regardless of political party in power (Freeman, 1998). On the other hand, Light (2000) argues that the promotion of competition in health care is primarily guided by political and ideological considerations and is in fact not supported by any scientific evidence. 'The myth of efficiency, productivity, and accountability trumps the myth of trustworthy expertise applied altruistically to the needs of patient . . . It is the master myth of modern society' (Light, 2000, p. 971). We further discuss the theoretical underpinnings and recent evidence below, mainly from an economic point of view, and henceforth leave the political and sociological debates behind.

The understanding of choice is complex both because it touches on a number of academic disciplines and because it can be assessed from a number of dimensions such as its impact on efficiency, quality and equity, and has its philosophical base in intrinsic arguments of individual autonomy. We here highlight the core arguments from this heterogeneous literature, starting with a discussion of the different aspects of choice in health care, followed by an outline of the intrinsic and extrinsic motivations driving the introduction of choice. A brief overview of specific choice policies enacted in Western Europe provides context for the final section, briefly surveying current evidence on the outcomes in terms of efficiency, equity and quality. The conclusion highlights the key arguments, motivations and challenges for the introduction of choice in health care.

2.   DEFINING CHOICE

The nature of choice in health care is complex in so far as it is dependent on the institutional structure and traditions of each specific health system. Further, the option to choose can be presented on different levels and in different types of choice settings. Broadly speaking, user choice can be applied to two aspects of health care – the provision and the financing. Regarding the provision of health care, there is a range of choices potentially available to users: first the choice of provider – the choice of hospital, general (or primary care) practice, or other medical facilities; second, the choice of professional for providing care, and the choice of service – such as different forms of medical treatment. The time of treatment can sometimes be a point of choice, as well as the access channel or method of communication with the health services. This has traditionally taken place face to face, but is increasingly being carried out over the phone or through the internet (Le Grand, 2007). Choice of financing, the question of 'who pays', is commonly a choice between insurance funds, either exclusively public or a combination of private and public funds (Thomson et al., 2009). The choice can also concern the option of substitutive or supplementary private health insurance, ensuring access to private health care provision not covered by statutory health insurance or tax-based provision. Finally, it is noteworthy that one choice may constrain other choices; for example, the choice of physician determines the location for care. Similarly, choosing what treatment to receive often dictates which physician or location a patient attends.

The link between choice and competition is not entirely straightforward. Not all choice policies imply increased competition between providers or financers, and the level of competition induced is highly dependent on payment structure and regulations for entry and exit of the market. This is particularly important to take into account when considering the potential extrinsic effects of choice as it is often by virtue of creating competition that choice-based reforms inject incentives for efficiency and quality improvements into the supply of health care. A system where money follows the patients' choices is necessary; however, the specific implementation varies between systems. Finally, we note that, arguably, the ideas and values behind choice are different from those behind competition. Competition is generally implemented as a way of cutting costs, similar to the various forms of cost sharing for basic services and co-payments for additional services that allow for constraining demand in line with individuals' capacity and willingness to pay. Choice on its own, on the other hand, often has idealistic connotations stemming from liberal ideology, cultural values and, as we discuss further below, an intrinsic value of its own (Feldman and Zaller, 1992).

3. THE INTRINSIC ARGUMENTS FOR CHOICE

The literature on choice in public services often mentions choice as something that is *intrinsically valuable*, desirable as an end in and of itself. However, it is still useful to dig deeper into the character of this intrinsic value and explicate why it is desired (Dowding and John, 2009). Interestingly, the UK government highlighted intrinsic desirability when motivating the introduction of choice, and this has been a common feature in other countries seeking to implement choice policies. The idea is here articulated by former UK Prime Minister Tony Blair in 2001:

> We are backing investment with reform around four key principles: First, high national standards and full accountability. Second, devolution to the front-line to encourage diversity and local creativity. Third, flexibility of employment so that staff are better able to deliver modern public services. Fourth, the promotion of alternative providers and greater choice. All four principles have one goal – to put the consumer first. We are making the public services user-led; not producer or bureaucracy led, allowing far greater freedom and incentives for services to develop as users want. (Blair, 2001)

The speech manifests the role of choice and consumerism as the core goal of the New Labour welfare policy and emphasises that public services should be 'user-led', which leads us to the role of choice for individual autonomy. The autonomy argument has a philosophical origin, and among others Dworkin (1988) has argued that choice is a necessary condition for individual autonomy. In fact, arguments in favour of the intrinsic value of choice often stem from understandings of the broader benefits of individual autonomy. While choice and autonomy are surely not analogous, choice is seen as a necessary condition for autonomy both because it is through choosing their own course (and hence having choices) that individuals express their autonomy and because the process of choosing well and hence effectively expressing their autonomy is a learned skill that is acquired only through making various choices throughout life (Dworkin, 1988).

There is also a broader libertarian argument for extending choice, and this line of argument has a narrower focus of the role of the state in allowing choice. As Hargreaves writes,

> Other things being equal, choice is preferable to lack of choice. It is the essence of a libertarian and common-sense democratic position that the state should not deny choice to those who want it unless there are very powerful and well documented grounds for doing so. Diversity and choice is the desirable state unless and until 1) some convincing argument and evidence can be adduced that the costs greatly outweigh the benefits, and 2) it can be shown that costs cannot be reduced or overcome by limited state intervention. (Hargreaves, 1996, p. 133)

Traditionally, most conventional conceptions of libertarian theory assume that the government should play no role in provision of services, or the redistribution of wealth or resources (Brighouse, 2002). However, Hargreaves's stance can be viewed as 'common-sense' libertarianism, or as Brighouse writes, 'a more intuitive sense of libertarianism in which it just asserts the prima facie desirability of individual choice' (Brighouse, 2002, p. 33). This definition is softer than traditional libertarianism and still affords government a role in public service provision, as long as users have choice of provider. The desirability of choice is further debated, and even with softer definitions of libertarianism, there are still some who reject the role of choice along ideological lines. Hargreaves further discusses anti-libertarians, who openly reject choice and diversity, and argue that there are other more central goals for the state such as distributive justice, which they believe are not compatible with choice. In contrast, quasi-libertarians do not reject the presence of choice, but rather they are committed to a set of principles that do not accord any intrinsic value to choice (Hargreaves, 1996).

The welfarist argument in favour of more choice states that individuals are more likely to maximise their welfare and get an optimal consumption bundle if they may select the items and services they consume (Krugman and Wells, 2006). As Dworkin argues, choice 'increases the probability that they [individuals] will satisfy their desires. People want various things – goods and services, status, affection, power, health, security – and their chances of getting these things are often enhanced if they have more options to choose among' (Dworkin, 1988, p. 78). These arguments reflect the possible instrumental arguments for choice, and build on assumptions of the individual's capacity to maximise welfare from the choice offered. Schwartz (2004) offers a different view on the benefits of choice – while accepting the welfarist argument that more choice is likely to satisfy individual preferences, Schwartz argues that too many, and particularly important choices, may have the opposite effect for individual welfare. An overload of choice causes stress and feelings of regret, increased transaction costs and potentially unnecessary time spent on collecting information. The libertarian paternalistic literature argues that due to the behavioural difficulties connected with choice, the role of the state is important. However, this does not exclude possible benefits from choice, and it is argued that the state should define a default option in order to make the choice easier and minimise transaction costs for 'choice-averse' individuals (Thaler and Sunstein, 2003).

4.   THE EXTRINSIC VALUES OF CHOICE

In addition to the argument that choice is a desirable end, in and of itself, a core motivation for expanding user choice is that it will yield extrinsic or instrumental benefits. This argument stems from traditional microeconomic theory, which predicts efficiency improvements and effects on quality of service from consumer choice in a market setting. Further, the effects of choice on equity are debated, for example in the UK, where it has been argued that choice actually improves the equity of provision. In this section we discuss the debate on the extrinsic benefits in terms of efficiency, quality and equity.

Efficiency

Efficiency is assumed to increase as individuals express their preferences, which puts competitive pressure on health care providers and, as in private markets, the providers are incentivised to improve in order to attract business (Propper et al., 2006). Health care systems are denoted by two kinds of efficiency considerations. Technical efficiency denotes a procedure that for a given service provides equal quality at a lower cost or higher quality at a lower cost. Second, allocative efficiency considers provision of the optimal combination of services (Bevan et al., 2010). In perfectly competitive markets both types of efficiency are achieved when consumers maximise their utility through choosing between competing providers, and in turn consumers' choices drive providers to further improve technical efficiency in order to stay in the market. However, the assumptions behind perfectly competitive markets are inherently problematic for the financing and provision of health care. Here we discuss the assumptions of perfect information, and unlimited entry and exit as the main divergences from a perfect market situation.

Information asymmetry between health care providers, the financers and patients carries implications for the efficiency of health care markets. Providers, often represented by the physician, are in reality making most of the decisions for the patients, based on a higher level of medical knowledge, which places them in a dominant position. Information access has increased in recent years, and patients are more likely to seek information for example on the internet, but due to the complex nature of medicine the asymmetry of information often persists. This constrains efficiency effects as the individual lacks the bargaining power to force the provider to improve the efficiency, as the individual is in essence not fully aware of the actual efficiency of service. Further, it is argued that the information asymmetries in relation to the financing party induce excess demand as neither the patient nor the physician is affected by the price of the service. Two common economic solutions are user charges and co-payments, but these are only partly effective as the information asymmetry between doctor and patient means that doctors, rather than patients, make decisions on amount of treatment (Evans, 1987).

Information problems are also prevalent on the supply side, which affects both the behaviour of individual hospitals and the cooperation between different providers. Competing hospitals may not be willing to share patient information, which induces unnecessary work of generating background information before treatment. This problem is amplified if individuals tend to move between providers. Even if hospitals willingly share information, the 'doctor hopping' is likely to reduce efficiency due to the time and effort spent sharing information, and the transaction costs of introducing a new relation with a provider. Lack of patient information may also lead to overprescription of medication and treatments, implying both an efficiency problem and a quality problem due to potential negative impact on health outcomes. Finally, the information asymmetries provide opportunity for health care providers to select 'cheaper' patients in order to benefit from what is known as 'cream skimming'. This implies a less efficient allocation of care as the decision on where patients receive care is not based on where the most appropriate care is available. The potential 'cream skimming' also represents a problem when considering equity effects, as we discuss further below.

The payments structure, as we discuss in more detail when surveying the evidence, has an important role in creating efficiency-enhancing incentives for providers. It is argued that payment systems where money follows individuals' choices are most conducive for efficiency improvements. One example often cited is payments based on diagnosis-related groups (DRG), under which hospitals are paid a fixed amount based on the patient's diagnosis, not on their actual cost of treatment. DGRs can be understood as 'benchmark' competition, where providers are incentivised to provide a certain treatment cost-efficiently in relation to the fixed price and where any additional treatment time or cost is borne by the provider (Street and Maynard, 2007).

Finally, efficiency outcomes are influenced by the fact that health care markets have considerable barriers to both entry and exit of suppliers. Free entry and exit is a basic assumption of a perfectly competitive market, but in reality, the entry and exit of providers into and out of the health care market is more or less constrained. The entry of new hospitals is often constricted by heavy regulation and close monitoring of new facilities providing a minimum standard of care, and for most providers the capital cost of setting up a new facility is likely to be a constraining element. The exit, for example closing, of underperforming hospitals is on the other hand a politically sensitive issue, as it commonly faces public opposition. Having hospitals locally is viewed as an important part of society, both to ensure safety and to provide hospitals as large employers. However, the opposition against closure depends on the public's understanding of the deteriorating quality of the underperforming unit (Le Grand, 2009).

Quality

The introduction of choice and competition in health services is argued to create incentives not only for increased efficiency but also for improving quality and responsiveness. However, not only are incentives for improved quality complex to establish, but there is debate on how to conceptualise and measure quality empirically. Quality in health care can be defined in terms of 'process quality' – capturing how the services are delivered, the responsiveness of hospital staff, the waiting times and whether the users felt that they were treated with respect and consideration, and 'outcome quality' – capturing whether the health services improved health outcomes (Le Grand, 2007). When considering health policy, the overall objective is generally improving health, but the particular character of health care provision calls for a broader approach to quality. For patients the process is important not only in its own right, but also as it is likely to help improve health outcomes.

The particularities of health care markets compared to 'textbook' competitive markets have implications for quality outcomes, due both to the challenges of calibrating the payments system, and to the considerable information problems discussed above. The structure of the payment system has significant impacts on the incentives of the market, and hence the impact of choice and competition on health care quality is likely to be highly dependent on the underlying market structure (Gaynor, 2004).

The information asymmetries attached to the provision and financing of health care discussed above – between patient and doctor as well as between purchasers and providers – influence the effects on quality (Arrow, 1963). Further, no two patients or procedures are exactly the same, which enhances the information asymmetries and weakens the link with quality. The information asymmetries also enable providers to inflate demand though informational advantages over purchasers – often the government. Accessible information is also crucial in enabling patients to make choices based on quality, but as we have noted, health care is a highly individualised service and useful quality indicators are hard to produce. Hospital ratings are the most common way to spread information on quality, but it is debated how aware patients are of indicators of quality (Marshall et al., 2000).

In the evidence section below we further discuss the role of prices for improving quality, and survey the available evidence.

Equity

The character of health care provision is often denoted by excess demand, requiring rationing by other indicators than price, often through waiting times and hence constrained and, problematically, unequal access. It is hence commonly argued that publicly financed health, which has the objective of being comprehensive, suffers from an intrinsic conflict between equity and high quality (Weale, 1998). The importance of equity as an objective for health care provision in public health care systems explains the prominence of the debate about the effects on equity of choice and competition policies. Conflicting arguments are put forward, in the literature as well as in the rhetoric of politicians and policy makers wanting to introduce market-based reforms in health care. Further, it is argued that choice and competition oppose the basic ideas of the collectivist nature of a publicly funded health system. Choice is argued to imply a more individualist approach to health care, and that this is inherently inequitable. The standard 'collectivist' idea is based on the assumption that, when there is no choice for users, the government can equalise the standard of care across the country and every user can have access to the same quality services (Dixon and Le Grand, 2006).

Equity has been particularly debated in the UK, and officials have extensively promoted the choice and competition policies as an equity-enhancing policy. This is highlighted in the following speech by John Reid, Health Secretary of the Labour government at the time:

These choices will be there for everybody . . . not just for a few who know their way around the system. Not just for those who know someone 'in the loop' – but for everybody with every referral. That's why our approach to increasing choice and increasing equity go hand in hand. We can only improve equity by equalising as far as possible the information and capacity to choose. (Reid, 2003)

The idea put forward by the UK government was that in a system where 'money follows the patient's choices', patients can switch providers, and as a result, incentivise providers to treat all patients well, irrespective of a patient's ability to negotiate, voice their displeasure with their care, or somehow manage to game the health care system (Department of Health, 2003). It was argued that in systems without formalised choice mechanisms, choice still existed for middle and upper classes that have the ability to negotiate with their providers for better care or pay to enter the private sector. Creating formalised choice mechanisms would give every patient the ability to choose irrespective of their socioeconomic status (Cooper and Le Grand, 2008).

The UK emphasis on the potential of choice to improve care for the underserved ran contrary to the traditional notion that giving patients choice could have negative effects on equity (Cooper and Le Grand, 2008). Choice is commonly argued to potentially harm equity in two ways: first by exacerbating inequalities that stem from differences in users' capacities to choose. The well-off are often thought to be better equipped to make choices through a higher level of education and be more used to advocate for themselves in relations with the physician. This may be true, but if choices are properly assisted, then benefits should arise equitably from a health service with choice. In order to provide assistance to patients in their choice, provider quality information should be easily accessible, and assigned staff needs to be available to help users choose the most appropriate providers and care options. Second, choice can create incentives for providers to 'cream-skim' – to avoid treating individuals with more severe health problems, where users from the lower socioeconomic groups are overrepresented. 'Cream skimming' is more likely if providers are paid per episode of care they deliver; hence they are incentivised to select patients who are cheaper to treat. As well-off patients are generally healthier, the system may result in providers avoiding the treatment of patients from lower socioeconomic groups.

5.   POLICIES TO INTRODUCE PATIENT CHOICE INTO HEALTH SYSTEMS ACROSS EUROPE

The ideas outlined above, in which choice and market-oriented health care reforms are argued to increase the system's efficiency, quality and responsiveness, while maintaining equal access, have gained great recognition across European countries. The timing and variation in type of choices offered, and the level of marketisation, can be explained by the traditions of the respective health care system, public opinion, as well as the ideological intentions of the political leaders (Cabiedes and Guilleen, 2001). At one extreme we find the USA, with a long tradition of extensive reliance on competitive market solutions in the provision of public services, however currently reformed in favour of a more universal solution. On the other hand, reformation of European health care systems tends to move in the opposite direction. Choice and competition policies resonate with the new role of the welfare state – and the modernisation agenda of the European Union

Table 5.1   Overview of choice and competition in European health care systems

	Financing	Provision	Competition	Key reform objective
Bismarck				
Belgium	Public and private insurance	Long tradition of choice of GP	Competition in 1990s	Cost containment, expenditure control
France	Public and private health insurance	Long tradition of choice of GP	No extended competitive elements	Administrative improvement
Germany	Choice of insurance fund	Long tradition of choice of GP	Managed competition among payers	Cost containment, expenditure control
Netherlands	Choice of insurance fund	Long tradition of choice of GP	Managed competition in 2006	Curb increasing health care expenditure
Southern Rim				
Italy	Tax-based financing, private insurance options	Free choice of provider in 1990s	Quasi-markets	Modernisation
Spain	Tax-based financing, private insurance options	Choice of GP and specialist doctors in 1990s	No competition of provider or financing, but has been discussed	Cost containment and improving efficiency
Beveridge				
Sweden	Tax-based financing, private insurance options	Freedom of choice of public and certain private practitioners	Consumerist approach	Efficiency issues
UK	Tax-based financing, private insurance options	Choice of hospital in 2006	Quasi-markets	Cost containment

(Schelkle et al., 2010). As we can see from Table 5.1, the approaches to choice policies are diverse in both timing and scope; the following section discusses the reformation of a selection of European countries in more detail.

The health care systems in European countries tend to follow two main archetypal trajectories of development; first the Beveridge model, which is the system of the UK, Denmark and Sweden. It is denoted by a single payer, financed by national taxation, with a National Health Service in which providers of publicly financed services are owned publicly, and access to hospital specialists is typically by referral via a general practitioner (GP). Countries of the Beveridge model have been relatively successful at controlling total expenditure and have traditionally given limited choice to their patients, while relying on GPs as gatekeepers, guides and coordinators of health care. In this set of countries, the emphasis has recently been on increasing choice of hospital for elective care (Bevan and Van De Ven, 2010). Much of the debate on choice in health care has concerned the UK and Sweden, and these Beveridge model countries strongly promoted choice policies in the 1990s. Particularly in the UK, the choice policies were denoted by a view of the citizen as a consumer, and the reforms in the UK, and to some extent in Sweden, have served as a role model for the introduction of choice policies in other European countries (Cabiedes and Guilleen, 2001).

Second, the Bismarck model, found in Germany, France and the Netherlands, is denoted by multiple insurer financing, employer-based schemes supplemented by the state, a mixed public and private provision in which patients have direct access to specialists. In the Bismarck-style countries, controlling total expenditure on health care has been problematic, and choice of specialist or GP has been free whereas choice of insurer has been limited or none. The reform aim in these countries is to reduce choice of specialists by types of 'soft' gatekeeping in order to control expenditure (Or et al., 2010). The countries have recently introduced choice and competition also in financing of health care to alleviate expenditure problems. The Netherlands is a particular example among the Bismarck model countries, as it has been relatively successful at constraining total expenditure on health care. Part of the success is due to the introduction of choice of insurer combined with more information for patients on choice of provider (Bevan et al., 2010).

Finally, Mediterranean models of health care such as those in Italy and Spain, once they have consolidated their health systems, have introduced policies to increase patients' choice. This is particularly the case of Italy, whilst in Spain choice and competition are only observed in Catalonia, where the competition between providers is incentivised by prospectively defined payments (Lopez-Casanovas et al., 2009). Finally, separate from the 'stylised' models, many Eastern European countries have as a part of the transition introduced market elements in health care. These are not covered in detail here, but the introduction of choice and competition as part of public service reforms highlights the importance of this type of policy in current public policy making.

6.   EVIDENCE ON THE EFFECTS OF CHOICE

While there is significant interest in expanding the role of choice of health care, there is still need for further accumulation of substantive empirical evidence from European countries of the impact on efficiency, quality and equity. To a large extent, the scarcity of evidence is due to the rather recent introduction of this type of policy, and to the empirical challenges of measuring particularly quality and equity. However, early evidence from the recent, and heavily debated, English patient choice reforms has generally been positive. We here discuss the current evidence concerning efficiency, quality and equity effects of choice and competition in health care.

Efficiency

As discussed at length above, consumer choice is seen as a major driver for efficiency in the market and this logic has been transferred to health care and the provision of public services in general. The approaches to measuring efficiency vary; in this limited space we focus on two approaches applied to a cross-section of countries and to the UK.[1]

Siciliani and Hurst (2005) take decreasing excessive waiting times to be an 'efficiency goal', and decreasing waiting times are also an often mentioned *driver* for choice reform. As 'The new policies reward reductions in waiting, on the assumption that lower waiting times are a signal of better management and higher efficiency', we can expect efficiency improvements (2005, p. 213). Siciliani and Hurst find that the level of choice and financial incentives have a positive effect on waiting times on both the supply and demand side in 12 OECD countries. On the other hand, a study on Denmark and Sweden, where the rationale for choice was to reduce waiting times by allowing patients to seek care outside the local area, found the opposite results. The study reveals that the incentives for hospitals to accept patients from outside their area have been weak and only a small proportion of patients went out of area under the schemes (Williams and Rossiter, 2004).

Using length of stay as a proxy for efficiency, Cooper et al. (2010) analyse the impact of patient choice and hospital competition on efficiency in the English NHS. Pre-surgery length of stay was argued to be a better proxy for efficiency than post-surgery length of stay because it is less sensitive to patient characteristics. In assessing the effects of the introduction of choice of hospital in 2006, Cooper et al. (2010) find that hospitals located in markets with more choice shortened the pre-surgery component of their length of stay with no measurable impact on the post-surgery length of stay, suggesting that hospitals facing competition were able to become more efficient without compromising patient outcomes.

Quality

The issue of how to measure quality in health care is both longstanding and contentious. Various potential proxies for quality have been put forward, including length of stay and mortality rates. In general, evidence suggests that the impact of choice and competition on health care quality is highly sensitive to whether or not hospitals can compete on price (Gaynor, 2004). In general, patients (and purchasers) seem to be significantly more reactive to price than they are to quality. As a result, in markets where providers can compete on both price and quality, evidence suggests that prices tend to drop, but so too does quality (Propper et al., 2008). In contrast, in markets where prices are fixed and providers can only differentiate themselves on quality, higher competition tends to lead to better quality (Kessler and McClellan, 2000; Kessler and Geppert, 2005).

Starting with the evidence from the USA, where choice is an inherent aspect of the health care system, Kessler and McClellan (2000) found lower mortality when studying the impact of hospital competition on acute myocardial infarction (AMI) mortality,[2] in a fixed price market with increasing competition, for Medicare beneficiaries from 1985 to 1994, with the results being strongest for the 1990s. However, as Gowrisankaran and Town (2003) highlight, in US markets with variable prices, competition alone does not improve quality unless coupled with the appropriate reimbursement rates. Higher competition in California led to an increase in mortality, but during the period hospitals were underpaid for Medicare patients (Gowrisankaran and Town, 2003). Also, Shen (2003) found that, particularly in competitive markets, lower Medicare reimbursement rates led to an increase in mortality. Further, Sari (2002) found that higher competition in a variable-priced market led to a significant improvement in hospital quality. Interestingly, Sari used a range of hospital complication measures, for example the number of obstetric complications, iatrogenic complications, wound infections and the provision of inappropriate services instead of the common AMI mortality.

The majority of the English literature on hospital competition concerns the 1990s NHS internal market reforms. Overall, researchers appear to be in agreement that the English internal market established neither strong incentives for hospitals nor a significant degree of competition between providers (Le Grand et al., 1998; Klein, 1999; Le Grand, 1999). Hence it is not surprising that the evidence of quality effects is mixed. Hamilton and Bramley-Harker (1999) found that waiting times for hip replacements fell and so too did patients' average length of stay after the NHS internal market reforms. On the other hand, Propper et al., in two separate studies, found that in a variable-price market setting, higher competition led to a statistically significant increase in 30-day AMI mortality that was larger than the mortality decline attributed to technological innovation during the same period (2004; Propper et al., 2008).

Interestingly, regarding the later wave of reforms in the English NHS, there is strong evidence that higher patient choice and hospital competition can improve quality. Bloom et al. (2010) found that hospital competition fostered higher management quality, and that higher management quality was associated with lower mortality from AMI. Further, again investigating the 2006 reform, Cooper et al. (2010) found that hospitals located in regions where patients had more choice improved their quality faster than hospitals located in monopoly markets. As discussed above, the approaches to the measurement of quality are diverse, and the indicator may affect the results. Dixon et al. (2010) found 'no evidence that the choice policy was resulting in significant changes for the patient or to patient's pathways', suggesting that it was not driving improvements in quality by provider competition. The argument builds on the assumption that if hospitals are able to compete on quality, then patients will choose to go to hospitals with higher ratings, and this would appear as changes to patients' pathways.

Equity

When empirically analysing the impact of choice on equity, the general question is whether different socioeconomic groups are likely to benefit to the same extent from having choice. Equity of benefits is analysed in a variety of ways, for example in terms of access to care, amount of medical attention, coverage of preventive medicine and equal health outcomes, which can be analysed in terms of morbidity. We here survey some recent, albeit scarce, evidence from England, where the debate on the effects of choice on equity has been particularly strong.

The UK government, as discussed above, as well as influential scholars, have listed equity as a major positive aspect of the introduction of choice (see, e.g., Cooper and Le Grand, 2008). Barr et al. (2008), on the other hand, survey the evidence and criticise the statements by the government, arguing that the claim is not based on an analysis of the evidence on the causes of health care inequity, and that it lacks a consistent normative definition of equity. Further, Dixon and Le Grand (2006) carried out a detailed survey of the evidence on the equity of the English NHS and found varying evidence of the effects of choice on equity, which we shall now discuss in more detail.

Depending on the scope and framework of study, among other explanations, the results of studies into the effects of choice on equity vary. Dixon and Le Grand (2006), while surveying the evidence, identify a range of potential reasons why extending user choice may not improve equity. They argue that unequal information, unequal capabilities and unequal patient mobility as well as the differing proportions of income spent on, for example, travelling costs, can cause inequity from the introduction of choice. They find, first, that extending patient choice may leave equity unchanged because of differences in health beliefs; this, as choice, does not affect health beliefs directly. Second, they find that choice may increase inequity due to unequal resources if, by making use of choice, patients may need to travel further, which benefits relatively more those who have more spending power. Finally, they argue that choice can improve equity because of unequal capabilities. They argue that without formalised choice mechanisms, more articulate and educated users can often negotiate with their providers, and gain choice or speedier access to the system. In contrast, when choice is formalised, all patients have the opportunity to choose irrespective of their socioeconomic status and choice is not as directly contingent on negotiations with patients' GPs. Finally, they argue, based on the London Patient Choice Pilot (LPCP), that it is crucial for lower socioeconomic groups to get the proper assistance in the opportunity to choose. This argument is shared by Barr et al. (2008), who further highlight the need to establish independent auditing in order to assess the effects on equity of the new choice policies.

7.   CONCLUSION

This chapter has sought to examine the conceptual underpinning for the introduction of choice across health systems in Europe. As we have discussed, arguments made for promoting patient choice are often centred on promoting patient autonomy and creating financial incentives for efficiency and quality. The motivations for, and evidence of, the effects of choice are context dependent and often vary based on the manner in which choice was introduced in a particular setting. Indeed, the effects of choice interact with different dimensions of the institutional design of the health system, its financing and the prevailing culture of the country where choice policies are being introduced.

The intrinsic value of choice can be argued to be a matter of ideology, particularly when it is coupled with competition and privatisation of health care. Choice and competition policies are often met with the argument that people do not want choice; they simply want a good local service. However, recent evidence suggests that an impetus for choice should be that it can potentially serve as a policy tool in order to drive up the quality of local services alongside the widely accepted goals of increasing overall efficiency and the responsiveness of health systems.

Ultimately, because they are so recent, there has been limited evidence thus far on the efficacy of choice policies. The evidence tends to vary considerably, depending on the scope, time frame and approach to measuring the benefit of interest. We have seen that, in terms of efficiency, quality and equity, numerous approaches to conceptualisation and measurement result in diverse conclusions on the effects of choice policies. In the future, more research needs to be carried out to determine how these types of policies impact quality, efficiency and equity. In addition, more empirical and theoretical work needs to be carried out, which examines the impact of choice on perceptions of responsiveness and patient satisfaction.

NOTES

1. For a survey of efficiency studies in the USA, see Hussey et al. (2009).
2. 30-day acute myocardial infarction (AMI) in-hospital mortality rate.

REFERENCES

Arrow, K.J. (1963), 'Uncertainty and the welfare economics of medical care', *The American Economic Review*, **53**(5), 941–73.
Barr, D.A., L. Fenton et al. (2008), 'The claim for patient choice and equity', *Journal of Medical Ethics*, **34**, 271–4,
Bevan, G., J.-K. Helderman et al. (2010), 'Changing choices in health care: implications for equity, efficiency and cost', *Health Economics, Policy and Law*, **5**(Special Issue 03), 251–67.
Bevan, G. and W. Van De Ven (2010), 'Choice of providers and mutual healthcare purchasers: can the English National Health Service learn from the Dutch reforms?', *Health Economics, Policy and Law*, **5**, 343–63.
Blair, T. (2001), Prime Minister's speech on public service reform.
Bloom, N., Carol Propper et al. (2010), 'The impact of competition on management quality: evidence from public hospitals', Centre for Economic Performance Discussion Paper.
Brighouse, H. (2002), *School Choice and Social Justice*, Oxford: Oxford Scholarship Online.
Cabiedes, L. and A. Guilleen (2001), 'Adopting and adapting managed competition: health care reform in Southern Europe', *Social Science & Medicine*, **52**, 1205–17.
Cooper, Z., S. Gibbons et al. (2010), 'Does hospital competition improve efficiency? An analysis of the recent market-based reforms to the English NHS', Centre for Economic Performance Discussion Paper.
Cooper, Z. and J. Le Grand (2008), 'Choice, competition and the political left', *Eurohealth*, **13**(4), 18–20.
Department of Health (2003), *Building on the Best – Choice, Responsiveness and Equity in the NHS*, London: HMSO.
Dixon, A. and J. Le Grand (2006), 'Is greater patient choice consistent with equity? The case of the English NHS', *Journal of Health Services Research & Policy*, **11**(3), 162–6.
Dixon, A., R. Robertson et al. (2010), 'The experience of implementing choice at point of referral: a comparison of the Netherlands and England', *Health Economics, Policy and Law*, **5**, 295–317.
Dowding, K. and P. John (2009), 'The value of choice in public policy', *Public Administration*, **87**(2), 219–33.
Dworkin, G. (1988), *The Theory and Practice of Autonomy*, Cambridge, Cambridge University Press.
Evans, R.G. (1987), 'Public health insurance: the collective purchase of individual care', *Health Policy*, **7**, 115–34.
Feldman, S. and J. Zaller (1992), 'The political culture of ambivalence: ideological responses to the welfare state', *American Journal of Political Science*, **36**(1), 268–307.
Freeman, R. (1998), 'Competition in context: the politics of health care reform in Europe', *International Journal for Quality in Health Care*, **10**(5), 395–401.
Gaynor, M. (2004), 'Competition and quality in hospital markets. What do we know? What don't we know?', *Economie Publique*, **15**(2), 3–40.
Gowrisankaran, G. and R.J. Town (2003), 'Competition, payers, and hospital quality', *Health Services Research*, **38**, 1403–22.
Hamilton, B.H. and R.E. Bramley-Harker (1999), 'The impact of the NHS reforms on queues and surgical outcomes in England: evidence from hip fracture patients', *The Economic Journal*, **109**(July), 437–62.
Hargreaves, D.H. (1996), 'Diversity and choice in school education: a modified libertarian approach', *Oxford Review of Education*, **22**(2), 131–41.
Hussey, P.S., H.D. Vries et al. (2009), 'A systematic review of health care efficiency measures', *Health Services Research*, **44**(3), 784–805.
Kessler, D.P. and J.J. Geppert (2005), 'The effects of competition on variation in the quality and cost of medical care', *Journal of Economics and Management Strategy*, **14**(3), 575–89.
Kessler, D.P. and M.B. McClellan (2000), 'Is hospital competition socially wasteful?', *The Quarterly Journal of Economics*, **115**(2), 577–615.

Klein, R. (1999), 'Markets, Politicians and the NHS', *British Medical Journal*, **319**(7222), 1383–84.

Kreisz, F.P. and C. Gericke (2010), 'User choice in European health systems: towards a systematic framework for analysis', *Health Economics, Policy and Law*, **5**, 13–30.

Krugman, P.R. and R. Wells (2006), *Economics*, New York: Worth Publishers.

Le Grand, J. (1999), 'Competition, cooperation, or control? Tales from the British National Health Service', *Health Affairs*, **18**(3), 27–39.

Le Grand, J. (2007), *The Other Invisible Hand: Delivering Public Services Through Choice and Competition*, Princeton, NJ: Princeton University Press.

Le Grand, J. (2009), 'Choice and competition in publicly funded health care', *Health Economics, Policy and Law*, **4**, 479–88.

Le Grand, J., N. Mays et al. (1998), *Learning from the NHS Internal Market*, London: King's Fund.

Light, D.W. (2000), 'Sociological perspectives on competition in health care', *Journal of Health Politics, Policy and Law*, **25**(5), 807–13.

Lopez-Casanovas, G., J. Costa-Font et al. (2009), 'Decentralisation and management autonomy? Evidence from the Catalonian hospital sector in a decentralised Spain', *International Public Management Review*, **10**(2), 1–17.

Marshall, M.N., P.G. Shekelle et al. (2000), 'The public release of performance data', *Journal of the American Medical Association*, **283**, 1866–74.

Or, Z., C. Cases et al. (2010), 'Are health problems systemic? Politics of access and choice under Beveridge and Bismarck systems', *Health Economics, Policy and Law*, 1–25.

Propper, C., S. Burgess and D. Gossage (2008), 'Competition and quality: evidence from the NHS internal market 1991–1996', *The Economic Journal*, **118**(1), 138–70.

Propper, C., S. Burgess and K. Green (2004), 'Does competition between hospitals improve the quality of care? Hospital death rates and the NHS internal market', *Journal of Public Economics*, **88**(7–8), 1247–72.

Propper, C., D. Wilson et al. (2006), 'Extending choice in english health care: the implications of the economic evidence', *Journal of Social Policy*, **35**(4), 537–57.

Reid, J. (2003), 'Speech to the New Health Network', 16 July. Accessible at http://www.newhealthnetwork.co.uk/Content.asp?ID=181, 3 March 2011.

Sari, N. (2002), 'Do competition and managed care improve quality?', *Health Economics*, **11**, 571–84.

Schelkle, W., J. Costa-Font et al. (2010), 'Consumer choice, welfare reform and participation in Europe. A framework for analysis', RECON Online Working Papers Series.

Schoen, C., R. Osborn et al. (2005), 'Taking the pulse of health care systems: experiences with health problems in six countries', *Health Affairs*, W5 Web Exclusive: 510–23.

Schwartz, B. (2004), *The Paradox of Choice: Why More is Less*, New York: HarperCollins.

Shen, Y.C. (2003), 'The effect of financial pressure on the quality of care in hospitals', *Journal of Health Economics*, **22**(2), 243–69.

Siciliani, L. and J. Hurst (2005), 'Tackling excessive waiting times for elective surgery: a comparative analysis of policies in 12 OECD countries', *Health Policy*, **72**, 201–15.

Street, A. and A. Maynard (2007), 'Activity based financing in England: the need for continual refinement of payment by results', *Health Economics, Policy and Law*, **2**, 419–27.

Thaler, R. and C. Sunstein (2003), 'Libertarian paternalism', *The American Economic Review*, **93**(2), 175–9.

Thomson, S., T. Foubister et al. (2009), *Financing Health Care in the European Union – Challenges and Policy Responses*, Copenhagen: World Health Organization on behalf of the European Observatory on Health Systems and Policies.

Weale, A. (1998), 'Rationing health care: a logical solution to an inconsistent triad,' *British Medical Journal*, **316**, 410.

Williams, J. and A. Rossiter (2004), *Choice: The Evidence*, London: Social Market Foundation.

6   A million years of waiting: competing accounts and comparative experiences of hospital waiting-time policy

Alec Morton and R. Gwyn Bevan

1.   INTRODUCTION

Waiting time for hospital care is one of the most easily measured dimensions of performance of a health care system, and one of the few dimensions that patients can assess unambiguously. Perhaps for that reason, it has been one of the most contentious and politically sensitive issues in health policy in many countries (although, arguably, patients should be more worried about variations in access and outcomes). The capacity for hospital waiting times to create acute political embarrassment can be seen in the headlines from various UK national newspapers during the period 2001–02 when popular concern about waiting times was running high (see Box 6.1). As a result of the high degree of exposure of this issue, waiting times have become an issue on which everyone has an opinion. At the roughest, rawest level, it is possible to distinguish two stances in lay and policy discussions about waiting times:

- policy action to improve waiting times is impossible, impractical, expensive and ineffectual, and has adverse effects on other hard-to-measure dimensions of quality of care;
- policy action to improve waiting times is possible, practical, desirable, and may even save money.

We call the former stance the 'miserabilist stance' and the latter stance the 'meliorist stance'.

Yet understanding the consequences of policy action requires getting beyond these stances, and understanding how and why health care systems generate waits. A central observation of the current chapter is that there are differing accounts of why waiting takes place, which find expression both in media reporting and political rhetoric, and indeed, which frame various social scientific research programmes. The accounts differ according to the disciplinary and professional background of the commentator, the nature of his/her role and/or 'stake' in the health care system and, perhaps, his/her general disposition and outlook on life. These various accounts do not necessarily conflict, in the sense that one or the other must be true; indeed all the accounts contain at least an element of truth, which accounts for their popularity. In so far as different accounts do conflict, empirical evidence and theoretic analysis have a role to play in adjudicating between them; however, all accounts of the world are to some extent underdetermined by the evidence (Kuhn, 1970), and so we would expect to see these various accounts continuing to play a role in ongoing debate around the waiting-time phenomenon. Our four generic

---

BOX 6.1   HEADLINES FROM UK NATIONAL NEWSPAPERS, 2001–02

HOSPITAL WAITING LISTS GROW
The Express, 30 August 2002

HOSPITAL WAITING NUMBERS RISE
The Sun, 13 September 2002

HOSPITAL WAITING LIST NUMBERS CONTINUE TO RISE
The Times, 10 August 2002

HOSPITAL WAITING IS SLAMMED
The Mirror, 0 September 2002

EXTRA CASH FAILS TO HALT RISE IN NHS WAITING LISTS
The Guardian, 6 October 2001

SCANDAL OF THE 'HIDDEN' HOSPITAL WAITING LISTS
Daily Mail, 10 August 2002

MINISTERS ACCUSED OF RIGGING HOSPITAL WAITING LIST FIGURES
Daily Mail, 20 December 2001

WAITING SHAME: STUNNED OAP GETS HOSPITAL APPOINTMENT FOR MARCH 2003
The Mirror, 27 December 2001

---

accounts of waiting are dubbed here the 'production account', the 'patient behaviour account', the 'process account' and the 'provider incentive account'. Our discussion reflects our reading of the relevant health economics and operational research/management science ('OR/MS') literatures. For alternative classifications, the reader is referred to Pope (1991), Cullis and Jones (1985), and Yates (1987).

Internationally, there is considerable diversity in the actions that particular countries have taken in order to address the issue of hospital waiting times: Hurst and Siciliani (2003) and, more recently, Willcox et al. (2007), and Pomey et al. (2009) provide excellent surveys. There is also diversity in the actions that have been taken, both between and (in the case of federal nations such as Canada) within countries. Some nations or regions are strongly associated with particular approaches: for example, waiting-list prioritisation methods have been pioneered in Western Canada and New Zealand. Of course, deriving lessons that are generally valid across different countries is challenging: command-and-control approaches that are possible in countries with centrally funded 'Beveridge' systems may simply be drastically culturally inappropriate in countries with social insurance or 'Bismarck' systems. And even within Beveridge systems there are crucial

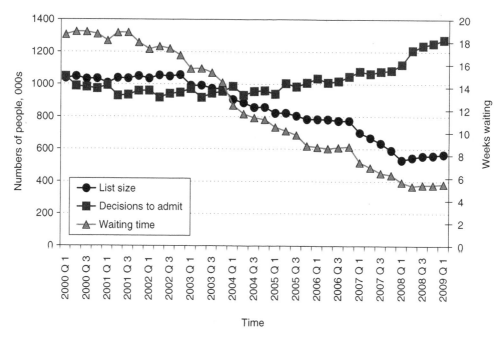

Figure 6.1   Inpatient waiting times in England, 2000–2009

differences: in the UK, hospital doctors are essentially salaried employees, whereas in Canada they are essentially small businessmen, and so the micro-politics of achieving waiting-time reductions may play out differently in the two countries. Nevertheless we hope and intend that our accounts are sufficiently general that they are recognisably applicable to any normal developed-country health care system.

Despite this aspiration to international relevance, we shall focus on recent UK experience. For insight into why this might be of interest to those not resident in the UK, see Figure 6.1 (the data are from the Department of Health[1]). This figure shows that despite an increase in the number of patients in England joining the waiting list for inpatient care in a given quarter (patients for whom there has been a 'decision to admit'), waiting lists and average waiting times have been in steady decline. The reader should note that, in this figure, the average waiting time is the time of everyone on the list up to a census date rather than the completed journey. While this is a somewhat unusual definition of waiting time, it has the advantage that data returns are available up to almost the end of the first quarter of 2009, by which time the English NHS was required to achieve a maximum wait of 18 weeks from referral to treatment. This performance improvement is particularly remarkable as ever-growing waiting lists and waiting times have been a feature of the NHS since its inception in 1948.

In this chapter, we shall:

- outline and comment on four accounts of waiting that provide a framework for organising a diverse and international literature and a general lens through which to view policy discussions;

- review and contrast recent history in the various UK countries, and identify lessons learned;
- consider whether investment in reducing waiting times in the UK has been value for money.

The remainder of our chapter is structured as follows. In Section 2, we present our competing accounts of waiting; in Section 3, we outline some recent policy history in the UK's four countries through the lens of these accounts; in Section 4, we discuss the value-for-money question, and in Section 5 we conclude. In a chapter of this length, it is impossible to do justice to the richness and depth of research on this topic, and we refer the interested reader to Cullis et al. (2000), Harrison and New (2000), Appleby et al. (2005a), Siciliani and Hurst (2005), National Audit Office (2001), and Pomey et al. (2009) for a range of alternative perspectives.

2. FOUR ACCOUNTS OF WAITING

In this section, we outline our four accounts of waiting:

- a production account, in which waiting lists are viewed as a signal of underinvestment;
- a patient behaviour account, in which waiting lists are viewed as an inevitable consequence of state provision of health care free at the point of delivery;
- a process account, in which waiting lists are viewed as a signal of poor design and management;
- a provider incentive account, in which waiting lists are viewed as arising from producer capture of the health care system.

In the remainder of this section, we present the key ideas of each of these accounts and outline some questions they raise.

2.1 The Production Account

One commonly cited reason for the existence of waiting times is that the health care system simply is not resourced to deliver timely care. For example, the Wanless report claims that 'One of the main reasons why people have to wait is that the health service faces significant capacity constraints, in terms of its workforce, its capital estate and infrastructure, reflecting past inadequate investment in the NHS' (Wanless, 2002, p. 17). This captures the essence of what we call the 'production account' of waiting times: the problem, basically, is not enough money. Wanless's text also captures a variant on the production account, which we call the 'backlog account'; in the past (typically, during the previous government) funding was inadequate and as a result there is a legacy of problems, either in terms of infrastructure or in terms of pent-up demand for health care. This means that waiting lists will persist for a period even when underinvestment is addressed.

From international comparisons, it does seem to be the case that countries that invest more in their health care systems have lower waits (Siciliani and Hurst, 2004). But the

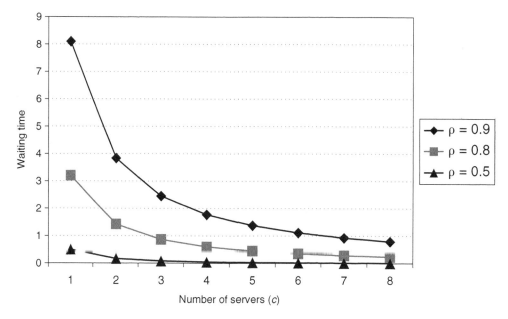

Figure 6.2   Average waiting times in the M/M/c *queue*

central question raised by this account is 'How much extra funding is enough?' and, valuable as international comparisons are, the relationships are noisy and national idiosyncrasies in data collection and clinical and management practice can make direct comparison difficult. Within a country, tying variations in performance back to variations in levels of resourcing can be still more difficult, even in the case of relatively simple facilities such as Accident and Emergency (A&E) Departments (Healthcare Commission, 2005; Morton and Bevan, 2008). Indeed, the use of funding formulas designed to allocate monies in rough proportion to need (Smith, 2003) means that intranational variations in funding may be rather small and any effects may be swamped by variations due to managerial practice.

An alternative way to tackle the 'how much is enough' question is through modelling methods. The OR/MS technique of queueing theory provides a modelling framework for studying such questions. Queueing theory is a formal framework for investigating the properties of systems in which 'customers' arrive and are processed by operatives referred to as 'servers'. Customer arrivals typically follow a stochastic process, such as a Poisson process; service times can also be random. For many queueing systems, analytic results are available, which characterise system performance for particular arrival and service processes. An example of a queueing system is the so-called *M/M/c* queue, a queue in which each customer arrives according to a Poisson distribution and is served by one of *c* servers (service time is assumed to follow a negative exponential distribution). Formulas exist for steady-state waiting time performance for such systems, and indicative values are shown in Figure 6.2 as the number of servers increases. Calculations were done using the software QTSPlus.[2] The reader is referred to a standard textbook on queueing theory, such as Gross and Harris (1998), for precise mathematical details and proofs.

Interpretation of Figure 6.2 is as follows. We suppose that we are dealing with an acute surgical specialty with one through to eight doctors, who do nothing but treat patients (i.e. they do not undertake research, private practice, administrative tasks etc.). The specialty receives in a time-unit (e.g. a day) on average one patient for each doctor. It takes each doctor on average ρ days to perform surgery on a patient: obviously $\rho < 1$, otherwise the waiting list will grow without limit. Although any serious queueing-theoretic model of a hospital would be much more complex than the $M/M/c$ queue, this simple model demonstrates some counterintuitive characteristics that are also found with more complex models. The first characteristic is illustrated by the length of the queue with a single server (the simplest model of all). This shows that as ρ increases from 0.5 to 0.9 the expected waiting time increases from 0.5 to 8.1. When ρ equals 1 (i.e. when the rate of service equals the rate of arrival), the expected waiting time becomes infinite. This highlights the vulnerability of a single server to stochastic variation. The second characteristic is illustrated by the way in which the expected waiting time diminishes dramatically for multiple servers: there is a sharp fall in waiting time in moving from a system with a single to two servers even though the ratio of rates of service to rates of arrival is constant. With six or more servers, fluctuations in the value of ρ (provided it remains less than 1) has little impact on the expected waiting time. There are hence three messages from Figure 6.2: intuition is a poor guide to managing stochastic processes; to have reasonable expected waiting times we require capacity to exceed demand and the price of low waiting times will be low utilisation of capacity; and there are economies of scale, because larger systems are better able to cope with variability in demand (Morton and Bevan, 2008).

2.2   The Patient Behaviour Account

The patient behaviour account, in contrast, is predicated on the notion that waiting lists for services that are free at the point of delivery play the same role as a price does in markets, discouraging would-be patients who would otherwise flood the system with frivolous demands. A consequence of this view is that low waiting times induce demand, and so reducing waiting times, as Enoch Powell recounted in his recollections of his unhappy time as Secretary of State for Health, 'is an activity about as hopeful as filling a sieve' (cited in Harrison and Appleby, 2005, p. 5). To address this concern, a tradition has developed of extensive and detailed econometric studies (Lindsay and Feigenbaum, 1984; Propper, 1995; Martin and Smith, 1999; Gravelle et al., 2003). The overall tendency of this line of research has been to show empirically that the phenomenon of induced demand, while real, is nevertheless rather modest. On the basis of this evidence, Martin and Smith have argued that initiatives to reduce waiting times are practicable: 'the ambitious waiting time target that is contained in the NHS plan . . . is in itself unlikely to lead to large increases in demand for NHS surgery and is therefore achievable provided that adequate additional resources are made available' (2003, p. 384).

   To expand on this notion, we outline the patient choice model that typically underlies econometric models. Suppose that the value of treatment is V (assumed to be positive), relative to a 0 of no treatment. The value of treatment decays (exponentially) at a rate d. This decay may be because of the patient's myopic disregard for her own future health, or it may be because treatment is less effective after the disease has progressed. Thus, if the patient has to wait t time periods, the value of the treatment is Ve^{-td}.

On the basis of this analysis, the value of this treatment so far is positive, and therefore care will be sought. However, it is conventional to suppose that there is a cost of joining the waiting list, C. If $Ve^{-td} > C$, the patient will join; otherwise she will 'baulk'. How plausible it is to assume a positive C will depend on the precise nature of the wait: for example, in waiting for emergency care, the waiter has to pay a time cost, spending part of her day in the uncomfortable surroundings of her local A&E, while in the case of elective care, the cost of joining may be rather small. A second factor in this analysis to be taken into account is if private care is available. In this case, the patient has to make a three-way comparison, checking first whether $Ve^{-td} - C > 0$, for the list-joining decision, and second whether $V - P > \max(Ve^{-td} - C, 0)$, where P is the price of private care (assumed to be delivered instantaneously): if so, private care will be purchased. To get a feel for numbers, consider a treatment that produces a single quality-adjusted life year (QALY), for which a patient will have to wait 18 weeks (comparable to the highest waiting times shown in Figure 6.1) and for a patient with a decay rate of 5 per cent a week. Assuming a rate of £30 000 per QALY, Ve^{-td} is about £12 000, so unless the cost of seeking treatment exceeds this amount, it would seem well worth the patient's while to seek care. At the same time, the benefit of going private is worth £18 000 and so if the patient is of average income, private treatment could be quite attractive.

This formalisation is a plausible first-cut approximation of decision behaviour, and is quite sufficient to drive the econometric models that provide the framework for empirical enquiry. But it is natural to ask for a more detailed, nuanced account of how patients make decisions, which would give insight into how far these results can be generalised as the economic and social context changes. From the empirical evidence that exists, it is clear that waiting times are only one dimension of hospital performance in patients' minds and may interact with other dimensions in complex ways (Burge et al., 2005; Burge et al., 2006). Even in favourable circumstances, people have significant difficulties in making choices that involve weighing up benefits realised in different time periods (Frederick et al., 2002), and list-joining decisions tend not to be made when people are at their best. People often make decisions using rather primitive heuristics, rather than performing a detailed decision analysis (Kahneman et al., 1982; Payne et al., 1993) – in the case of the joining decision, a plausible heuristic might be 'take private care if I can afford it' irrespective of the degree of benefit obtained. One of the limitations of econometric studies (or indeed any backward-looking statistical analyses) is that they provide relatively weak information about how the system will respond to a wholesale transformation (as depicted in Figure 6.1) and knowing more at the micro-level about how patients make these decisions, as a complement to macro-level studies, seems a worthwhile direction for future research.

2.3   The Process Account

Our third account is what we call the process account, which stresses the importance of proper work design in the management of care. In this account, NHS hospitals are often portrayed as rather sluggish, backward organisations, in contrast with other industries (Young et al., 2004), or with private sector health care (Ham et al., 2003). In a typical statement of the process account, and in direct contrast to what we have called the production account, Silvester et al. (2004) claim that 'a lack of capacity is not the main issue' and propose that the real need is 'to properly understand and manage patient flow' (p. 109). A common claim of proponents of the process account is that 'quality is free' (Crosby, 1979) in the sense that interventions that reduce waiting times may also save money, for example by eliminating duplication of effort or unnecessary bureaucratic procedures.

To understand the scope of opportunities for process improvement, it is important to take a systems view of the hospital. Processing patients is more complex than the simple model of the $M/M/c$ queue of Section 2.1 (Appleby et al., 2005a; Vissers and Beech, 2005). For one thing, the outpatient journey often involves multiple iterations, as patients require possibly multiple diagnostic tests before treatment. In contrast to the simplified world of the $M/M/c$ queue, the elective inpatient system operates on a booked admission basis and scheduled admission dates may not be adhered to if patients are unable to attend or hospitals are unable to accommodate. A particular challenge facing the smooth management of elective care is the existence of emergency demand from the hospital's A&E Department or elsewhere; from time to time the volume of emergency demand may require the cancellation of elective admissions if a bed is unavailable, or elective operations if a theatre is unavailable. Successful and safe conduct of surgical operations requires that the appropriate staff (including, e.g., anaesthetists as well as surgeons) and equipment be in place. Complications may lead to patients moving between specialties, as when a patient admitted for a gastro-intestinal complaint subsequently develops pneumonia. Discharge planning is difficult if patients (so-called 'bed-blockers') need care arrangements to be put in place before they leave the hospital. Post discharge, patients may continue to attend outpatient clinics. As these activities may be separated in time, managed by different parties, and linked by imperfect information flows, there are multiple opportunities for coordination failures.

A considerable amount of practical knowledge now exists on how to undertake process improvement and the sorts of benefits that can be realised. In particular, the Institute for Healthcare Improvement in the USA and the Modernisation Agency (latterly the Institute for Innovation and Improvement) in England have championed process improvement approaches and developed practical tools for implementation. In particular, the Modernisation Agency's document, *10 High Impact Changes* (Modernisation Agency, 2004) describes evidence-based ways in which health care service delivery can be improved. Many of these proposed changes draw on basic queueing-theory intuitions. For example, Change 8, reducing the number of queues, exploits economies of scale in queueing as depicted in Figure 6.2: the insight is that, where possible, capacity should be pooled. Experience shows that this intuition is counterintuitive to many in health service management, who often respond to local problems with waiting times in particular specialties by 'carving out' dedicated capacity, a response that leads, with mathematical certainty, to greater overall waiting times.

The critical question here is how managers should develop and prioritise a programme of action that makes sense in the context of their particular organisation. One well-established management technology that has the potential to help get a grip on this sort of complex system with multiple interacting resources, actors and flows of demand, and to understand quantitatively the effects of different management actions, is 'discrete event simulation' (Banks et al., 2000; Law and Kelton, 2000; Pidd, 2004). Discrete event simulation is a management science technique that seeks to model systems using the same basic framework and concepts as queueing theory, but with the capacity to capture a richer and more complex set of structures (e.g. booked admission systems), and more complex interactions, such as those between the outpatient, inpatient and emergency parts of the hospital. Unlike queueing theory, the technique is essentially computational, and so users of modelling are not limited to the tightly defined class of models for which mathematical results are available. Although several simulations of A&E Departments, outpatient clinics and so on exist (e.g. Worthington, 1987, 1991; Bagust et al., 1999; Harper and Shahani, 2002; Fone et al., 2003; Fletcher et al., 2007), there seem to be hardly any simulations that seek to capture the systemic complexity of the entire hospital; one example we are particularly aware of (having been personally involved in it) is that of the project DGHSIM (Gunal and Pidd, 2007; Pidd et al., 2008; see also the project website at http://www.hospitalsimulation.info).

2.4   The Provider Incentive Account

Our fourth and final account stresses the role of provider incentives generated by government policies as directed at waiting lists and times. This is a relatively recent theme in waiting-time discourse. Historically, it has been argued that health care workers – and public servants more generally – have been seen as 'knights': 'politicians, civil servants, state bureaucrats, and managers were supposed accurately to divine social and individual needs in the areas concerned, to be motivated to meet those needs and hence operate services that did the best possible job from the resources available' (Le Grand, 2003). In health care, it is natural to suppose that this means that all those involved in the delivery of elective care would naturally aim to keep waiting as low as possible without any incentives for them to do so. However, Iversen (1993) has shown, in the context of a Stackelberg game between a provider and government in which budgets are endogenous, that even when health care workers are altruistic, they may generate excessive waits for patients as a way of attracting additional funding for their institutions.

Moreover, some have suggested that health care workers may have less honourable motives. In particular, the medical profession has come to be perceived as the culprit (or the scapegoat) as far as waiting times are concerned. In the UK NHS, a source of particular concern has been the nature of professionals' contracts of employment, agreed as part of the political deal to bring hospital consultants into the NHS (Yates, 1995). Surgeons could opt for a maximum part-time contract that allowed them to work part time in the NHS and practise privately. The incentives for consultants were described by Le Grand (2002, p. 126):

> A consultant confronted with an NHS patient who needs an operation has an incentive to encourage the patient to 'go private.' For if the patient remains in the NHS, the consultant will have to do the operation without any extra reward, whereas if the patient sees the consultant privately, the consultant will be paid. It is hardly surprising, therefore, that the longest NHS waiting lists occur in the specialties in which specialists have the highest private earnings.

Despite the *prima facie* plausibility of this account, empirical analysis of five high-volume surgical specialties by Bloor et al. (2004) found that surgeons with a maximum part-time contract (and the strongest perverse incentives to conduct fewer operations), had *higher* absolute rates of operating among NHS surgeons. The Department of Health's experiences in negotiating a new consultant contract, intended to bring greater transparency about work planning and to raise productivity, illustrate the danger of making careless assumptions about doctor behaviour and motivation. The new contract turns out to involve spending about 25 per cent more to cover the extra work that consultants had done willingly in the old relational contract. Despite these payments, consultants were alienated and worked fewer hours under the new contract; hence the intended gains in productivity did not materialise (National Audit Office, 2007; Public Accounts Committee, 2007).

We emphatically do not take the message from Bloor et al. (2004) that incentives do not operate, and that hospitals and doctors should be left to their own devices – there is considerable unexplained variability in the consultant workload even with adjustment for case-mix, which is an unsatisfactory state of affairs. Nevertheless, it is important to understand the subtle ways in which waiting-time-related goals and incentives operate in hospital organisations. Hospitals are not monoliths, and clinical staff retain considerable *de facto* power. Perhaps the essence of management is the translation of the higher-level objectives of the organisation as goals for the individual staff member. Clearly there is an interpretative, sociological dimension to this translation activity, a shaping of what people feel are valid goals and appropriate behaviour. But there is also a game-theoretic aspect. For example, an externally imposed waiting-time target may strengthen the hand of a chief executive who favours change and reform, since if her continued employment is on the line, no one can doubt her resolve to see the job through, and cooperation may be more forthcoming. A deeper, genuinely multidisciplinary analysis of how hospitals are able to effect changes in attitude and behaviour towards waiting would be a useful direction for further research.

3.   CROSS-COUNTRY COMPARISON

In this section, we contextualise our account by discussing recent UK experience. The UK makes a particularly interesting case study because of differing styles of health policy in the devolved UK countries. The incoming Labour government of 1997 inherited a crisis brewing in the NHS, with waiting lists reaching record highs, but also a Britain in which two of the parties in the Union, Scotland and Wales, were smarting under an extended period of Conservative dominance. In an attempt to placate nationalist tendencies, the new government established devolved administrations in these two countries, with Scottish and Welsh (and subsequently Northern Irish) electorates electing parliaments or assemblies with control over domestic policy, such as health, education, environment and so on.

In order to organise our discussion of the various national responses, we observe that the four accounts offered above lead naturally to different policy recommendations:

- the implication of the production account is that funding should be increased;
- the implication of the patient behaviour account is that demand should be controlled;

- the implication of the process account is that developmental support should be provided to help organisations improve and develop;
- the implication of the provider incentive account is that rewards and sanctions should be brought to bear.

We describe the differing national responses through the framework of these four accounts.

3.1   The Production Account

All the countries identified 'underfunding' as an explanation for long waiting times. Certainly, the UK had spent less on the NHS than had been invested in other systems in comparative countries (Appleby and Boyle, 2000; Propper, 2001). That rationale was removed after the 'most expensive breakfast in British history', when on 20 January 2000, following a television interview, the prime minister committed the government to unprecedented and sustained massive increases in NHS funding in England: of 5 per cent in real terms over the six years from 2001 to 2002 (Smee, 2005). Spending in the other UK countries has also been on a growth path in recent years (Alvarez-Rosete et al., 2005).

3.2   The Patient Behaviour Account

Demand management does play a role in the various UK health care systems, most notably through the National Institute for Clinical Excellence (NICE), which promulgates guidance on appropriate treatment (Sorenson et al., 2008). However, the central focus of NICE is cost control rather than waiting list control: NICE's core criterion is the incremental cost-effectiveness ratio, and does not include considerations related to the length of the waiting list, although, as Harrison and Appleby (2005) remark (p. 38), the decline in non-evidence-based procedures such as tonsillectomies can only have helped waiting-list management. The idea of an appropriateness threshold specifically as a device to control waiting lists did attract some government and parliamentary support in the 1990s, although not to the point of actual implementation (see Harrison and New, 2000, pp. 10–12) and the use of a waiting-list prioritisation scheme of the sort deployed in New Zealand or parts of Canada has also been studied by several UK analysts (Mullen, 2003; Goddard and Tavakoli, 2008; Gravelle and Siciliani, 2008). However, this idea does not seem to have found favour in policy circles in the UK.

3.3   The Process Account

In terms of developmental support, the UK countries have all established in the last few years some sort of improvement agency charged with identifying and sharing good practice, particularly around waiting-time management. At the time of writing, these improvement agencies are: the Institute for Innovation and Improvement[3] in England; the Health Delivery Improvement Support Team[4] in Scotland; and the National Leadership and Organisation Agency[5] in Wales. Additional, targeted developmental

No. per 1000 waiting >6 months

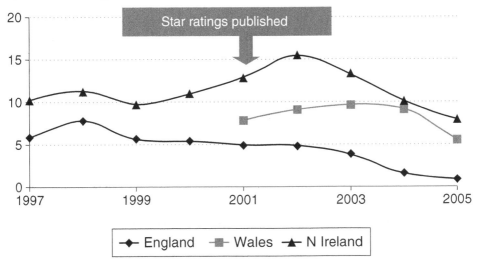

Figure 6.3   Waiting for elective hospital admission following decision to admit

support has been available from Departments of Health centrally, most notably in the shape of the English and Scottish 18-week wait initiatives.[6]

3.4   The Provider Incentive Account

A distinctive feature of the response of the English Department of Health (in contrast to the other UK countries) was the importance it placed on rewards and sanctions. In the initial phase, this was done through the radical and controversial regime of annual 'star rating' of NHS organisations, between 2001 and 2005 (Bevan and Hood, 2006; Bevan and Hamblin, 2009). This regime 'named and shamed' the 'failing' zero-rated hospitals; and offered 'earned autonomy' to the 'high-performing' three-star hospitals. Achieving annual reductions in waiting times was vital to doing well in the 'star rating' system. After 2005, the English NHS has continued to stress accountability, but now through a reformed system of hospital financing whereby funding is dependent on volume of service delivered, and an emphasis on patient choice: the idea is that patients, rather than central government or regulators, will punish providers who fail to provide timely care.

Figures 6.3 and 6.4 show comparative results by giving ratios (per 1000 population) of those waiting more than six months for an elective admission following a decision to admit, and more than three months to be seen in outpatients following referral by a GP in the run-up to and in the immediate aftermath of the star rating experience. These figures show sustained improvement in England with reductions in both those ratios from 1999; in Wales and Northern Ireland waiting ratios for inpatients increased after 1999, but then declined, but this improvement was offset by dramatic increases in those waiting to be seen in outpatients following referral by a GP. Scottish figures are not comparable, because they exclude patients with a waiting guarantee exception code, which constitutes some quarter to a third of all waiting patients (Audit Scotland, 2006):

No. per 1000 waiting >3 months

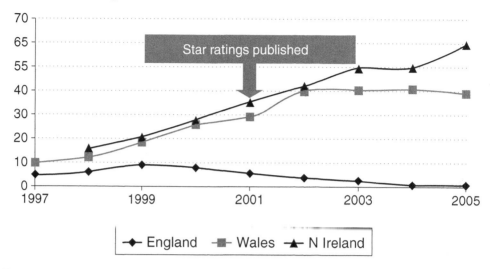

Figure 6.4   Waiting from GP referral to first appointment

Propper et al. (2008a) show that when the figures are put on a comparable basis, the marked improvement in the English data is not replicated in the Scottish data, and so, in this sense, the Scottish story is the same as in Wales and Northern Ireland.

Since 2005, England has continued to lead the pack in terms of waiting-time perform-ance. In the last quarter of 2008, England met its target of having 90 per cent of patients requiring admission, and 95 per cent of patients not requiring admission, waiting 18 weeks or less from referral to treatment, that is, from the beginning to the end of the acute pathway.[7] Scotland aims to achieve this level of performance in December 2011.[8] Wales's achievement of a target of 10 weeks for outpatients and 14 weeks for inpatients by March 2009 does not seem to be sustainable,[9] and the Welsh Assembly government also has an outstanding 26-week referral to treatment target for the end of the year.[10] Northern Ireland's most recent target is 13 weeks for an outpatient appointment and 20 weeks for an inpatient appointment.[11]

What can we learn from this natural experiment? Clearly, it provides qualified support for the central insight of the production account; additional investment can reduce waiting times, but does not do so on its own. As systematic, centralised demand man-agement strategies in the service of waiting-time management were not implemented in any of the UK countries, the natural experiment provides no evidence on the relevance or otherwise of the patient behaviour account to guiding action. In the absence of strik-ing differences between the developmental activities undertaken by the improvement agencies in the different countries, we, broadly in line with other commentators such as Alvarez-Rosete et al. (2005), Bevan and Hood (2006), Hauck and Street (2007), Propper et al. (2008a, 2008b), Willcox et al. (2007) and Harrison and Appleby (2009), conclude that the experience of England provides strong support for giving serious heed to the producer incentive account, and making available rewards and sanctions to ensure that increases in funding produce improvements in patient experience.

4.   WERE THE WAITING-TIME REDUCTIONS VALUE FOR MONEY?

A natural question is whether the effort and expense associated with waiting-time reduction in England have been value for money. A common approach in economics is to attempt an overall assessment of the welfare consequences of some action. Economists acknowledge that if the market for some particular goods or services is seriously dysfunctional for one reason or another – for example, in the case of health care, there are significant information asymmetries, with customers unable to reliably assess the quality of the product with which they are provided (Arrow, 1963) – then it may make sense for government to step in as provider. However, the core of the welfarist idea is that this provision should be assessed *as if* a market were operating, in the sense that the benefits to (and recognised and assessed by) patients should exceed the costs of the system (for an interesting discussion of the merits of this idea in a waiting time context, see Cullis et al., 2000).

Wanless et al. (2007) observe that 'it is surprising, given that waiting times are such a major strand of government health policy, that there is no readily available data on the costs and benefits of meeting successive waiting time targets' (p. 193). Yet while it is impossible (or very difficult) to identify precisely the costs and benefits to the NHS of the improvement in waiting-time performance, it *is* possible to make a few broad-brush estimates to get a feel for orders of magnitude. Spending in 2007–08 on UK NHS was about £97 billion, of which, based on England in 2006–07, about a third of spending goes directly into acute and general hospital services (Department of Health, 2008, ch. 9). After adjusting for general and NHS-specific inflation, about £24.3 billion of the total is new since 2002 (Wanless et al., 2007, pp. 13–14). If this growth is proportionally distributed between sectors, it is plausible to suppose that acute and general hospitals at time of writing (2009) consume about £8.1 billion more than they did in 2002. Between 2002 and 2008, demand (expressed as decisions to admit – see Figure 6.1) has grown by about 20 per cent, so if one takes the view that spending would have to have grown proportionately to 120 per cent of 2002 spending as a result of this increased demand, this reasoning suggests that slightly more than £3 billion incremental recurring spend for the UK as a whole, and slightly less than £3 billion for England alone, is not accounted for, and is thus an upper bound on the expenditure on waiting times.

We now weigh this investment against the benefits. We do not have a long time series for outpatient waits, so we consider only inpatient waits, from the decision to admit onwards. According to the Hospital Episode Statistics,[12] mean waiting times per admission peaked in 2002/03 at 99 days, and after hovering at that level, subsequently declined steadily, reaching 60 days in 2007/08. To get a first feel of scale, assume that patients had continued to wait 99 days throughout the five years to 2007/08 – this would have led to an incremental 480 million days of waiting, or 1.3 million years (hence our title). Now we discuss how to value this avoided 39 days of waiting per patient, assuming that this represents a sustainable level of performance. The benefits of this avoided waiting are at least twofold – they comprise avoided time in a degraded health state (with a resulting burden on the economy and the sufferer's family as well as pain and discomfort), and improved response to treatment and reduced mortality from timely intervention. Propper (1995) describes a contingent valuation study (conducted in 1987) in which subjects are asked to assess their willingness to pay to avoid time in a degraded health state (in Propper's experimental design, there is no change in response to treatment with time) and estimates a mean value of waiting of £37 a month. Dawson et al. (2005), in the context of productivity measurement, use £3.13 per day (based on the Propper study inflated to 2002/03 prices), £10 per day (which seems to us intuitively reasonable), and an extreme value of £50 per day (described as 'likely to be at the high end of any willingness to pay for a reduction in waiting time for most elective care') as valuations of waiting time. Adjusting this value for inflation, and grossing up to the 4.9 million or so patients who were admitted in 2007/08, leads to valuations of the avoided waiting as £0.7 billion, £2.2 billion or £10.1 billion. Thus, these figures are clearly on the same scale as the $3 billion cited in the previous paragraph, but it is not clear whether the benefits outweigh the costs or vice versa.

The reader can surely list several important elements that are missing from this quick and dirty calculation. On the cost side, we have ignored the costs of central government time and the investment in developmental support and regulation, and the opportunity cost of the attention from those at the very top of government. On the benefit side, we have ignored outpatient waits, and benefits associated with improved health outcomes from earlier treatment (including avoided deaths on the waiting list). There is a popular perception within and outside the health care professions that targets have led to quality failures; how far this is due to vivid instances of gaming reported in the media and generalised distrust of government, and how far it is due to actual experience, is difficult to tell. Despite instances of truly appalling quality failures linked to targets (see para. 52 of Public Administration Select Committee, 2002–2003; Healthcare Commission, 2009), there is a dearth of systematic evidence that targets have impacted negatively on quality across the system as a whole, although Bevan and Hood (2006) note that audit of reported performance to detect distortions or outright fraud was rather limited, and observe that this absence of 'hard looks' may have been in the interest of both providers and government. Appleby et al. (2005b) and Dimakou et al. (2009) report evidence of changes in admission pattern as a result of targets but do not take a view on whether the overall impact on clinical quality was positive or negative. Propper et al. (2008b) present evidence that key dimensions of quality actually have improved in England over the target period. In any case, our calculations do not include changes in quality of care, positive or negative. Our main take-home message, however, is that, although the investments have been substantial, in England at least, the benefits seem to have been on a comparable scale.

There are, however, further – and perhaps more compelling – reasons for investment in improving waiting times, beyond this narrow reckoning of the costs and benefits. A very reasonable concern – for which there is some empirical support (see Besley et al., 1999; Propper, 2000; Costa-Font and Jofre-Bonet, 2008) – is that high waiting times may lead the middle classes to exit the state-funded system and this in turn may weaken taxpayer commitment to a system that is free to all comers at the point of delivery. If one believes (as we do) that such a system is desirable for reasons of social justice and solidarity, then the investment in reducing waiting times, irrespective of its performance as a near-term investment, looks like foresighted long-term strategic positioning.

5. CONCLUSION

In this chapter, we have contrasted meliorist and miserabilist stances on waiting and summarised four different accounts of why people wait for health care, and have outlined recent experience in the various UK countries. We consider that recent history in England convincingly refutes the miserabilist view, in that it shows that substantial improvement is possible if provider incentives are aligned, and funding and support are provided to organisations that wish to improve.

We also outlined four stylised accounts of the mechanism underlying waiting for health care: a 'production account' in which waiting is viewed as a signal of inadequate resource input; a 'patient behaviour account' that stresses the role of patient behaviour in generating waits; a 'process account' that focuses on the importance of appropriate work design, and a 'producer incentive account' that views provider capture as the main determinant of waiting times. All these accounts have some element of truth, and, underscoring this, our main policy lesson from the recent UK (and particularly English) experience is the importance of a coordinated response to waiting-time problems, involving increases in financing, support for process improvement and, crucially, meaningful incentives for providers to improve.

It is, however, worth noting that recent UK experience has been rather expensive. As most health care systems face either stable or decreasing budgets in the next few years, we see questions of value for money looming increasingly large: policy makers fortunate enough to be in a position to invest in waiting-time reductions will have to make a value-for-money case with greater rigour than previously; policy makers under pressure to find efficiency savings will have to find ways to do so without driving up waiting times to unacceptable levels. Indeed, as financial pressures bite, countries that have historically not experienced waiting times for health care should perhaps be asking themselves whether this is a signal of overcapacity in their systems. Addressing such questions will, we think, involve drawing on a range of social-science disciplines (in no particular order, OR/MS, health economics, medical sociology, decision psychology and political science), and using a range of empirical and modelling methods along the lines we have sketched out in this chapter.

ACKNOWLEDGEMENTS

A preliminary version of this chapter was presented at the Workshop on Determinants of Wait Time Management Strategies in Healthcare Organisations in Ottawa, and we would like to thank attendees for their helpful comments, and Marie-Pascale Pomey for the invitation to speak at this event. We are grateful to Seán Boyle and the editors for comments, as well as feedback from members of LSE Health. Particular gratitude goes to Tony Harrison for several extremely helpful suggestions.

NOTES

1. See the historical time series data at http://www.dh.gov.uk/en/Publicationsandstatistics/Statistics/
    Performancedataandstatistics/HospitalWaitingTimesandListStatistics/index.htm (provider-based series).
    Mean waiting times are averaged over the three months in the quarter to yield a quarterly figure; for
    waiting-list length, the list in the last month of the quarter is taken.
2. Available at ftp://ftp.wiley.com/public/sci_tech_med/queueing_theory/.
3. http://www.institute.nhs.uk/
4. http://www.scotland.gov.uk/Topics/Health/NHS-Scotland/Delivery-Improvement.
5. http://www.wales.nhs.uk/sitesplus/829.
6. http://www.18weeks.nhs.uk and http://www.18weeks.scot.nhs.uk/.
7. http://www.18weeks.nhs.uk/Content.aspx?path=/News-and-Comment/news-archive/on-track/.
8. http://www.18weeks.scot.nhs.uk/timetable/.
9. http://www.statswales.wales.gov.uk/TableViewer/document.aspx?ReportId=10403.
10. http://new.wales.gov.uk/docrepos/40382/dhss/reportsenglish/safftargets06-07-e.pdf?lang=en.
11. http://www.dhsspsni.gov.uk/waiting-lists.
12. http://www.hesonline.nhs.uk.

REFERENCES

Alvarez-Rosete, A., G. Bevan, N. Mays and J. Dixon (2005), 'Effect of diverging policy across the NHS',
   British Medical Journal, **331**, 946–50.
Appleby, J. and S. Boyle (2000), 'Blair's billions: where will he find the money for the NHS?', *British Medical
   Journal*, **320**, 865–7.
Appleby, J., S. Boyle, N. Devlin, M. Harley, A. Harrison, L. Locock and R. Thorlby (2005a), *Sustaining
   Reductions in Waiting Times: Final Report to the Department of Health*, London: King's Fund.
Appleby, J., S. Boyle, N. Devlin, M. Harley, A. Harrison and R. Thorlby (2005b), 'Do English NHS waiting
   time targets distort treatment priorities in orthopaedic surgery?', *Journal of Health Services Research and
   Policy*, **10**, 167–72.
Arrow, K.J. (1963), 'Uncertainty and the welfare economics of medical care', *The American Economic Review*,
   53, 941–73.
Audit Scotland (2006), *Tackling Waiting Times in the NHS in Scotland*, Edinburgh: Audit Scotland.
Bagust, A., M. Place and J. Posnett (1999), 'Dynamics of bed use in accommodating emergency admissions:
   stochastic simulation model', *British Medical Journal*, **319**, 155–8.
Banks, J., J.S. Carson, N.L. Nelson and D.M. Nicol (2000), *Discrete-Event System Simulation*, Englewood
   Cliffs, NJ: Prentice Hall.
Besley, T., J. Hall and I. Preston (1999), 'The demand for private health insurance: do waiting lists matter?',
   Journal of Public Economics, **72**, 155–81.
Bevan, G. and R. Hamblin (2009), 'Hitting and missing targets by ambulance services for emergency calls:
   effects of different systems of performance measurement within the UK', *Journal of the Royal Statistical
   Society A*, **172**, 161–90.
Bevan, G. and C. Hood (2006), 'What's measured is what matters: targets and gaming in the English public
   health care system', *Public Administration*, **84**, 517–38.
Bloor, K., A. Maynard and N. Freemantle (2004), 'Variation in the activity rates of consultant surgeons and
   the influence of reward structures in the English NHS', *Journal of Health Services Research and Policy*, **9**,
   76–84.
Burge, P., N. Devlin, J. Appleby, F. Gallo, E. Nason and T. Ling (2006), *Understanding Patients' Choices at
   the Point of Referral*, London: King's Fund.
Burge, P., N. Devlin, J. Appleby, C. Rohr and J. Grant (2005), *London Patient Choice Project Evaluation: A
   Model of Patients' Choices of Hospital from Stated and Revealed Preference Choice Data*, London: King's
   Fund.
Costa-Font, J. and M. Jofre-Bonet (2008), 'Is there a "secession of the wealthy"? Private health insurance
   uptake and national health system support', *Bulletin of Economic Research*, **60**, 265–87.
Crosby, P.B. (1979), *Quality is Free: The Art of Making Quality Certain*, New York: Mentor.
Cullis, J.G. and P.R. Jones (1985), 'National Health Service waiting lists: a discussion of competing explana-
   tions and a policy proposal', *Journal of Health Economics*, **4**, 119–35.

Cullis, J.G., P.R. Jones and C. Propper (2000), 'Waiting lists and medical treatment: analysis and policies', in A.J. Culyer and J.P. Newhouse (eds), *Handbook of Health Economics*, Amsterdam: Elsevier, pp. 1201–49.

Dawson, D., H. Gravelle, M. O'Mahony, A. Street, M. Weale, A. Castelli, R. Jacobs, P. Kind, P. Loveridge, S. Martin, P. Stevens and L. Stokes (2005), *Report RP6: Developing New Approaches to Measuring NHS Outputs and Productivity*, York: University of York, Centre for Health Economics.

Department of Health (2008), *Department of Health: Departmental Report 2008*, London: Department of Health.

Dimakou, S., D. Parkin, N. Devlin and J. Appleby (2009), 'Identifying the impact of government targets on waiting times in the NHS', *Health Care Management Science*, **12**, 1–10.

Fletcher, A., D. Halsall, S. Huxham and D. Worthington (2007), 'The DH Accident and Emergency Department model: a national generic model used locally', *Journal of the Operational Research Society*, **58**, 1554–62.

Fone, D., S. Hollinghurst, M. Temple, A. Round, N. Lester, A. Weightman, K. Roberts, E. Coyle, G. Bevan and S. Palmer (2003), 'Systematic review of the use and valuation of computer simulation modelling population health and healthcare delivery', *Journal of Public Health Medicine*, **25**, 325–35.

Frederick, S., G. Loewenstein and T. O'Donoghue (2002), 'Time discounting and time preference: a critical review', *Journal of Economic Literature*, **40**, 351–401.

Goddard, J. and M. Tavakoli (2008), 'Efficiency and welfare implications of managed public sector hospital waiting lists', *European Journal of Operational Research*, **184**, 778–92.

Gravelle, H. and L. Siciliani (2008), 'Is waiting-time prioritisation welfare improving?', *Health Economics*, **17**, 167–84.

Gravelle, H., P. Smith and A. Xavier (2003), 'Performance signals in the public sector: the case of health care', *Oxford Economic Papers*, **55**, 81–103.

Gross, D. and C.M. Harris (1998), *Fundamentals of Queueing Theory*, Chichester, UK: Wiley.

Gunal, M.M. and M. Pidd (2007), 'Interconnected DES models of Emergency, Outpatient, and Inpatient Departments of a hospital', in S.G. Henderson, B. Biller, M.-H. Hsieh et al. (eds), *Proceedings of the 2007 Winter Simulation Conference*, pp. 2663–8.

Ham, C., N. York, S. Sutch and R. Shaw (2003), 'Hospital bed utilisation in the NHS, Kaiser Permanente, and the US Medicare programme: analysis of routine data', *British Medical Journal*, **327**, 1257–60.

Harper, P.R. and A.K. Shahani (2002), 'Modelling for the planning and management of bed capacities in hospitals', *Journal of the Operational Research Society*, **53**, 11–18.

Harrison, A. and J. Appleby (2005), *The War on Waiting for Hospital Treatment: What has Labour Achieved and What Challenges Remain?*, London: King's Fund.

Harrison, A. and J. Appleby (2009), 'Reducing waiting times for hospital treatment: lessons from the English NHS', *Journal of Health Services Research and Policy*, **14**, 168–73.

Harrison, A. and B. New (2000), *Access to Elective Care: What Really Should be Done About Waiting Lists*, London: King's Fund.

Hauck, K. and A. Street (2007), 'Do targets matter? A comparison of English and Welsh national health priorities', *Health Economics*, **16**, 275–90.

Healthcare Commission (2005), *Acute Hospital Portfolio Review: Accident and Emergency*, London: Healthcare Commission.

Healthcare Commission (2009), *Investigation into Mid Staffordshire NHS Foundation Trust*, London: Healthcare Commission.

Hurst, J. and L. Siciliani (2003), 'Tackling excessive waiting times for elective surgery: a comparison of policies in twelve OECD countries', OECD Health Working papers, Paris: OECD.

Iversen, T. (1993), 'A theory of hospital waiting lists', *Journal of Health Economics*, **12**, 55–71.

Kahneman, D., P. Slovic and A. Tversky (eds) (1982), *Judgement under Uncertainty: Heuristics and Biases*, Cambridge, UK: Cambridge University Press.

Kuhn, T.S. (1970), *The Structure of Scientific Revolutions*, Chicago, IL: University of Chicago Press.

Law, A.M. and W.D. Kelton (2000), *Simulation Modelling and Analysis*, Boston, MA: McGraw-Hill.

Le Grand, J. (2002), 'Further tales from the British National Health Service', *Health Affairs*, **21**, 116–28.

Le Grand, J. (2003), *Motivation, Agency and Public Policy: Of Knights and Knaves, Pawns and Queens*, Oxford: Oxford University Press.

Lindsay, C.M. and B. Feigenbaum (1984), 'Rationing by waiting lists', *American Economic Review*, **74**, 404–17.

Martin, S. and P.C. Smith (1999), 'Rationing by waiting lists: an empirical investigation', *Journal of Public Economics*, **71**, 141–69.

Martin, S. and P.C. Smith (2003), 'Using panel methods to model waiting times for National Health Service Surgery', *Journal of the Royal Statistical Society: Series A*, **166**(3), 369–87.

Modernisation Agency (2004), *10 High Impact Changes for Service Improvement and Delivery: a guide for NHS leaders*, Leicester, UK: Modernisation Agency.

Morton, A. and R.G. Bevan (2008), 'What's in a wait?: Contrasting management science and economic perspectives on waiting for emergency care', *Health Policy*, **85**, 207–17.

Mullen, P.M. (2003), 'Prioritising waiting lists: how and why?', *European Journal of Operational Research*, **150**, 32–45.

National Audit Office (2001), *Inpatient and Outpatient Waiting in the NHS*: London: The Stationery Office.

National Audit Office (2007), *Pay Modernisation: A New Contract for NHS Consultants in England. HC: 335 2006–2007*, London: National Audit Office.

Payne, J.W., J.R. Bettman and E.J. Johnson (1993), *The Adaptive Decision Maker*, Cambridge, UK: Cambridge University Press.

Pidd, M. (2004), *Computer Simulation in Management Science*, Chichester, UK: Wiley.

Pidd, M., M.M. Gunal and A. Morton (2008), 'DGHPSIM: performance modelling of general hospitals', 4th Operational Research Society Simulation Workshop, Worcestershire, UK, Operational Research Society.

Pomey, M.-P., P.-G. Forest, C. Sanmartin, C. DeCoster and M. Drew (2009), *Determinants of Waiting Time Management for Health Service – A Policy Review and Synthesis*, Montreal, Canada: Groupe de recherche interdisciplinaire en santé, Université de Montréal.

Pope, C. (1991), 'Trouble in store: some thoughts on the management of waiting lists', *Sociology of Health and Illness*, **13**, 193–212.

Propper, C. (1995), 'The disutility of time spent on the United Kingdom's National Health Service waiting lists', *Journal of Human Resources*, **30**, 677–700.

Propper, C. (2000), 'The demand for private health care in the UK', *Journal of Health Economics*, **19**, 855–76.

Propper, C. (2001), 'Expenditure on healthcare in the UK: a review of the issues', *Fiscal Studies*, **22**, 151–83.

Propper, C., M. Sutton, C. Whitnall and F. Windmeijer (2008a), 'Did "targets and terror" reduce waiting times in England for hospital care?', *BE Journal of Economic Analysis and Policy*, **8**(2), Article 5.

Propper, C., M. Sutton, C. Whitnall and F. Windmeijer (2008b), *Incentives and Targets in Hospital Care: Evidence from a Natural Experiment*, Bristol, UK: Centre for Market and Public Organisation, University of Bristol.

Public Accounts Committee (2007), *Pay Modernisation: A New Contract for NHS Consultants in England. HC 506*, London: House of Commons.

Public Administration Select Committee (2002–03), *On Target? Government By Measurement*, London: House of Commons.

Siciliani, L. and J. Hurst (2004), 'Explaining waiting-time variations for elective surgery across OECD countries', *OECD Economic Studies*, **38**, 95–123.

Siciliani, L. and J. Hurst (2005), 'Tackling excessive waiting time times for elective surgery: a comparative analysis of policies in 12 OECD countries', *Health Policy*, **72**, 201–15.

Silvester, L., R. Lendon, H. Bevan, R. Steyn and P. Walley (2004), 'Reducing waiting times in the NHS: is lack of capacity the problem?', *Clinician in Management*, **12**, 105–11.

Smee, C. (2005), *Speaking Truth to Power: Two Decades of Analysis in the Department of Health*, Oxford: Radcliffe Press.

Smith, P.C. (2003), 'Formula finding of public services: an economic analysis', *Oxford Review of Economic Policy*, **19**, 301–22.

Sorenson, C., M. Drummond and P. Kavanos (2008), *Ensuring Value for Money in Healthcare: The Role of Health Technology Assessment in the European Union*, Copenhagen: European Observatory on Health Systems and Policies.

Vissers, J. and R. Beech (eds) (2005), *Health Operations Management*, London: Routledge.

Wanless, D. (2002), *Securing Our Future Health: Taking a Long-Term View*, London: HM Treasury.

Wanless, D., J. Appleby, A. Harrison and D. Patel (2007), *Our Future Health Secured? A Review of NHS Funding and Performance*, London: King's Fund.

Willcox, S., M. Seddon, S. Dunn, R.T. Edwards, J. Pearse and J.V. Tu (2007), 'Measuring and reducing waiting times: a cross-national comparison of strategies', *Health Affairs*, **26**, 1078–87.

Worthington, D.J. (1987), 'Queueing models for hospital waiting lists', *Journal of the Operational Research Society*, **38**, 413–22.

Worthington, D. (1991), 'Hospital waiting list management models', *Journal of the Operational Research Society*, **42**, 833–43.

Yates, J. (1987), *Why are we Waiting? An Analysis of Hospital Waiting Lists*, Oxford: Oxford University Press.

Yates, J. (1995), *Private Eye, Heart and Hip: Surgical Consultants, the National Health Service and Private Medicine*, Edinburgh: Churchill Livingstone.

Young, T., S. Brailsford, C. Connell, R. Davies, P. Harper and J.H. Klein (2004), 'Using industrial processes to improve patient care', *British Medical Journal*, **328**, 162–4.

7 Measuring access to health care in Europe
Sara Allin and Cristina Masseria

1. INTRODUCTION

European governments seek to ensure that their citizens have access to safe and effective health care. Most countries have achieved universal coverage of health care for their populations. They have also made efforts to reduce barriers to accessing care for vulnerable groups and to more equitably distribute health services across the population. Moreover, at the EU level, improving access to health care is among the priority objectives for promoting social inclusion and equal opportunities for all (Atkinson et al., 2002; European Commission, 2005, 2007). Numerous studies have evaluated the extent to which equitable access to health care has been achieved, although there is no consensus on how to conceptualise and measure access.

The aim of this chapter is to examine one indicator of access to health care: self-reported unmet need. First, it reviews some health system features that affect the accessibility of health care, and describes some of the challenges in defining and measuring access. Next, it presents unmet need and forgone care as indicators of access, reviewing their prevalence across countries, and examining the association between forgoing health care and both utilisation and health, drawing on the first two waves of the Survey of Health, Ageing and Retirement in Europe. Finally, the chapter concludes with a discussion of the policy relevance of this indicator and areas for future research.

2. WHAT AFFECTS ACCESS TO CARE?

Access to care is a complex concept that relates to the health system, to the patients themselves, and to the interactions between them. There is general agreement among scholars and policy makers that the provision and collective financing of health services is not sufficient to ensure their accessibility. In contrast, a multitude of factors affects accessibility above and beyond the simple presence of a facility and the removal of direct cost barriers. In other words, accessibility depends on services being available, affordable and acceptable (McIntyre et al., 2009), and it relates to quality, convenience and information (Goddard and Smith, 2001).

The availability of services depends on a number of supply-side factors, many of which are commonly measured both within and across countries. These include design of statutory health care coverage and public benefits packages, the volume and distribution of human resources and capital, cost-sharing requirements, waiting times, referral patterns, booking systems and hours of operation, how individuals are treated within the system (continuity of care), and quality of care (Aday and Andersen, 1974; Whitehead, 1991; Starfield, 1993; Gulliford et al., 2002; Healy and McKee, 2004). These can be constituted as different 'hurdles' or 'barriers' that need to be overcome in order to achieve universal access to care (Gulliford et al., 2002; Wörz et al., 2006).

Because of variations in the financing and organisation of health care across countries, supply-side factors that affect access also vary. For example, some countries require patients to either register with a gatekeeping doctor or to get a referral to access a specialist (as in Denmark, Italy, the Netherlands and Spain). Referral rates may differ across population groups (Kikano et al., 1996; Chan and Austin, 2003; Dixon et al., 2007), which may reflect systemic barriers to accessing specialist care for some patients. Moreover, some countries base entitlement to statutory coverage on residence (as in Greece, Sweden, Denmark, Italy and France), while others require individuals to enrol in an insurance fund (as in Austria, Belgium, the Netherlands, Switzerland and Germany). However, there might be some groups who do not have coverage, and face substantial financial barriers to accessing care (Foubister and Wörz, 2006). For all those legally resident in the country, these barriers have largely been removed.

In addition to supply-side factors, there are a number of individual-level characteristics that affect the accessibility of services; these factors not only vary across countries but also within countries across different sub-populations. Characteristics of patients, such as their age, gender, socioeconomic status, past experiences with health care, their perceptions of the benefits and quality of care, cultural identity, and level of health literacy may also affect their decisions to seek care and the acceptability of services (Aday and Andersen, 1974; Mitchell and Schlesinger, 2005; Dixon et al., 2007; Fernandez et al., 2008; McIntyre et al., 2009).

These individual characteristics interact with the supply-side factors in determining access (McIntyre et al., 2009). For instance, the affordability of a service depends on both the user charges or exemptions at the point of use and the individuals' ability and willingness to pay. Communication between providers and patients also affects the quality of care and adherence; effective communication will depend on, among other things, the time a physician can spend with the patient, as well as the level of education and health literacy of the patient.

Clearly, the numerous factors that affect each of these dimensions of access, and the way they interact, raise many challenges for measuring access. While health care use is often seen as evidence of accessibility, and a number of studies have identified systematic differences in health care use across socioeconomic groups (van Doorslaer et al., 2004; Allin et al., 2009), the use of services does not capture the different dimension of access, nor does it explain the reasons for non-use. In addition, the extent to which different patterns of utilisation reflect individuals' choices (Le Grand, 1991) as opposed to policy-relevant concerns such as service availability, or personal, organisational or financial barriers to access (Gulliford et al., 2002) is not easily understood.

One relatively straightforward tool is the direct questioning of individuals as to whether there was a time when they needed health care but did not receive it, or whether they had to forgo health care. Individuals are in a unique position to estimate their health status (Idler and Benyamini, 1997), as well as their experiences with health care. If an individual experienced difficulties in accessing care, or experienced suboptimal care, then this information could be elicited directly. This approach could also help to disentangle the reasons for different patterns of health care utilisation.

3.   UNMET NEED AS AN INDICATOR OF (POOR) ACCESS

Self-reported unmet need for health care in the past 12-month period is included in two international surveys. The Survey on Health, Ageing and Retirement in Europe (SHARE) includes individuals aged 50 years and older in ten European countries plus Switzerland, and from the second wave also Poland and Israel. The EU Survey of Income and Living Conditions (EU-SILC) looks at residents of private households aged 16 years and older in all EU countries. These surveys present opportunities for cross-country comparative research on access to health care. However, the survey questions on unmet need differ, as do the samples. The phrasing of the question in EU-SILC is as follows: 'Was there any time during the last 12 months when, in your opinion, you personally needed a medical examination or treatment for a health problem but you did not receive it?' Follow-up questions include the reasons for unmet need. Among these possible reasons for 'unmet need' are those that are important from a policy perspective, such as the individual could not afford to (costs), waiting lists, and travelling related problems, but also those that are less clearly relevant to policy makers, such as that the respondent wanted to wait to see if the problem got better on its own, didn't know any good doctor, fear of care, and could not take time off work.

In SHARE the question focuses on forgone care that is due either to costs or unavailability of care. Specifically, the questions are: 'During the last twelve months, did you forgo any types of care because of the costs you would have to pay?' and 'During the last twelve months, did you forgo any types of care because they were not available or not easily accessible?' Follow-up questions then focus on the type of care (e.g. physician, medicine, dental) that the individual reported to forgo.

3.1   Prevalence of Unmet Need

Across Europe there is heterogeneity in the proportion of the population who report an unmet need or who report to have forgone care in the past 12 months. Any unmet need (in the adult population) varies from less than 1 per cent in Slovenia and Belgium to 26 per cent in Latvia followed by Poland, Sweden and Hungary (Figure 7.1). However, the diverse set of reasons for reporting unmet need (in EU-SILC) necessitates its disaggregation in order to gain meaningful information. For example, as shown in Figure 7.1, the prevalence of unmet need in 2007 in Sweden is 14.4 per cent when all reasons are included (7.4 per cent on average across all EU countries surveyed), but it falls to 1.9 per cent (3.3 per cent on average across countries) when only reasons related to costs and availability (defined as waiting-time and travelling-related reasons) are included. Similarly, in Hungary it decreases from 14 per cent to 2.3 per cent. However, in Latvia, the percentage of the surveyed population reporting unmet needs remains relatively high, 14.5 per cent, also when only costs and availability are considered.

The population aged 50 and over that is surveyed in SHARE should lead to higher estimates of access problems, given the strong relationship between age and health. Self-reported forgone care in this population subgroup ranges from 2.6 per cent in the Netherlands to 16 per cent in Israel (Figure 7.2). Austria and Denmark remain among the countries with the lowest reported access problems, and Greece, France and Italy

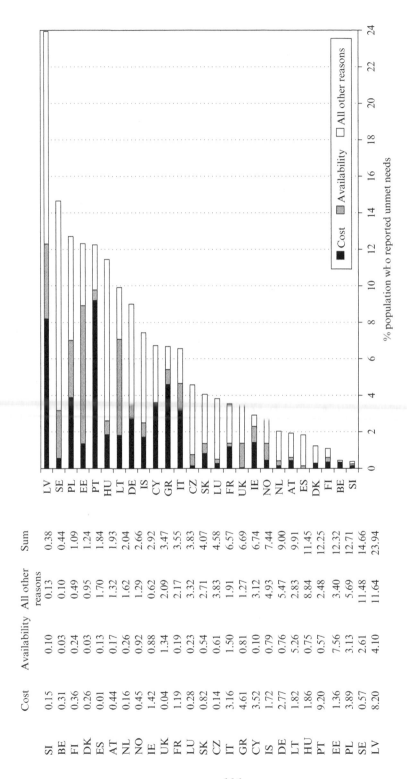

	Cost	Availability	All other reasons	Sum
SI	0.15	0.10	0.13	0.38
BE	0.31	0.03	0.10	0.44
FI	0.36	0.24	0.49	1.09
DK	0.26	0.03	0.95	1.24
ES	0.01	0.13	1.70	1.84
AT	0.44	0.17	1.32	1.93
NL	0.16	0.26	1.62	2.04
NO	0.45	0.92	1.29	2.66
IE	1.42	0.88	0.62	2.92
UK	0.04	1.34	2.09	3.47
FR	1.19	0.19	2.17	3.55
LU	0.28	0.23	3.32	3.83
SK	0.82	0.54	2.71	4.07
CZ	0.14	0.61	3.83	4.58
IT	3.16	1.50	1.91	6.57
GR	4.61	0.81	1.27	6.69
CY	3.52	0.10	3.12	6.74
IS	1.72	0.79	4.93	7.44
DE	2.77	0.76	5.47	9.00
LT	1.82	5.26	2.83	9.91
HU	1.86	0.75	8.84	11.45
PT	9.20	0.57	2.48	12.25
EE	1.36	7.56	3.40	12.32
PL	3.89	3.13	5.69	12.71
SE	0.57	2.61	11.48	14.66
LV	8.20	4.10	11.64	23.94

Source: EU Survey of Income and Living Conditions, 2007.

Figure 7.1 Proportion of the population who reported unmet need, 2007

116

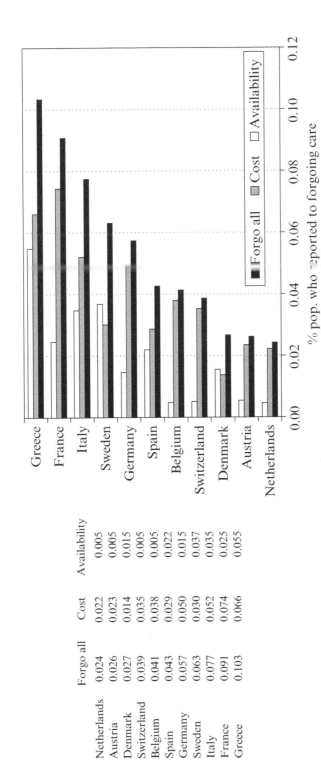

	Forgo all	Cost	Availability
Netherlands	0.024	0.022	0.005
Austria	0.026	0.023	0.005
Denmark	0.027	0.014	0.015
Switzerland	0.039	0.035	0.005
Belgium	0.041	0.038	0.005
Spain	0.043	0.029	0.022
Germany	0.057	0.050	0.015
Sweden	0.063	0.030	0.037
Italy	0.077	0.052	0.035
France	0.091	0.074	0.025
Greece	0.103	0.066	0.055

Source: Survey on Health, Ageing and Retirement in Europe, 2004.

Figure 7.2   Self-reported forgone care, forgone care due to costs, and forgone care due to unavailable/inaccessible care

remain among the countries with higher prevalence of access problems (over 6 per cent in SHARE; over 4 per cent in EU-SILC).

Some national studies have revealed higher estimates of forgone care than those reported in cross-country surveys. Swedish studies of the 20–65 age group identified higher rates of forgone physician visits in the past three months, with 24 per cent of those surveyed having refrained from a visit when needed (Westin et al., 2004), and even higher estimates among the unemployed population of the same age (42 per cent) (Ahs and Westerling, 2006). The latter clearly reflects the relationship between being unemployed and in poorer health. Similarly, an earlier Swedish study found a high proportion (22 per cent) of individuals who reported forgoing primary health care due to the cost (Elofsson et al., 1998). Also in France, 4 per cent of adults reported unmet need due to financial reasons for general health care services over the past 12 months, but the proportion was much higher, at 12 per cent, for dental care (Bocognano et al., 1999).

3.2   Who Reports Unmet Need and Forgone Care?

Perceived access problems would be expected to be greater among those with higher need for health care. People with health problems, whether acute or chronic, and worse self-assessed health are expected to have a greater prevalence of reported unmet need. Indeed, in all countries, there is a relationship between reported forgone care and self-assessed health status. On average, people who report an unmet need are more likely to be in poor health and to report limitations in daily activity (using SILC data), although the likelihood of having chronic conditions is higher among people without unmet needs. Moreover, using the SHARE data we can see differences across countries in the distribution of forgone care by level of health (Figure 7.3). For example, in some countries (Denmark, the Netherlands), almost all of those who report forgoing health care are in the worst general health, whereas in other countries (Spain, Germany, Sweden) there is a clear gradient in reporting forgone care by level of health.

The few studies that have been conducted to examine unmet need in Europe have identified a strong association with both income and health whereby people who report unmet need tend to be in worse health and with lower income, after controlling for other measurable characteristics. An early study of the EU-SILC found that unmet need was concentrated among those with lower income in all countries, and that after adjusting for health (which tends to be worse among those with lower income), the relationship with income persists in almost all countries (see Figure 7.4) (Koolman, 2007). The unadjusted association between income and unmet need for both medical and dental care can be seen in the more recent data and across a wider range of countries (Huber et al., 2008; de Looper and Lafortune, 2009). A recent analysis of income-related inequalities in medical and dental unmet needs (Hernández-Quevedo et al., 2010) found statistically significant pro-poor inequality by income in all European countries both for medical and dental unmet needs, with, on average, higher level of inequalities due to cost-related unmet needs than to availability-related unmet needs.

Analyses of SHARE also show an association between forgone care and income. One study found a higher likelihood of care forgone among individuals with lower income in

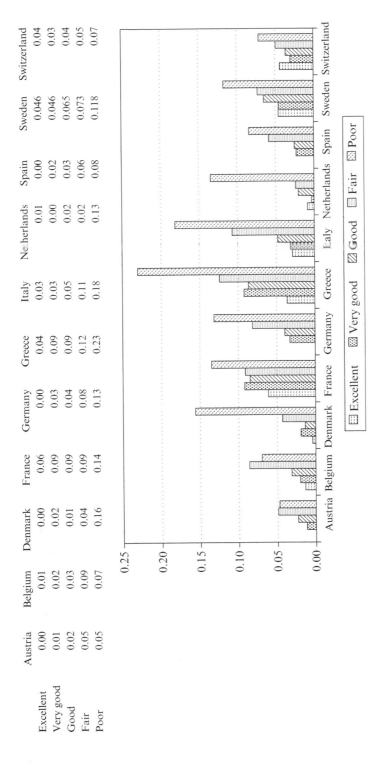

	Austria	Belgium	Denmark	France	Germany	Greece	Italy	Netherlands	Spain	Sweden	Switzerland
Excellent	0.00	0.01	0.00	0.06	0.00	0.04	0.03	0.01	0.00	0.046	0.04
Very good	0.01	0.02	0.02	0.09	0.03	0.09	0.03	0.00	0.02	0.046	0.03
Good	0.02	0.03	0.01	0.09	0.04	0.09	0.05	0.02	0.03	0.065	0.04
Fair	0.05	0.09	0.04	0.09	0.08	0.12	0.11	0.02	0.06	0.073	0.05
Poor	0.05	0.07	0.16	0.14	0.13	0.23	0.18	0.13	0.08	0.118	0.07

☒ Excellent ☒ Very good ☒ Good ▦ Fair ▨ Poor

Source: Survey on Health, Ageing and Retirement in Europe, 2004.

Figure 7.3   The proportion of the population who report forgoing health care by level of health, by country, 2004

119

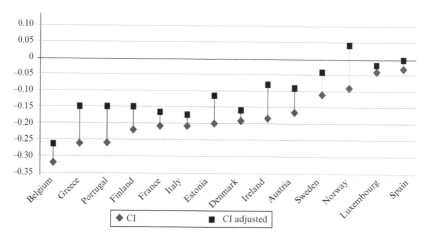

Source: Adapted from Koolman (2007)

Figure 7.4   Concentration indices (CI) of the concentration of unmet need by income, and the CI after adjusting for differences in health status

all countries studied (Mielck et al., 2007), although the highest income groups in Sweden, and to a lesser extent in Greece, had a higher prevalence than the middle-income groups. Another study focused on forgone care due to costs and found younger age (50–59), worse health, greater out-of-pocket spending and perceived income inadequacy significantly increased the likelihood of forgone care, with some variations across countries (Litwin and Sapir, 2009).

3.3   Do Individuals Who Report Forgoing Care Use Fewer Services or Experience Worse Health Outcomes?

People who report either forgoing care or an unmet need tend on average to be in worse health than those who do not report either of these problems. However, do these people use more or less health care? After adjusting for differences in health status, one may expect that those who report forgoing care use fewer services than those who do not report these problems, but who are at similar levels of health. Studies from Canada show different patterns of health care utilisation according to the different reasons for reporting an unmet need (Hurley et al., 2008; Allin et al., 2010). For instance, individuals who report an unmet need due to system-related factors such as unavailable care or high costs appear to use the health system differently, on average, from those who report unmet needs due to reasons such as personal choices. These studies underscore the importance of examining the different types of unmet need separately.

The SHARE data allow us to examine the significance of forgoing health care either because of costs or availability[1] for both the use of health services[2] (using cross-sectional data from 2004), and future health status[3] (using the longitudinal sample of individuals who were surveyed twice) in 11 countries.[4]

To measure the extent to which reported forgone health care is associated with the actual and future use of health services, we ran a series of regressions on a comprehen-

Table 7.1   Models of utilisation, 2004 and 2006 (marginal effects from probit)

	Likelihood of a GP visit		Likelihood of a specialist visit		Likelihood of hospital admission	
	Clustered model	Nested model	Clustered model	Nested model	Clustered model	Nested model
Forgone care 2004						
Availability	**0.03**	0.03	**0.12**	−0.11	0.01	0.01
Cost	0.02	0.02	0.03	0.03	−0.01	−0.01
Forgone care 2006						
Availability	0.00	0.00	**0.08**	**0.35**	**0.05**	**0.05**
Cost	−0.02	−0.02	−0.02	−0.02	−0.01	−0.02

Note.   Partial models adjust standard errors for clustering by country; full models include interactions between country dummies and all independent variables. Bold indicates significant at *p* < 0.05.

Table 7.2   Models of the likelihood of worse reported health in 2006 (marginal effects from probit, and standard errors)

	Cluster model		Nested model	
	Marginal effect	Standard error	Marginal effect	Standard error
Forgone care 2004				
Availability	0.02	0.03	0.02	0.04
Cost	**0.05**	0.02	0.05	0.03
Pseudo *R²*	0.12		0.13	

Note: Bold indicates significant at *p* < 0.05.

sive set of demographic and health indicators including age, gender, self-assessed health, limitations in activities due to health and the presence of a chronic condition. Also included in the regressions was individual-level information on socioeconomic status including education, income and employment status. Because the analysis pools all 11 countries, we included dummy variables to represent the country of residence to control for country-level variations in utilisation and access (Austria is the reference country).[5] A simple cluster model as well as a nested model (with country interaction terms) were estimated for GP, specialist and hospital care for the two waves of the SHARE survey.

The results of these analyses paint a mixed picture (see Table 7.1). Those who reported forgoing care due to availability in 2004 are more likely to use GP and specialist care both in the same year (but only when the cluster model is used[6]), and in the future (2006) than those who do not report forgoing care. People who report forgoing care due to costs are neither less nor more likely to use current and future health services than those who do not report this access problem, with the exception of specialist care, where the nested model shows significant country differences. In Greece, the Netherlands and Sweden, people who reported forgoing care because of costs in 2004 are less likely to use specialist care in 2006 (results not reported). Therefore, although it is likely that people who reported forgoing care due to costs may have reduced the use of a particular service that was too costly, on average, this access problem did not appear to affect their likelihood of receiving physician or hospital care when compared to individuals who did not report forgoing care due to costs.

However, when we examine the factors that lead to worse health in the second survey wave, we find that people who report forgoing care due to costs, but not due to availability, are significantly more likely to report worse health in the following year. In other words, when costs deter individuals from seeking care, there may be deleterious effects on their health. This finding is in contrast with studies from the USA that found delayed or forgone care did not have any significant effect on adverse health measured more objectively in terms of functional decline and survival (Franks et al., 1996; Rupper et al., 2004).

4.   DISCUSSION

The measurement of access with unmet need or forgone care presents opportunities for capturing the interaction between individuals' characteristics and the health system. In this chapter, we document some of the differences in perceived access problems across countries, and provide a preliminary analysis of the associations between forgone care, health care use and health status. In doing so we reveal some of the challenges associated with interpreting these measures. It is unlikely that accessibility can be summarised in a single indicator, and in order to gain a comprehensive understanding of accessibility, self-reported unmet need and forgone care should be presented alongside other measures. Forgoing care due to costs represents an interaction between the supply side characteristics – the organisation of cost sharing in the system and the limits to the public benefits package – and the individuals, such as their ability and/or willingness to pay and their calculations of the benefits to costs ratio. Therefore the policy responses that are needed in order to improve accessibility along this dimension will aim to achieve a greater degree of balance between these two perspectives.

The decision to forgo care because of unavailability similarly reflects an interaction between the provision of services and the level of personal inconvenience. From a policy perspective this information could be combined with waiting-time data in order to determine whether these access problems are considered acceptable on the basis of agreed standards or not.

Several studies have examined variations in waiting times across socioeconomic groups. One study used the SHARE data on waiting times for specialist consultations and non-emergency surgery and found that individuals with more education experience significantly shorter waits than the less educated in most countries (Siciliani and Verzulli, 2009). A study from Rome, Italy, found patients with higher socioeconomic status waited significantly less time for emergency surgery following hip fractures than those with lower socioeconomic status, as defined by a geographically derived index of deprivation (Barone et al., 2009). In England there also appear to be differences across ethnic groups in reported waiting times for physician care that relate to differences in perceived quality of care (Mead and Roland, 2009). Using hospital administrative data in England, it appears that there has been a reduction over time in the extent of the differences in waiting times for elective surgery across socioeconomic groups (Cooper et al., 2009).

A better understanding of the relationship between unmet needs and other indicators of access is indispensable to designing *ad hoc* policies able to reduce access problems. This is important as a policy objective *per se* and also as a way to reduce inequalities given the relationship between unmet needs and income. Disadvantaged people are on average more likely to report unmet needs. However, the research that investigates the relationship between unmet needs and health care utilisation is so far inconclusive, and better and longer-term data are necessary to be able to disentangle the determinants of this relationship.

ACKNOWLEDGEMENTS

This chapter uses data from SHARE release 2.2.0, as of 19 August 2009. SHARE data collection in 2004–07 was primarily funded by the European Commission through its 5th and 6th framework programmes (project numbers QLK6-CT-2001-00360; RII-CT-2006-062193; CIT5-CT-2005-028857). Additional funding by the US National Institute on Aging (grant numbers U01 AG09740-13S2; P01 AG005842; P01 AG08291; P30 AG12815; Y1-AG-4553-01; OGHA 04-064; R21 AG025169) as well as by various national sources is gratefully acknowledged (see http://www.share-project.org for a full list of funding institutions).

NOTES

1. The questions are: 'During the last twelve months, did you forgo any types of care because of the costs you would have to pay?' and 'During the last twelve months, did you forgo any types of care because they were not available or not easily accessible?' Follow-up questions then focus on the type of care (e.g. physician, medicine, dental) that the individual reported to forgo. Total forgone care is reported by 7 per cent of the total sample of 11 countries. Across all countries, dental care accounts for 46 per cent of the reported care forgone due to costs, and specialist care accounts for 38 per cent of the care forgone due to availability.
2. We measure health care utilisation using three separate indicators: the likelihood of a visit to a GP, a specialist, and an admission to a hospital.
3. 'Compared with your health when we talked with you in [month and year of previous interview], would you say that your health is better now, about the same, or worse?' About 30 per cent of those who were interviewed in both years report their health to be worse over the period. The proportion with worse health over the two-year period is higher in some countries (e.g. 69 per cent in Greece, 50 per cent in Switzerland and Belgium) and lower in others (e.g. 30 per cent in Germany, 32 per cent in Spain).
4. The sample totalled 28 517 individuals in the first wave (2004), and 18 741 individuals who were surveyed in both 2004 and 2006. After dropping observations with missing values we end up with a sample of 26 690 individuals in 2004 and 14 716 individuals in both years. Detailed information on the survey methodology is available elsewhere; see Borsch-Supan and Jurges (2005).
5. In addition we run two sets of models, clustered probit models (clustering by country) and nested probit models with country interaction terms. The nested model allows us to account for differences across countries by including interaction terms for each independent variable multiplied by the country dummy.
6. Although the coefficients of the nested model are the same as those of the cluster model, they are not statistically significant.

REFERENCES

Aday, L. and R. Andersen (1974), 'A framework for the study of access to medical care', *Health Services Research*, **9**, 208–20.
Ahs, A. and R. Westerling (2006), 'Health care utilization among persons who are unemployed or outside the labour force', *Health Policy*, **78**, 178–93.
Allin, S., M. Grignon et al. (2010), 'Subjective unmet need and utilization of heatlh care services in Canada: what are the implications for equity?', *Social Science and Medicine*, **70**(3), 465–72.
Allin, S., C. Masseria et al. (2009), 'Measuring socioeconomic differences in use of health care services by wealth versus by income', *American Journal of Public Health*, **99**(10), 1849–55.
Atkinson, A., B. Cantillon et al. (eds) (2002), *Social Indicators: The EU and Social Inclusion*, Oxford: Oxford University Press.
Barone, A.P., D. Fusco et al. (2009), 'Effects of socioeconomic position on 30-day mortality and wait for surgery after hip fracture', *International Journal for Quality in Health Care*, **21**(6), 379–86.
Bocognano, A., S. Dumesnil et al. (1999), 'Santé, soins et protection sociale en 1998', Questions d'économie de la santé IRDES no. 24, Paris: IRDES.
Borsch-Supan, A. and H. Jurges (eds) (2005), *The Survey of Health, Aging, and Retirement in Europe – Methodology*, Mannheim: Mannheim Research Institute for the Economics of Aging (MEA).
Chan, B.T. and P.C. Austin (2003) 'Patient, physician, and community factors affecting referrals to specialists in Ontario, Canada: a population-based, multi-level modelling approach', *Medical Care*, **41**(4), 500–511.
Cooper, Z.N., A. McGuire et al. (2009), 'Equity, waiting times and the NHS reforms', *British Medical Journal*, **339**, b3264.
de Looper, M. and G. Lafortune (2009), 'Measuring disparities in health status and in access and use of health care in OECD countries', OECD Health Working Papers No. 43, Paris: OECD.
Dixon, A., J. Le Grand et al. (2007), 'Is the British National Health Service equitable? The evidence on socio-economic differences in utilisation', *Journal of Health Services Research and Policy*, **12**(2), 104–9.
Elofsson, S., A.-L. Undén et al. (1998), 'Patient charges – a hindrance to financially and psychosocially disadvantaged groups seeking care', *Social Science and Medicine*, **46**(10), 1375–80.
European Commission (2005), 'Working together, working better: a new framework for the open coordination of social protection and inclusion policies in the European Union', Brussels, Communication from the Commission, COM(2005)706.
European Commission (2007), 'Joint report on social protection and social inclusion', Brussels, SEC(2007)329.
Fernández, J.-L., D. McDaid et al. (2008), 'Inequalities in the use of services among older people in England. A rapid review of the literature for Age Concern', PSSRU Discussion Paper DP2610, Canterbury, Kent: PSSRU.
Foubister, T. and M. Wörz (2006), 'Access to health care: illegal immigrants and asylum seekers', *Euro Observer*, **8**(2).
Franks, P., M.R. Gold et al. (1996), 'Use of care and subsequent mortality: the importance of gender', *Health Services Research*, **31**(3), 347–63.
Goddard, M. and P. Smith (2001), 'Equity of access to health care services: theory and evidence from UK', *Social Science and Medicine*, **53**, 1149–62.
Gulliford, M., J. Figueroa-Munoz et al. (2002), 'What does "access to health care" mean?', *Journal of Health Services Research and Policy*, **7**(3), 186–8.
Healy, J. and M. McKee (eds) (2004), *Accessing Health Care: Responding to Diversity*, Oxford: Oxford University Press.
Hernández-Quevedo, C. Masseria and E.A. Mossialos (2010), Methodological issues in the analysis of the socioeconomic determinants of health using EU-SILC data', Eurostat, Methodologies and Working Papers.
Huber, M., A. Stanciole et al. (2008), *Quality in and Equality of Access to Healthcare Services*, Brussels: European Commission, DG Employment, Social Affairs and Equal Opportunities.
Hurley, J., T. Jamal et al. (2008), 'The relationship between self-reported unmet need for health care and health care utilization', Report for the Ontario Ministry of Health and Long Term Care, Hamilton, McMaster University.
Idler, E.L. and Y. Benyamini (1997), 'Self-rated health and mortality: a review of twenty-seven community studies', *Journal of Health and Social Behaviour*, **38**(1), 21–37.
Kikano, G.E., M.A. Schiaffino et al. (1996), 'Medical decision making and perceived socioeconomic class', *Archives of Family Medicine*, **5**, 267–70.
Koolman, X. (2007), 'Unmet need for health care in Europe', *Comparative EU Statistics on Income and Living Conditions: Issues and Challenges. Proceedings of the EU-SILC Conference*, Helsinki, Eurostat, pp. 183–91.

Le Grand, J. (1991), *Equity and Choice: An Essay in Economics and Applied Philosophy*, London, HarperCollins Academic.

Litwin, H. and E.V. Sapir (2009), 'Forgone health care due to cost among older adults in European countries and in Israel', *European Journal of Ageing*, **6**(3), 167–76.

McIntyre, D., M. Thiede et al. (2009), 'Access as a policy-relevant concept in low- and middle-income countries', *Health Economic, Policy and Law*, **4**, 179–93.

Mead, N. and M. Roland (2009), 'Understanding why some ethnic minority patients evaluate medical care more negatively than white patients: a cross sectional analysis of a routine patient survey in English general practices', *British Medical Journal*, **339**, b3450.

Mielck, A., R. Kiess et al. (2007), 'Association between access to health care and household income among the elderly in 10 western European countries', in *Tackling Health Inequalities in Europe: An Integrated Approach*, Rotterdam, Erasmus MC Department of Public Health, pp. 471–82.

Mitchell, S. and M. Schlesinger (2005), 'Managed care and gender disparities in problematic health care experiences', *Health Services Research*, **40**(5, Pt 1), 1489–513.

Rupper, R.W., T.R. Konrad et al. (2004), 'Self-reported delay in seeking care has poor validity for predicting adverse outcomes', *Journal of the American Geriatrics Society*, **52**, 2104–9.

Siciliani, L. and R. Verzulli (2009), 'Waiting times and socioeconomic status among elderly Europeans: evidence from SHARE', *Health Economics*, **18**(11), 1295–306.

Starfield, B. (1993), *Primary Care: Concept, Evaluation and Policy*, Oxford: Oxford University Press

van Doorslaer, E., C. Masseria et al. (2004), *Income-related Inequality in the Use of Medical Care in 21 OECD Countries*, Paris: OECD.

Westin, M., A. Ahs et al. (2004), 'A large proportion of Swedish citizens refrain from seeking medical care – lack of confidence in the medical services a plausible explanation?', *Health Policy*, **68**, 333–44.

Whitehead, M. (1991), 'The concepts and principles of equity and health', *Health Promotion International*, **6**, 217–28.

Wörz, M., T. Foubister et al. (2006), 'Access to health care in the EU Member States', *Euro Observer*, **8**(2), 1–4.

PART III

INSURANCE AND EXPENDITURES

8 How are rising health care expenditures explained?
Alistair McGuire, Victoria Serra-Sastre and Maria Raikou

1. INTRODUCTION

Health systems continue to grow in both absolute and relative terms. This holds true not only for the high-income countries but also for middle-income countries, as well as some low-income ones. This has been an historical fact and looks set to continue into the future. That this is the case is well accepted. Why this is the case is less well understood. This chapter focuses on trends in health care expenditures and the main driving forces of these trends. While a number of potential explanations can be forwarded, it is argued that the continuing impact of new health care technology is the major component of health care expenditure growth. The chapter outlines recent trends in expenditure across a number of countries, discusses the common explanatory factors associated with this increase in health care expenditure and concludes with a discussion of whether future cost containment is necessary or indeed will prove effective.

2. HEALTH CARE EXPENDITURE

It is well recognised that health care expenditure growth has exceeded national income in all the high-income countries for most of the past 30 years; for some like the USA this has been the case for over 50 years. Table 8.1a shows the average annual growth rates in five-year periods for health care expenditure in a number of the wealthier OECD countries beginning in 1970 and contrasts this with the average annual growth rates of GDP (Table 8.1b). Both health expenditure and GDP are controlled for population size (they are expressed as health expenditure per capita and GDP per capita) and are converted into a common currency (the US$) using purchasing power parity rates that take account of differences in relative prices across the different countries. As can be seen in all countries, and this is generally true although Finland is a marginal exception, the health care system is taking an increasing share of the resources of each individual country. The current trends in health care expenditure in a group of these high-income countries are given in Figure 8.1. As can be seen, health expenditure as a percentage share of GDP is, with some periods of stability or downturn, in general continuing to increase. This trend is not just confined to high-income countries. The OECD (2010) projects that for the middle-income countries Korea and Mexico health and long-term care expenditure will rise from 3.3 per cent to 9 per cent of GDP over the period 2005 to 2050 in the absence of any cost containment policies and will of course be higher without such policies (estimated at 1.9 per cent of GDP in this case).

Table 8.1a   Per capita total health care expenditure growth (%)

Countries	1970–75	1975–80	1980–85	1985–90	1990–95	1995–2000	2000–2005
Australia	6.3	1.1	2.6	2.3	3.5	5	3.3
Canada	2.9	2.7	4.7	3.3	0.9	2.7	3.8
Finland	6.2	3.1	4.6	4.7	−1.4	2.6	5.8
France	6.7	5	3.7	3.6	4.1	1.8	4.0
Germany	9.0	3.6	2.4	1.4	2.7	2.3	1.2
Ireland	11.3	5.7	−0.2	0.5	6.2	7.0	9.3
Sweden	4.3	4.6	0.9	1.4	−0.6	3.9	4.5
UK	5.9	2.4	2.7	3.5	4.4	3.8	4.5
USA	4.1	4.9	5.1	5.8	3.4	2.9	4.2

Note: 1970 figure for Australia corresponds to 1971; 2000 GDP price level.

Source: OECD Health Data, 2008.

Table 8.1b   Per capita GDP growth (%)

Countries	1970–75	1975–80	1980–85	1985–90	1990–95	1995–2000	2000–2005
Australia	0.8	1.9	1.5	1.3	2.1	2.7	2.1
Canada	2.7	2.5	1.7	1.5	0.6	3.2	1.5
Finland	3.9	2.7	2.2	3.0	−1.2	4.5	2.3
France	3.1	2.9	1.1	2.7	0.7	2.4	1.0
Germany	2.0	3.5	1.3	2.0	−1.3	1.9	0.3
Ireland	3.4	3.1	1.7	4.9	4.1	8.3	3.7
Sweden	2.2	1.0	1.8	2.0	0.1	3.2	2.2
UK	1.9	1.7	1.9	3.0	1.4	2.9	2.0
USA	1.8	2.6	2.3	2.3	1.2	2.9	1.3

Note: 2000 GDP price level.

Source: OECD Health Data, 2008.

3.   THE ROLE OF INCOME (AND PRICES)

Generally, income elasticities for health care are estimated to be greater than one at the aggregate level. Table 8.2 reproduces the elasticities found empirically in a number of studies. Commonly, it is argued that this reflects the fact that higher health care expenditure is a natural consequence of increased income. While there are some statistical issues surrounding the validity of these results, the findings are common and highly reproduced with a fairly accepted average elasticity at the aggregate level of around 1.3, implying that a 10 per cent increase in GDP will increase health expenditures by 13 per cent.

These aggregate effects are somewhat surprising. First, they do not hold at lower levels of aggregation. Examination of income elasticities at the regional level, normally defined across US states, generally reveal income elasticities of less than unity, and at

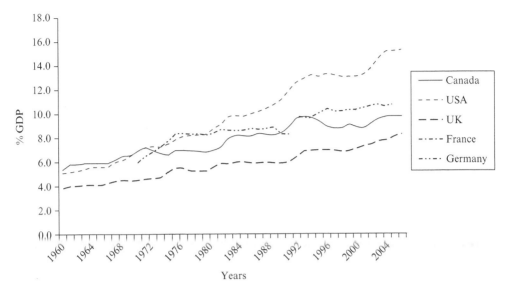

Figure 8.1   Health expenditure as a percentage of GDP

Table 8.2   Income elasticities: the empirical evidence

Individual (micro)	Income elasticity
Insured	
Newhouse and Phelps (1976)	≤0.1
Hahn and Lefkowitz (1992)	≤0.0
Less insured/uninsured	
Falk et al. (1933)	0.7
Andersen and Benham (1970) – dental	1.2
AHCPR (1997) – dental	1.1
Regions (intermediate)	
Fuchs and Kramer (1972) – 33 states, 1966	0.9
Di Matteo and Di Matteo (1998) – 10 Canadian provinces, 1965–91	0.8
Freeman (2003) – US states, 1966–98	0.8
Nations (macro)	
Newhouse (1977) – 12 countries, 1972	1.3
Getzen (1990) – USA, 1966–87	1.6
Schieber (1990) – 7 countries, 1960–87	1.2
Gerdtham and Löthgren (2000, 2002) – 25 OECD countries, 1960–97	Co-integrated
Dreger and Reimers (2005) – 21 OECD countries	Unitary elasticity not rejected

Source: Authors' own calculation.

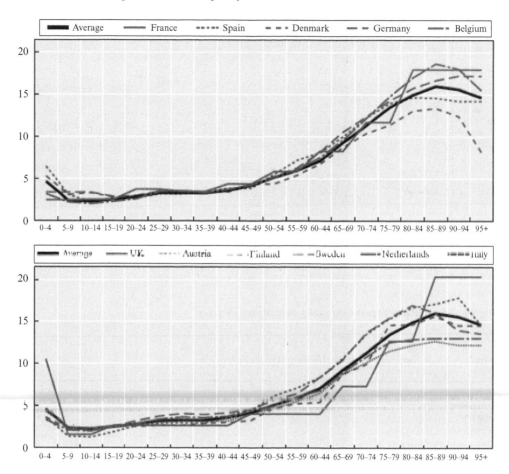

Source: Draws on S. Bjomerud and J.O. Martins, 2005 presentation at OECD Workshop, Brussels.

Figure 8.2   Average expenditure per capita as a percentage of GDP by age group

the individual level this is generally also true, although not for US dental care, where the elasticity is estimated to be above unity. Moreover, the studies of the relationship between health expenditure and GDP per capita generally find that over 85 per cent of the variation in health expenditure per capita can be explained by GDP per capita alone (see Figure 8.2). Not only was this correlation robust to time and across different groups of countries; it leaves little scope for the influence of other factors such as demographics, form of health care system and financing or increasing use of health care technology. In further studies these factors were found to be statistically insignificant, apart from in Leu (1986), where the share of public expenditure and degree of health system centralisation were found to be significant. Such factors could operate indirectly through increasing GDP levels, of course. Technological take-up might be easier with rising income, for example. Moreover, the relationships examined between health expenditures and GDP are generally statistical correlations rather than examination of causal mechanisms; if health expenditure and income co-vary over time, correlations between health expenditure and income are unlikely to reveal any causal relationship, particularly if no statistical account is taken of this co-variation.

These income elasticities are normally defined as the proportionate change in the quantity of health care consumed as income changes; health care is a 'luxury good' such that expenditure on it rises disproportionately as a country's income increases. The elasticities reproduced in Table 8.2 are the result of examining the proportionate change in the expenditure on health care as income changes, where expenditure is defined as price times quantity, and are therefore not precisely income elasticities. There is an obvious relationship between quantity consumed and expenditure, but this will be mediated through price levels. For the estimated empirical elasticity to be interpreted as an income elasticity, prices have to be held constant across countries.

Of course relative prices may be taken account of to some extent if the statistical relationship between health expenditures and GDP per capita is converted into a common currency using purchasing power parity (PPP) exchange rates. PPP exchange rates attempt to take account of price differences across countries, reflecting the fact that the cost of living varies across countries (a person can buy fewer cups of coffee for $1 in the USA than in India, for example, even if the dollar–rupee exchange does not fluctuate). However, PPP exchange rates still suffer from distortions caused by exchange rate fluctuations, so that the basket of goods, particularly health care, to which PPPs are attached may vary in composition markedly and, more importantly, PPP prices will normally be lower where incomes are lower. Thus PPP exchange rates will be correlated with GDP, and it is clear that PPP exchange rate conversion will not establish price effects.

It should also be noted that in most health care systems the price of health care is subsidised, with the price to the consumer at the time of consumption being close to or even zero. Technically, as the price of a commodity tends to zero, income elasticity will also tend to zero. That is, with a commodity price that is close to zero, income no longer acts as a constraint and should play less of a role in determining expenditure at the individual level. Of course the elasticities reported in Table 8.2 have been estimated at the aggregate country level, where again income would form less of a constraint, although countries would face the 'full price' of health care and therefore a much stronger relationship between expenditure and income might be expected at this level of aggregation (Parkin et al., 1987; Gerdtham and Jönsson, 2000).

To the extent that the price of health care is important, it should of course be controlled for in any examination of the relationship between income and health expenditure. Indeed, if it is not and a statistical regression relationship is specified between these two variables, then the coefficient determining the statistical response of one variable to the other, which determines the elasticity, will be biased. The bias entailed from omitting a price variable will be larger, the larger the relationship between price and expenditure, and will be positive if income and price are positively related, as would be the case in dealing with health expenditures. Health care is an inherently labour-intensive sector and if labour is more costly in high-income countries, as would be expected, then the price of health care and income will be highly correlated.

Moreover, the defined empirical elasticity is heavily dependent on the precise relationship deemed to hold. The estimated elasticity of health care is the ratio of the marginal propensity to spend on health care to the average propensity to spend on health care, where the marginal propensity is the rate of spending on health care as small changes are seen in income and the average propensity is health care expenditure divided by GDP at any given level of GDP. In general, a linear relationship is held to hold between health care expenditure per capita (HE) and GDP per capita of the following form: HE = α + β GDP + ε, where ε is the error term reflecting a statistical rather than mathematical relationship, α is the intercept term and β is the given specified relationship between health care expenditure and GDP, and is also slope of the linear line formed by the statistical relationship, as well as a representation of the marginal propensity to spend on health care. If the intercept term, α, is negative (as it normally is, as determined empirically in the studies referred to in Table 8.2), it follows by definition that the marginal propensity, reflecting a positive relationship between expenditure and GDP, will be greater than the average propensity. So the ratio of the marginal propensity to spend on health care to the average propensity to spend on health care, that is the income elasticity, must be greater than unity, due to the statistical relationship assumed.

Price components of expenditure growth can also be considered. This is important as health expenditure comprises prices and quantity, and increased quantities, estimated after taking account of price movements (inflation), reflect increased consumption. Table 8.3 outlines the health-specific inflation rates over and above economy-wide inflation in a number of OECD countries. Although there are general difficulties regarding definitions of the health care sector and methods in calculating inflation, the general trend is clear: health sector price inflation generally outpaced general price inflation, in some cases substantially. Moreover, it has been suggested that at least for France the health care price deflators may be erroneous (Schieber et al., 1994). As such, price increases partly explain the growing share of health expenditures in most countries,

Why are prices rising faster in the health sector? A number of dimensions could be at work here. First, price indices, which form the basis of this type of comparison, are measured with respect to a given basket of goods. If the composition of these goods changes or the quality of these goods changes over time, then like-for-like comparisons are not made through time. Second, such price indices are likely to be cost-based and as such, price indices must have limited application in the analysis of health care expenditure when the actual price of health care is heavily subsidised and near to zero in most countries. Costs may increase in any manner of ways in such an environment, even after accounting for quality changes. In particular, cost-increasing technological change may be a specific route, of which more later.

Leaving these issues aside, some have proposed a specific mechanism through which price inflation may be higher in the health care sector. Alternatively, relative price could be a reflection of productivity in the health care sector, differing from that in other sectors. Some economists, including Fuchs (1967) and Baumol (1968), have argued that productivity growth in the service sectors, such as the health care sector, is likely to be lower than in the manufacturing sectors of the economy. The basis of this argument is that technology changes that allow the substitution of capital for labour provide the main source of productivity growth and that the scope for such changes is limited in the service sector, and this sector is labour rather than capital intensive. Therefore productivity in the service sector will lag behind that in the manufacturing sector.

This lower-than-average-growth in labour productivity in the health care sector will

Table 8.3   Annual average health care price inflation relative to general inflation

	1970–80	1980–90	1990–2000
Australia	0.60	0.46	0.40
Austria	3.10	1.51	2.97
Belgium	0.28	0.59	2.30
Canada	0.16	1.06	0.23
Denmark	−0.16	−0.20	−0.16
Finland	−0.51	1.40	1.09
France	−1.14	−0.86	−0.16
Germany	0.60	0.52	n/a
Greece	n/a	n/a	n/a
Hungary	n/a	n/a	n/a
Iceland	2.32	0	1.42
Ireland	−3.82	2.50	1.48
Italy	n/a	n/a	0.17
Japan	n/a	0.14	0.88
Korea	−0.17	−0.99	−0.37
Luxembourg	0.42	1.20	4.39
Netherlands	3.71	0.35	0.30
Norway	n/a	n/a	n/a
Portugal	n/a	n/a	n/a
Spain	1.07	−0.54	−0.13
Sweden	n/a	n/a	n/a
Switzerland	2.33	0.36	0.95
UK	−0.54	1.07	1.36
USA	0.83	3.07	1.47

Note: n/a = data not available.

Source: Authors' own calculation.

mean higher-than-average costs as labour costs keep pace with those in the manu-facturing sector. If the demand for health care is relatively price inelastic, then as the economy expands the service sector's share of total employment will increase. Coupled with relatively high average costs, this means increasing expenditure on health care over time. That said, the differences in relative prices in the health care sector and the rest of the economy appear to be small, such that any growth in health care expenditure is not fully explained by relative price movements. The relative growth in expenditure has not been dominated by relative price movements. Consequently, the conclusion is that any increase in expenditure has been real rather than nominal, and the impact of lower productivity gain has not led, in line with the arguments forwarded by Fuchs (1967) and Baumol (1968), to excessive price increases in the sector.

Moreover, this small increase in health care prices over general prices could be fully explained by increases in the quality of health care over time. Some recent studies have highlighted the difficulties of controlling for quality in constructing price indices for health care (see Triplett, 1999). While this remains a difficult and contentious issue, cer-tainly the aggregate price differences found over time and reproduced within Table 8.3

would seem to be well within ranges that could be fully explained by quality improvements over time.

Finally, in discussing relative price differences and the Baumol effect, we should mention the work by Hartwig (2008), who explicitly tests the Baumol effect on health care expenditure using estimates of relative growth rates and productivity. He concludes that there is evidence of a Baumol effect, with the implication that productivity does lag in the health care sector, pushing up relative prices in this sector. He suggests that this supports Pauly's (1993) conclusion that it is higher labour costs, maintained through monopoly supply, that leads to increasing health expenditures over time. Pauly notes that expenditure is merely income when defined from another perspective. Health care expenditure is equal to income earned by those factors of production, mainly labour, that provide health care. If monopoly power is held by these suppliers of health care, then the prices paid for their services will not represent merely the cost of providing these services but also the rent or surplus gained from exploiting this monopoly power. Given the barriers to entry in most health care professions, and the subsequent monopoly gained over service provision, it can at least be speculated that labour in this sector earns above-normal income. Expenditure will encompass some element of monopoly return and expenditure growth will be driven partly by this mechanism. Pauly provides some empirical evidence to support this argument.

Thus there is some support for relative price increases fuelling health expenditure growth through mechanisms consistent with a Baumol effect and expression of monopoly power. It must nevertheless be concluded that the relative price effect is so small that this impact is secondary. Moreover, it is equally the case that such a relative price impact may be associated with increasing quality of provision.

4.   INCREASING VOLUME AND ITS CAUSES

If price relativities are small, then greater expenditure growth in health care relative to GDP must be explained by greater utilisation. Table 8.4 gives health care expenditure growth relative to GDP growth. As can be seen, for the majority of countries these relative growth rates are positive and in some cases relatively high. Examining the information from Tables 8.3 and 8.4 shows that the combined effect of prices and volumes has given rise to substantial growth in health care expenditures, and given that the total growth is generally much greater than relative price growth, the largest push historically appears to have been through increasing volume, for which we can read utilisation, rather than relative prices.

A number of factors have been forwarded as possible explanatory variables for this increasing utilisation. The most obvious is demographic pressure. Most wealthier countries are experiencing ageing populations. This is held to present at least two problems for health care expenditures: first, a declining tax revenue base, and second, increasing demands placed on the system. Bains and Oxley (2004) report the pattern of age-related public per capita expenditure for a number of countries. Not surprisingly, health care costs increase with age. However, it would be a mistake to state that as health expenditures increase with age and ageing, population will increase health expenditures. The reason is that health expenditures tend to be concentrated in the last year of life; while

Table 8.4   *Annual average relative growth in health care expenditure relative to GDP growth*

	1970–80	1980–90	1990–2000
Australia	n/a	n/a	n/a
Austria	0.59	1.09	1.50
Belgium	3.87	−0.72	0.88
Canada	4.99	1.49	1.73
Denmark	0.22	2.40	−0.08
Finland	−0.16	−0.71	−0.18
France	1.35	2.14	−1.61
Germany	2.91	1.90	0.87
Greece	3.57	−0.20	2.23
Hungary	0.89	1.16	2.78
Iceland	n/a	n/a	n/a
Ireland	3.01	2.58	1.42
Italy	5.21	−3.20	0.14
Japan	n/a	n/a	n/a
Korea	3.78	−0.94	2.48
Luxembourg	5.36	0.30	−1.07
Netherlands	1.06	0.64	0.19
Norway	4.92	1.09	−0.09
Portugal	8.03	1.10	4.13
Spain	4.34	2.17	1.14
Sweden	2.82	−0.79	0.06
Switzerland	3.10	1.24	2.35
UK	2.30	0.68	1.95
USA	2.32	3.27	1.01

Note: n/a = data not available.

Source: Authors' own calculation.

health care costs increase with age, the largest impact on costs is in the last year, some would argue the last months, of life. A number of studies have confirmed that it is the proximity to death, rather than age itself, that dictates ageing expenditures (Zweifel et al., 1999). Seshimani and Gray (2004) in an econometric model find a small but significant age effect over and above the proximity to death effect, but Zweifel et al. (2004) dispute this for a range of ages, in particular with respect to the elderly. The argument is that proximity to death matters, but for the surviving elderly health expenditures do still increase with age. Generally speaking, however, given that the proximity-of-death argument merely shifts expenditure rather than increases it, the overall demographic impact is held to be low. Newhouse (1992) holds it to be around 1 per cent per annum, which is consistent with the UK government's estimate of this effect.

Weisbrod (1991) and Newhouse (1992) state that increasing insurance coverage and the changing form of insurance coverage may account for some increase in the utilisation of health care. Weisbrod noted that the postwar era had seen significant rises in the level of health care expenditures across a number of countries with different health care systems. Focusing his attention on the USA, he concluded that while moral hazard might be a plausible influence on rising expenditure levels, a common factor across health care sectors might explain witnessed health care expenditure growth across a number of countries. His common factor was health care technology, but he hypothesised a two-way causal relationship between health care technology and health care insurance, particularly within the USA. Weisbrod documented the changing characteristic of health care insurance from reimbursement based on 'costs incurred' to one that was somewhat independent of the actual costs incurred, exemplified by health maintenance organisation (HMO) or diagnosis-related group (DRG) type systems where reimbursement was based on average treatment costs for specific case types, which allowed a certain openness in the funding system and provided incentives for health care providers to pursue cost-increasing health care technologies. At the same time this cost-increasing technology faced consumers with an incentive to broaden their insurance coverage as the pursuit of technology results in the average cost of treatment increasing for individual treatment, or the variance of the cost of certain treatments increasing or both. With both the average cost and variance increasing as new technology is taken up, the individual consumer has a strong incentive to demand higher insurance coverage against unpredictable higher-cost items.

The coupling of the changing characteristics of the insurance and the increasing demand for insurance provided a conceptual mechanism to support the argument that technology was a major driver of health care expenditure growth. This will be considered explicitly below, but can we say anything about a pure insurance influence on health care expenditure? Newhouse, drawing on elasticities of the demand for insurance in the range −0.1 to −0.2, and observing reductions in co-insurance rates over a 50-year period, finds that a pure insurance effect does exist but is relatively small, explaining at most one eighth of the increase in health expenditures in the USA over a 50-year period.

In summary, Newhouse contends that any combination of the factors discussed above, and including the impact of supplier-induced demand, could only account for approximately 50 per cent of the growth in health care expenditures in the USA over the previous five decades at most. Newhouse concludes that the growth in health care expenditure must therefore be driven by another factor, which he proposes is health care technology. The arguments are so generic and the empirical evidence used so transferable that this general conclusion can be held to extend to other OECD countries. Indeed, similar calculations have been undertaken by the Australian Productivity Commission (2005) to arrive at essentially the same conclusion.

That study examines the growth in Australian health care expenditure by once again decomposing expenditure growth into a number of components and then determining the residual growth in expenditures that is, as with the Newhouse study, attributed to health care technology. Specifically the study considers:

$$\Delta E = \sum_{i=1}^{n} \varepsilon_i g_i + R$$

where ΔE is the average annual growth rate of health care expenditure in Australia, ε_i is the elasticity of the ith growth factor, g_i is the average annual growth rate of the ith growth factor and R is the residual average annual growth rate that is attributed to technology. The growth factors included are demographic change, where again the actual ageing of the population is held to have minimal impact; the movement in the relative price of health care, where it is acknowledged that because of the normal difficulties faced in indexing quality improvements derived from improved technology there may be some influence of technological change on health care expenditure coming through the relative price movements; income, again a minimal influence; and the proportion of individuals with private insurance, where moral hazard arguments are held to apply but again with minimal force. Under a range of assumptions the study finds that the residual growth attributable to expenditure growth varies between approximately 17 per cent and just over 55 per cent, with some justification for accepting a range of between 35 per cent and 55 per cent.

Smith et al. (2009) generally support this impact of technological change on health expenditure growth, but state that income growth *per se* has an important influence, and that the role of insurance in allowing such technological growth to take place should be acknowledged. That said, the authors still find that technological growth fuels at least 30 per cent of health care expenditure growth. Two statistical studies, while not quantifying the impact of technology on health care expenditure growth, confirm the existence of a causal relationship between these variables. Okunade and Murthy (2002), using R&D expenditures to proxy technology, and Di Matteo (2005), using time trends as a proxy for technological uptake, confirm this relationship.

Technological change is therefore seen to be a prime mechanism in explaining health care expenditure growth in all these studies, but the mechanics through which it operates are not well understood, judging by the reliance in these studies on the definition of effect through the residual. Cutler and Huckman (2003) in a seminal work consider the empirical impact of the substitution effect across two types of surgery, coronary artery bypass graft (CABG) and percutaneous transluminal coronary angioplasty (PTCA), where the latter leads to a fall in input price for treatment of the same individuals. They argue that while substitution is extensive, there is also a patient expansion effect, which dominates the substitution effect and accounts for around 65 per cent to 75 per cent of the incremental impact of PTCA, which may be thought of as a combination of both the output and profit/surplus-maximising effect noted above. That is, the patient expansion effect may be thought of as more output being achieved with the same budget, but additionally and importantly it leads to budget expansion, as the surplus-maximising level of output is able to increase as the marginal cost of production falls and an increase in output and expenditure becomes achievable. Follow-up work by McGuire and Raikou (2010), which adopts a similar methodology to assess technological change associated with the replacement of CABG by PTCA in UK hospitals, found supporting evidence that the quantifiable level of substitution was around 30 per cent. Again the inference is that the vast majority of PTCA is used to expand the surgical patient population, thereby expanding health care expenditure. If a similar mechanism operates for other health care interventions, then unit-cost-reducing new technology may still be associated with increasing total costs to the extent that the 'demand' curve for health care is moved to the right with improved technology.

For new effective technologies that are associated with increases in unit costs, for example new pharmaceutical products or new expensive surgical interventions, given an ability to bundle such interventions into treatments, there may still be incentives to introduce these new technologies assuming that the overall price of the treatment bundle drops. Here once again the patient population expansion mechanism may still give rise to increased total expenditure.

5.   CONTROLLING EXPENDITURE

Health care expenditures cannot grow at rates 2 per cent or 3 per cent higher than GDP indefinitely. Accordingly, cost containment policies are increasingly being put in place to limit such growths in expenditure across different countries. As Donaldson and Gerard (1993) point out, expenditure is Σ $(p \times q)$, where p is price and q is quantity at the individual treatment level. Expenditure can be controlled through regulating prices, quantities or both. The different forms of cost containment, particularly as aimed at controlling the diffusion of technology, have different incentive properties and more or less efficient proportion in containing costs.

Efficient incentives are obviously not embedded in retrospective reimbursement where health care providers receive payment in full for past expenditures. To the extent that prospective payment means that providers are constrained to operate within a predefined budget, financial risk is passed from the funding body to the provider with a consequent increase in incentive to contain costs. The form of incentives will of course reflect the specific form of the prospective payment mechanism.

Generally, the literature finds little evidence that regulating price alone through fee-for-item of service schedules has much impact on containing health care costs. Ellis and McGuire (1986) and Chalkley and Malcolmson (1998) show theoretically why cost containment may be sacrificed if this restricts treatment quality and patient benefits, if physicians give positive weight to such concerns even if they do take account of financial surplus.

The most extensive use of price control is through DRG-type pricing, which is now commonly used across most OECD countries for some part of the hospital sector. DRG pricing utilises a basic form of game theory to motivate efficiency gains. Under certain conditions, including ownership of similar technologies, hospitals faced with fixed DRG prices for similar output bundles will reduce costs. Under an idealised scheme the funding body pays each individual provider the average cost returned by all other providers; individual providers who are 'inefficient' receive reimbursement below their average cost and therefore have an incentive to stop production or lower costs. Over time, if there is no gaming or cartelisation, hospital costs are driven down to the true average cost. One issue with DRG pricing is that costs are pushed down to the average, making the scheme statically efficient but potentially dynamically inefficient as it may be difficult to introduce new technologies, especially where DRG pricing is used within a global budget-setting arrangement. While DRG creep, the reclassifying of low-cost output into high-cost output, is possible, there has been remarkably little evidence of its existence (Carter et al., 1990). There is more evidence of cream skimming, where high-cost patients are turned away, but only in the US environment (Newhouse, 1987; Ellis and McGuire, 1986; Meltzer and Chung, 2002).

As DRG pricing tends to reimburse existing technology, it may be that the increasing use of health technology assessment (HTA) structures is to a degree complementary to this dampening impact on health care technology of DRG pricing. To the extent that HTA regulation uses cost-effectiveness to assess new technologies, this provides a channel through which new technologies are introduced into a health care system formally and may be incorporated into existing reimbursement schemes such as DRG pricing. Possibly the most extensive use of cost-effectiveness within an HTA setting has been in the UK through the operation of NICE, where the rationing of new technology has largely been through restricting volume of use in a manner that is entirely complementary to DRG pricing.

One specific question of interest is the impact of incentives and regulation on the diffusion of technology if it is believed that this has a major impact on driving expenditure growth. Beck et al. (2010), drawing on work by the TECH group, considered the impact of different incentive structures on the take-up and diffusion of three technologies in the treatment of coronary heart disease: catheterisation; CABG; and PTCA. They show that differences in the utilisation rates of three technologies for treating acute myocardial infarction (AMI) can be explained by country income and a number of institutional factors. Health care systems characterised as public contract or reimbursement systems have generally higher utilisation compared to public integrated systems. Funding of investments through a general remuneration scheme rather than through investment funds granted by third-party payers is associated with higher utilisation rates. The main effects of these influences seem, however, to diminish through time. Thus a positive main effect will typically have a negative interaction with the time trend, which means that income and institutional influences explain less and less of the variation as technologies mature. These empirical findings suggest that while different regulatory structures can affect technology diffusion, their influence is weakened over time. One implication is that technology diffusion adapts to the regulatory structure and that, if control of technology diffusion is used as an indirect control of expenditure level, optimal regulation ought to encompass some dynamic element, possibly through the type of 'risk-sharing' agreements used to regulate drug prices in a number of countries, where price setting is examined at different points in time. Such regulatory lag would enhance the incentive to reduce costs through innovation, although this may be offset by delaying benefits to consumers, of course. Moreover, the results also suggest that the impact of system regulation is different for different technologies.

6. CONCLUSIONS

If technology is the main driver of rising health care expenditures and the different incentives and regulations of different systems affect uptake and diffusion differently but with a time diminishing effect as shown by Beck et al. (2010), and higher-income countries are placing greater restrictions on costs, then it is likely that countries will find their health care expenditures converging. Indeed there is some evidence this is the case through the work of Barros (1998).

We have only considered expenditure and not the benefits of health care. Cost containment is only required if it is decided that the expenditure exceeds the benefits. It is probable that most countries are experiencing flat-of-the-curve health care in some parts of their system. It is not always clear what the return is to new health care technology. What is clear is that R&D expenditure, which underpins new technology, continues to increase across the OECD. R&D expenditure grew at just under 10 per cent per annum, albeit from a low base, across the OECD between 1995 and 2008, illustrating that new techno-logically motivated health care expenditure will not be a diminishing phenomenon.

What remains to be answered is what is the optimal level of health care expenditure for a country. Increasingly health care is financed through the public purse across most countries. Such expenditure averages 10 per cent of GDP in the OECD countries, appreciably higher than this average in a number of individual countries – most notably the USA where health care technology appears to be taken up and diffused quickly. In answer to the question, it must be recognised that, in part at least, the optimal level of funding is a normative question dictated by the aggregate tastes and preferences of society. While accepting this, it is also true that an appropriate understanding of what drives these tastes and preferences is critical to controlling growth rates of health care expenditure. Income levels, insurance coverage and the availability of health care tech-nology are important dimensions of this driving force. It is critical to gain greater under-standing of the way in which these forces push health care expenditure ever upwards. Ultimately, however, the level of expenditure will be determined by the preferences for health care displayed by individual countries.

REFERENCES

AHCPR (1997), *Trends in Personal Health Care Expenditures, Health Insurance and Payment Sources: Community-Based Population, 1987–1995*, National Medical Expenditure Survey, Public Health Service, Rockville, MD: Agency for Health Care Policy and Research.
Andersen, R. and Benham, L. (1970), 'Factors affecting the relationship between family income and medical care consumption', in H. Klarman (ed.), *Empirical Studies in Health Economics*, Baltimore, MD: Johns Hopkins.
Australian Productivity Commission (2005), *Impact of Advances in Medical Technology in Australia – Research Report, 09/2005*, Canberra: Australia.
Bains, M. and Oxley, H. (2004), 'Age-related spending projections on health and long-term care', in *Towards High Performing Health Care Systems Policy Studies*, OECD Health Policy Studies, OECD: Paris, pp. 319–31.
Barros, P. (1998), 'The black box of health care expenditure growth determinants', *Health Economics*, **7**, 533–44.
Baumol, W. (1968), 'Microeconomics of unbalanced growth', *American Economic Review*, **53**, 941–73.
Beck, M., Christensen, T., Dunham, K. et al. (2010), 'The influence of economic incentives and regulatory factors on the adoption of treatment technologies: a case study of technologies used to treat heart attacks', *Health Economics*, **18**, 1114–32.
Carter, G., Newhouse, J. and Relles, A. (1990), *How Much Change in the Case-Mix Index is DRG Creep?*, RAND Technical Report, Santa Monica: RAND Corporation.
Chalkey, M. and Malcolmson, J. (1998), 'Contracting for health services with unmonitored quality', *Economic Journal*, **108**, 1093–10.
Cutler, D.M. and Huckman, R.S. (2003), 'Technological development and medical productivity: the diffusion of angioplasty in New York State', *Journal of Health Economics*, **22**, 187–217.
Di Matteo, L. (2005), 'The macro determinants of health expenditure in the United States and Canada: assess-ing the impact of income, age distribution and time', *Health Policy*, **71**(1), 23–42.
Di Matteo, L. and Di Matteo, R. (1998), 'Evidence on the determinants of Canadian provincial government health expenditures: 1965–1991', *Journal of Health Economics*, **17**, 211–28.
Donaldson, C. and Gerard, G. (1993), *Economics of Health Care Financing: The Visible Hand*, Basingstoke: Macmillan.
Dreger, C. and Reimers, H.E. (2005), 'Health care expenditures in OECD countries: a panel unit root and cointegration analysis', *International Journal of Applied Econometrics and Quantitative Studies*, **2**(2), 5–20.
Ellis, R. and McGuire, T. (1986), 'Provider behavior under prospective reimbursement: cost sharing and supply', *Journal of Health Economics*, **5**, 129–51.
Falk, I.S. et al. (1933), *The Incidence of Illness and the Receipt and Costs of Medical Care Among Representative*

Families, Committee on the Costs of Medical Care, Publication number 26, Chicago: University of Chicago Press.

Freeman, M. (2003), 'Is health care a necessity or a luxury? Pooled estimates of income elasticity from US state-level data', *Applied Economics*, **35**, 495–502.

Fuchs, V. (1967), *The Service Economy*, New York: Columbia University Press.

Fuchs, V. and Kramer, M. (1972), 'Determinants of expenditures for physican services in the US, 1948–1968', NCHSRD, NBER Working Paper number 117.

Gerdtham, U. and Jönsson, B. (2000), 'International comparisions of health expenditure', in A.J. Culyer and J. Newhouse (eds), *The Handbook of Health Economics*, Vol. 1A, Amsterdam: North Holland, pp. 11–53.

Gerdtham, U. and Löthgren, M. (2000), 'On stationarity and cointegration of international health care expenditures and GDP', *Journal of Health Economics*, **19**, 461–75.

Gerdtham, U. and Löthgren, M. (2002), 'New panel estimates on cointegration of international health expenditure and GDP', *Applied Economics*, **34**, 1697–86.

Getzen, T. (1990), 'Macro forceasting of national health expenditures', *Advances in Health Economics*, **11**, 27–48.

Hahn, B. and Lefkowitz, J. (1992), *Annual Expenses and Sources of Payment for Health Care Services*, National Medical Expenditure Survey Research Findings, 14, AHCPR publication 93-0007, Public Health Service, Rockville, MD: Agency for Health Care Policy and Research.

Hartwig, J. (2008), 'What drives health care expenditures: Baumol's model of unbalanced growth revisited', *Journal of Health Economics*, **27**, 603–23.

Leu, R. (1986), 'The public–private mix and international health care costs', in A. Maynard and A. Ludbrook (eds), *Public and Private Health Services: Complementarities and Conflicts*, Oxford: Oxford University Press.

McGuire, A. and Raikou, M. (2010), 'Inferring the value of medical research to the UK', LSE Health Working Paper, Number 5, London: LSE Health, The London School of Economics and Political Science.

Meltzer, D. and Chung, J. (2002), 'Effects of competition under prospective payment on hospital costs among high- and low-cost admissions: evidence from California, 1983 and 1993', *NBER Frontiers in Health Policy Research*, **5**, 53–102.

Newhouse, J.P. (1977), 'Medical care expenses: a cross national survey', *Journal of Human Resources*, **12**, 115–25.

Newhouse, J.P. (1987), 'Cross national differences in health spending: what do they mean?', *Journal of Health Economics*, **6**, 159–62.

Newhouse, J.P. (1992), 'Medical care costs: how much welfare loss?', *The Journal of Economic Perspectives*, **6**, 3–21.

Newhouse, J.P. and Phelps, C. (1976), 'New estimates of price and income elasticities of medical care services', in R. Rossett (ed.), *The Role of Health Insurance in the Health Services Sector*, New York: NBER, pp. 261–312.

OECD (2010), *OECD Health Data*, Paris: OECD.

Okunade, A.A. and Murthy, V.N. (2002), 'Technology as a major driver of health care costs: a cointegration test of the Newhouse conjecture', *Journal of Health Economics*, **21**, 147–59.

Parkin, D., McGuire, A. and Yule, B. (1987), 'Aggregate health care expenditures and national income: is health care a luxury good?', *Journal of Health Economics*, **6**, 109–27.

Pauly, M. (1993), 'US health care costs: the untold true story', *Health Affairs*, **12**, 152–9.

Schieber, G. (1990), 'Health expenditures in major industrialised countries, 1960–1987', *Health Care Financing Review*, **11**, 159–67.

Schieber, G.J., Poullier, J.P. and Greenwald, L.M. (1994), 'Health system performance in OECD Countries, 1980–1992', *Health Affairs*, **13**(4), 100–112.

Seshimani, M. and Gray, A. (2004), 'A longitudinal study of the effects of age and time to death on hospital costs', *Journal of Health Economics*, **23**, 217–35.

Smith, S., Newhouse, J. and Freeland, M. (2009), 'Income, insurance, and technology: why does health spending outpace economic growth?', *Health Affairs*, **28**, 1276–84.

TECH (2001), 'Technological change around the world: evidence from heart attack care', *Health Affairs*, **20**, 25–42.

Triplett, J.E. (1999), *Measuring the Prices of Medical Treatments*, Washington, DC: Brookings Institution.

Weisbrod, B. (1991), 'The health care quadrilemma: an essay on technological change, insurance, quality of care and cost containment', *Journal of Economic Literature*, **29**, 523–52.

Zweifel, P., Felder, S. and Meiers, M. (1999), 'Ageing of the population and health care expenditure: a red herring?', *Health Economics*, **8**, 485–96.

Zweifel, P., Felder, S. and Werblow, A. (2004), 'Population ageing and health care expenditure: new evidence on the red herring', *Geneva Papers on Risk and Insurance: Issues and Practice*, **29**, 653–67.

9 Providing financial incentives for improved quality and efficiency: a literature review of the effects of payment for performance (P4P) policies
Irene Papanicolas

1. INTRODUCTION

Recent years have seen a growing interest in payment systems that specifically reward provider performance, also know as payment for performance (P4P) systems. These types of systems offer pay, usually in the form of bonuses, to doctors who meet special performance rates or reach target levels of cost or quality. The main driver behind such systems is to offer different rewards to physicians who provide excellent care and those who provide inadequate care. Moreover, economic theory predicts that by offering financial incentives linked to performance, physicians will become more motivated to provide high-quality care (Rosenthal and Frank, 2006; Young and Conrad, 2007). There is concern that under such systems there will be increased incentives for patient selection or gaming, causing providers to drop risky patients and opt for low-risk patients to maximise their payments (Banker et al., 1996; Doran et al., 2006; Smith and York, 2004). It is also possible that the performance of untargeted areas that are not measured may experience quite limited or even distorted quality effects (Holmstrom and Milgrom, 1991; Smith and York, 2004). Moreover, much of the literature on P4P mechanisms expresses the importance of implementation and system design, which could result in ineffective (Bokhour et al., 2006; Meterko et al., 2006; Young et al., 2007a) or harmful effects on quality of care (Berwick, 1995) if not performed correctly.

In the last few years, P4P systems have become increasingly common in health care. Health maintenance organisations (HMOs) in the USA now commonly use P4P systems (Rosenthal et al., 2006; Christianson et al., 2007a), and are increasingly attracting attention from other developed countries (Scott, 2007). The UK has been using P4P programmes since the 1990s for the remuneration of general practitioners (GPs), initially for child vaccinations, immunisations and cervical cytology (Health Departments of Great Britain, 1989), and expanded the use of P4P in the 2004 GP contract to cover 146 performance indicators for ten chronic diseases, patient experience and organisation of care (DoH, 2004). Data collected from the Commonwealth Fund international health survey indicate the presence of such systems in other developed countries such as Canada, New Zealand, Australia, Germany and the Netherlands (www.commonwealthfund.org).

The empirical evidence on the effectiveness of P4P programmes is still not conclusive, with findings from the literature reporting mixed results. Systematic reviews by Christianson et al. (2007b), Petersen et al. (2006) and Rosenthal and Frank (2006), as well as a literature synthesis by Conrad and Christianson (2004) noted the presence of few robust empirical studies to evaluate. From the studies that met their criteria, they found only weak empirical evidence to support the effectiveness of P4P systems in improving quality of care (Fairbrother et al., 1999; Fairbrother et al., 2001; Grady et al., 1997; Kouides et al., 1998; Rosenthal et al., 2005; Roski et al., 2003).

Part of the difficulty in assessing the effectiveness of P4P systems is that their design often varies along many parameters, and so different programmes are difficult to compare. This chapter will investigate four key design parameters, and how these can influence the effectiveness of P4P systems. These parameters are:

a) who payments are made to (e.g. individual physicians, groups of physicians, organisational systems);
b) the type of services the financial incentive is directed at (e.g. chronic care, acute care, preventive care, patient satisfaction, IT implementation, practice efficiency;
c) the magnitude and type of payment: the type of payment given (e.g. whether this reaches an absolute threshold of performance, improvement over a baseline of performance or each occurrence of a service);
d) data measurement systems: the type of performance indicators payments are attached to, and the clinical relevance and validity of data.

2.   UNIT OF ASSESSMENT

Theory

The literature on P4P programmes typically examines payments made to providers, where providers can be individual physicians, groups of physicians, or an institutional entity such as a hospital. Fundamental to the correct functioning of a P4P programme is holding the right entity accountable for the action being rewarded. In order for the optimal behaviour to be incentivised, it must be correctly targeted (Town et al., 2004). In practice, targeting any one of these groups may result in creating different incentive structures. The difficulty in designing a P4P programme with respect to this parameter is to make sure the incentive attached to meeting a performance target is made to the entity that has control of the necessary means to achieve that target (Young et al., 2005). Often achieving a quality target will be the result of teamwork as well as patient adherence and proper measurement systems; in deciding whom to direct the incentive at it is fundamental to take such factors into account.

Young et al. (2007b) identified physicians' concerns about their ability to control all the parts of the health system necessary to achieve the quality targets for which they were being incentivised, including the cooperation of other providers and personnel. If a payment is directed at an organisation with the aim of improving its procedures, it is expected that the payment will incentivise the hospital administration to take the appropriate steps to reach this desired outcome. However, it is not clear that the payment made will reach the physicians, nurses or other staff who deliver care to the patients; this is left to the administration of the hospital. Even if the payment does reach these parties, it may come bundled together with other payments so that it is not apparent that they are being rewarded for a specific target. On the other hand, if the payment is made directly to physicians, the effect of the reward may in part depend on whether the physician practises as part of a group or as an individual. If the reward is allocated to a group practice,

Table 9.1   Mechanisms for distribution of incentive dollars and impact on quality of care

Mechanism	Potential mode of impact on quality of care
Equal distribution to all providers	May enhance group work
	May remove power of incentive from individual physicians
Dependent on individual provider performance on payer's quality targets	Most powerful incentive to directly affected provider behaviour
Dependent on individual provider performance on practice-based incentive schemes	Reduces power of the incentive direct from payer. May affect performance in other ways
Money retained wholly by organisation	Least powerful incentives to physicians. May effect change in quality of care by implementing system-level changes
Hybrid approach (money directed towards individual physicians and also towards the organisation)	May effect change at provider level and at systems level to improve quality of care

Source: Bokhour et al. (2006).

the way the group decides to distribute the reward among themselves may influence the impact it has (Table 9.1).

Patients are also often responsible for the success of a treatment, given their adherence to treatment or lifestyle choices. Bokhour et al. (2006) found that some physicians felt the P4P programmes unfairly penalised them due to their lack of control over both process and outcome indicators, which depend largely on their patients' adherence to treatment or lifestyle choices. A literature synthesis by Christianson et al. (2007a) notes that in economically deprived areas, financial and other patient-related barriers limited the ability of physicians to increase the use of targeted services for their patients. In practice, P4P programmes should attempt to separate these effects from the payment either by attaching financial rewards to clinical process measures rather than outcomes, or even by including exemptions to take into account different patient populations. Yet such exemptions should be designed very carefully to ensure that they do not create adverse incentives such as patient selection or gaming.

Evidence

In practice, most P4P programmes are targeted at the group level. A 2004 survey carried out by MedVantage Inc. showed that in the USA, 14 per cent of physician P4P programmes targeted individual physicians alone, 61 per cent targeted groups alone and 25 per cent targeted both individual physicians and groups (Scott, 2007). While most reviews identify a lack of P4P targeted at hospitals, most of those that do target hospitals have been set up in the past five years and consist of non-competitive bonus programmes, often sponsored by health plans (Baker and Delbanco, 2007; Christianson et al., 2007b; Grossbart, 2006). In the UK the P4P payments attached to the new GP contract are made directly to the practice and not to individual physicians (Smith and York, 2004).

Qualitative work undertaken in the US setting by Bokhour et al. (2006) identified five broad mechanisms by which incentive money paid to groups was then distributed among physicians – and the potential effect on incentivising quality of care each of these mechanisms has (Table 9.1).

A systematic review by Petersen et al. (2006) investigated P4P programmes by level of incentive (individual, group or payment system). They reviewed 17 studies with incentives awarded at different levels (6 physician level, 9 group level, and 2 payment level). The results of the 17 studies largely confirmed the impacts predicted by the different payment mechanisms as laid out by Bokhour et al. (2006). A separate review by Armour et al. (2001) found incentives directed at the individual physician level to be the most effective. The survey by Bokhour et al. (2006) suggests that the effectiveness of the financial incentive will depend on the type of activity being incentivised (provider behaviour, group work, system-level changes), and small effects can be attributed to weakened incentives at the individual level (Petersen et al., 2006). Hillman et al. (1998, 1999) supports this with findings of ineffectual incentives at the group level due to its distribution among the two group members in such a way that over 40 per cent of the participants were unaware of the incentives.

While typically most individual and group-level incentives are attached to clinical process and outcome measures, system-level incentives are focused on the management and administration of organisations. Indeed, studies show that system-level incentives are effective in making structural changes within an organisation with respect to admissions and referral policies, which in turn also influence the quality of care provided (Berthiaume et al., 2006; Cameron et al., 1999; Norton, 1992). Investigations of the effectiveness of the Center for Medicare and Medicaid Services Premier Hospital Quality Incentive Demonstration indicate that P4P programmes can be successful in encouraging system-level changes by helping to identify areas of underperformance (Glickman et al., 2007; Grossbart, 2006; Lindenauer et al., 2007).

3.   TYPE OF SERVICE TARGETED

Theory

The pioneering P4P programmes were mostly targeted at preventive care, such as the administration of vaccinations. Later, financial incentives were attached to reward areas in primary care that were known to affect patient outcomes in the longer term (Christianson et al., 2007b; Sikka, 2007; Young and Conrad, 2007). This was in part the result of the increased availability of performance indicators in these areas (Christianson et al., 2007a), but also due to documented gaps in treatment, which, if covered, could yield considerable benefits. In recent years the number of P4P programmes in hospitals and directed towards specialists has grown, and continues to do so (Baker and Delbanco, 2007; Rosenthal et al., 2007; Sikka, 2007). There is some evidence on the effectiveness of P4P programmes targeting preventive and primary care, but little to none on those in the acute care or emergency care setting (Christianson et al., 2007b; Sikka, 2007). While most work reviews the clinical indicators in P4P programmes, other areas have been targeted such as patient satisfaction, IT implementation and some measures of efficiency

(Rosenthal and Adams Dudley, 2007). Often areas targeted are not only those with a policy priority, but areas where data are easily accessible and of high quality.

Evidence

Providing physicians with financial bonuses in order to incentivise the provision of preventive health care procedures (such as immunisations) is not a recent policy measure. The UK has paid their GPs for cervical cytology as well as certain immunisations since 1966. As a result, there has been more work done investigating the effectiveness of financial incentives in the delivery of preventive care than in other areas (Christianson et al., 2007b; Rosenthal and Frank, 2006). Achat et al. (1999) investigate the effectiveness of financial incentives in immunisations specifically. However, it was difficult to determine whether the financial incentives themselves were responsible for positive results, or a combination of other factors introduced at the same time. Town et al. (2005) conducted a systematic review of the financial incentives in the area (limited to immunisations and screenings), limiting their search only to randomised trials. They found that of the eight incentives reviewed, only one resulted in a significant change of services provided, although they note that this is likely to be a result of the small incentives provided, which may not be large enough to cause a change in behaviour.

Financial incentives have also been used to promote smoking cessation programmes. Roski et al. (2003) and Amundson et al. (2003) both investigated the effects of a financial incentive tied to smoking cessation and found mixed results. Roski and colleagues (2003) found the financial incentive to have had no significant effect on smoking cessation rates, despite increased adherence to guidelines; however, they suspect that this may have been because the incentive was too small to bring about change. Amundson et al. (2003) did find a significant change; however, due to the construction of the study where there was no control group, it is difficult to attribute this change entirely to the financial incentive as performance feedback for the medical groups was also adopted at the same time.

Another area that has been targeted is the management of chronic conditions such as diabetes or asthma (Levin-Scherz et al., 2006) in the primary care setting, where rewards were based mostly on clinical process measures. While more research has been done on diabetes than the other areas (Beaulieu and Horrigan, 2005; Ettner et al., 2006; Larsen et al., 2003; Levin-Scherz et al., 2006; Srirangalingam et al., 2006), the results as to the effectiveness of financial incentives are mixed. In most cases where there was an indication of positive change in treatment, this change could not be solely attributed to the financial incentive as other policies were implemented alongside (Beaulieu and Horrigan, 2005; Ettner et al., 2006; Levin-Scherz et al., 2006). Similar results were found for programmes addressed to asthma (Levin-Scherz et al., 2006) and epilepsy (Shohet et al., 2007). Recent findings from the English experience have further suggested that improvement in conditions targeted has been limited to the direct processes incentivised with little change in other behaviours, including those for the same condition which were not attached to the incentive (Doran et al., 2011; Steel et al., 2007).

In the past five years P4P programmes have been increasingly directed at emergency care, such as the Center for Medicare and Medicaid Premier Hospital Quality Incentive Demonstration. The evidence on the effectiveness of these incentives is still sparse, however (Sikka, 2007), with even fewer studies designed in a way that allows isolation of the financial incentive effect (Christianson et al., 2007a). Christianson et al. (2007b) identify five studies investigating the effectiveness of hospital incentives, with three specifically addressing the CMS programme. Four of the five studies identify a significant positive effect of the payments (Berthiaume et al., 2006; Cameron et al., 1999; Glickman et al., 2007; Grossbart, 2006; Lindenauer et al., 2007).

4. MAGNITUDE AND TYPE OF PAYMENT

Theory

The higher the amount of the physician's salary being supplemented through financial incentive schemes, the more likely physicians are to take account of the incentive and change their behaviour accordingly. While the size of the incentive alone is not enough to determine whether the provider will attempt to reach the quality target, it is generally agreed that as long as the reward exceeds the administrator's opportunity and administration costs, some effort to achieve the targets will be made (Beaulieu and Horrigan, 2005; Rosenthal and Adams Dudley, 2007; Young and Conrad, 2007). There are also concerns regarding the level of the payment and how this will influence the intrinsic motivation of providers. Social psychologist Edward Deci published results of a series of experiments indicating that the introduction of monetary awards to incentivise a task reduces the intrinsic motivation associated with it (Deci, 1971). While not much empirical work on intrinsic motivation has been conducted with regard to the medical profession, the question of whether extrinsic rewards undermine professional norms of autonomy is an ongoing debate in the health care sector (Conrad, 2009; Rothstein, 2008).

While the magnitude of the payment is important, the terms under which the reward is allocated will also influence the effectiveness of the incentive. Some programmes offer financial rewards based on the achievement of certain benchmarks, while others reward improved performance in general. Each of these designs has its benefits and drawbacks (Christianson et al., 2007b). If rewards are made for achieving a certain benchmark, deciding where to set the benchmark becomes problematic; if benchmarks are set too high, then low-performing physicians might not bother trying to meet them as they will require too much effort. However, if the benchmark is set too low, then high-performing physicians will not be incentivised to improve. Paying physicians for improvements in care does not reward already high-performing physicians and may distort incentives.

Similarly, deciding whether to award physicians based on a fixed or relative performance will influence behaviour. A fixed incentive will reward all physicians who meet the quality target (benchmark or improvement), while a relative payment will only reward the performers. A fixed payment provides physicians with the certainty of knowing they will reap the gains of their increased efforts to meet the quality targets set. However, it may be difficult for a payer to budget for this sort of P4P programme, or could end up being very costly if the targets are relatively simple to achieve. This was the case for the UK GP contract, where over 90 per cent of GPs were rewarded, costing the government much more than initially anticipated (Doran et al., 2006). A relative performance payment system can be set up so that only a top percentage of performers are paid, thus encouraging competition between physicians. However, there is the danger that the uncertainty of the reward may discourage physicians from putting in the effort to achieve the targets, especially if the reward is targeted at a group level or largely depends on patient-level factors.

Rosenthal and Adams Dudley (2007) suggest it may be more effective to vary the payment approach according to the stream of costs that the programme creates rather than offering a one-off bonus payment, such as achieving an 80 per cent screening rate. This will allow increased differentiation in the time and magnitude of payments to better reflect costs. For example, paying providers for each immunisation rate is logical as the equipment necessary is relatively inexpensive yet each injection is time consuming for the physician. In contrast, something such as updating records on an IT system has large initial costs (buying, installing and learning to use the necessary software) but then has much smaller subsequent costs (such as updating the software). In this case it would make more sense to pay a larger bonus in the first instance, and then smaller payments in the following years.

Evidence

One of the main design issues in creating a P4P programme is deciding on the magnitude of the payment that should be made. In practice the amount of physicians' incomes from these types of incentives varies considerably. The new GP contract in the UK awards up to 20 per cent of annual income (Doran et al., 2006) while other plans offer much more modest incentives, as little as $2 per patient (Rosenthal and Adams Dudley, 2007; Young and Conrad, 2007). Evidence indicates that small-scale financial incentives may have been unsuccessful in attracting much attention from physicians, given that the rewards they offered made up only a small proportion of total physician income (Rosenthal et al., 2005). Similarly, McLean et al. (2006) found that the incentives provided by the GP contract were stronger in practices with fewer sources of alternative income. It has been suggested that modest-sized incentives may be more appropriate in the early phases of a P4P programme in order to minimise the chance that the rewards 'crowd out' the provider's intrinsic motivation and reduce the incentive to game (Young and Conrad, 2007). However, as Felt-Lisk et al. (2007) demonstrate by comparing different size incentives for the same service, the initial incentive must be large enough at the starting point to encourage change.

The general payment framework into which an incentive scheme is adopted has also been shown to affect physician behaviour. Each payment scheme is likely to employ a variety of measures, and each to reward these measures in a different way. Depending on the complexity of the incentive scheme and the amounts of different payment schemes being implemented, physicians may be more or less likely to change their behaviour or even to become aware of the programme's existence. For example, two studies by Hillman et al. (1998, 1999) found no significant improvements in targeted areas offering financial reward, and attributed this mainly to poor implementation and communication with physicians, many of whom were unaware of the programme's existence. Felt-Lisk et al. (2007) emphasised the importance of good communication as well as timely feedback and support to the effectiveness of P4P programmes. Moreover, many P4P systems were implemented as part of greater changes, making it hard to draw conclusive results about their effect (Ashworth et al., 2005; Beaulieu and Horrigan, 2005). Similarly, while studies indicate that different P4P progammes use different types of payments, it is difficult to draw conclusive results as to the effect this has overall, given the variation in many other factors, such as magnitude of payment, organisation and unit of assessment. More case-control studies are needed to draw conclusive results in this design area, as in many of the others discussed.

5.   DATA AND MEASUREMENT SYSTEMS

Theory

One of the most important design issues in constructing a successful P4P system is ensuring the validity of the performance data used to award payments. Many physicians are concerned about the way in which their performance is measured (Bokhour et al., 2006). Most of the initial P4P systems in the USA emerged with the use of HEDIS data in the early 1990s, which is a collection of data from HMO surveys, medical charts and insurance claims. These data were largely limited in the areas they covered, mostly chronic diseases and the provision of preventive services (Bodenheimer, 1999). More recently there has been more demand for the increased adoption of electronic medical records that will allow for better-quality data. Concerns arise when practical differences in the information capabilities of payers and providers potentially raise data issues – where the metrics corresponding to payment are systematically under- or over-reported, as was the case in the Integrated Healthcare Associations (IHA) programme in California (Damberg et al., 2005; Young and Conrad, 2007).

Moreover, in order for P4P to operate correctly, it is vital that the information connected to financial systems is valid to avoid the possibility of unfairly rewarding providers for differences in case-mix or other confounding factors. If physicians have higher amounts of clinically complicated patients, or patients with multiple conditions, it may be more difficult for them to score well on the outcome or process indicators on which the financial incentive is based. For this reason it is important to risk-adjust data for patients' clinical characteristics as well as socioeconomic and other factors that may influence their response to treatment (Iezzoni, 2009). If this is not done, or not done properly, it could result in adverse behavioural incentives, such as adverse selection or dumping (McMahon et al., 2007). Physician surveys repeatedly indicate concerns that such incentives may lead to these eventualities (Casalino et al., 2007). However, when designing risk adjustment schemes or exception clauses for high-risk patients, policy makers must be extremely careful to ensure that other unintended effects are not incentivised, such as misreporting, gaming or fraud.

Another consideration is the clinical relevance of the data collected. While data such as HEDIS are clinically relevant, they focus on key areas that are not necessarily the areas that physicians feel they should prioritise in their practices. Many other performance-based systems have involved physicians in the selection of indicators, to ensure that the professional culture and values are taken into account (Duckett et al., 2008). Evidence suggests that providers' perception of the clinical relevance of the targets may be just as important as the magnitude of the financial incentive (Young et al., 2005). Involving practitioners in the selection of indicators may help to reduce the possible negative effects such schemes have on providers' intrinsic motivation. In addition to clinical indicators, many P4P systems attach financial incentives to measures of patient satisfaction and use of IT, indicating that these tasks are also important in achieving high-quality care.

Finally, there is the consideration of what types of indicators to attach to financial incentives. Following Donabedian (1966), indicators can be classified into three types: structural indicators, which consider factors such as the availability of facilities and staff; process indictors, which measure whether treatment adheres to agreed good practice; and outcome indicators, which consider the resulting changes in health status. While outcome measures are appealing due to their clear and easy interpretation, process measures are more feasible and controllable as they are less easily influenced by patient case-mix, and are often easier to measure, especially when faced with a small sample and a short time frame (Smith et al., 2009). Moreover, because of the attribution issues associated with outcome measures, they are most suitable in areas where procedures and/or populations are largely homogeneous, or where cases have a proven strong association between interventions and outcomes (Davies, 2005; Mant, 2001). In recognition of these differences, most P4P programmes attach financial incentives to both types of indicators. Rosenthal and Adams Dudley (2007) note that initially P4P programmes focused mostly on process measures, yet they have increasingly incorporated outcome measures.

Evidence

As past experience has indicated, not taking physician values into account for incentive mechanisms (whether financial or not) can result in creating mechanisms that are not aligned with professional values. This can result in backlash, ineffectual policy and in the worst case create unintended effects such as adverse selection (Scheider and Epstein, 1996). However, current performance measurement systems seem to acknowledge the importance of involving practitioners in the selection of indicators (Engels et al., 2006; Marshall et al., 2003; Steel et al., 2004). This helps to ensure a degree of acceptance among the entities being rewarded. A study by McDonald et al. (2007) found little evidence of the crowding out of intrinsic incentives in GP practices after the implementation of the quality of outcomes framework (QOF). They attributed this partly to the practitioners' acceptance of the indicators as incentivising what clinicians themselves already regarded as good clinical care.

While there are concerns about the possibility of adverse selection and gaming, evidence of such effects occurring is sparse. Shen (2003) identified an instance of adverse selection in a P4P programme where the design of the incentive attached the following year's funding to predetermined quality targets in the year measured. Failing to meet the quality targets set resulted in providers being penalised by lower funding, a shortened contract or 'special conditions' attached to their payments. In order to avoid these penalties, providers avoided treating high-risk patients after the introduction of the payment. In order to avoid problems of adverse selection, the QOF section of the UK GP contract is designed to allow physicians to exclude certain patients from the performance measurement scheme (see Box 9.1). However, this exemption design may create incentives for misreporting or gaming, as physicians can potentially increase their incomes by excluding patients for whom they missed targets (Doran et al., 2006).

It is partly the inclusion of administration and IT targets that have led to one of

---

BOX 9.1   PATIENT EXCLUSION CRITERIA FOR QOF SCHEME IN GP CONTRACT

The patient received at least three invitations for a review during the preceding 12 months but has not attended.

The indicator is judged inappropriate for the patient by the GP because of particular circumstances, such as terminal illness, extreme frailty, or the presence of a supervening condition that makes the specified treatment of the patient's condition clinically inappropriate.

The patient has recently received a diagnosis or has recently registered with the practice.

The patient is taking the maximal tolerated does of a medication, but the levels remain suboptimal.

The patient has an allergic or other adverse reaction to a specified medication or has another contra-indication to the medication.

The patient does not agree to investigation or treatment.

A specified investigative service is unavailable to the family practitioner.

---

the unexpected successes of P4P programmes: the improvement in data collection and administration of practices, which have in turn resulted in better quality of care for patients. However, in many cases improvements in these areas were not targeted, but necessary to improve performance in the other, targeted areas. More than one study has attributed large gains in quality due to better documentation in practices, which, while not an explicit target of the programme, emerged as a result of it (Fairbrother et al., 1999; Fairbrother et al., 2001; Roski et al., 2003). Beaulieu and Horrigan (2005) found that some physicians even applied the new documentation processes necessary to receive the financial reward to other areas of their practice that were not incentivised. Grady et al. (1997) found through a case control study that while better information and documentation proved to substantially increase quality of care, an added financial reward had no extra effect.

In conjunction with these findings, Doran et al. (2006) found UK GP practices employing more administrative staff and increasingly using electronic medical records in preparation for the 2004 contract, in addition to employing more nurses and establishing chronic-disease clinics. Similarly, Gulliford et al. (2007) found that while intermediate diabetic outcomes have improved since the introduction of the new GP contract, the degree or service organisation in GP practices was important in explaining variations in clinical outcome measures, and concluded that the financial incentives provided by the new contract would help to achieve this objective.

6.   DISCUSSION

One of the main issues raised by this review, and any other review of the literature in this area, is the lack of evidence with which to evaluate the effectiveness of P4P programmes. While there are hundreds of P4P programmes being administered in several countries, the studies evaluating what works in this area are limited. Moreover, most of the literature focuses on P4P programmes implemented in the US setting and the GP contract, while much of the experience in the rest of Europe remains undocumented. Most of the studies available in the literature are descriptive rather than analytical, and very few have robust case-control studies from which concrete conclusions can be drawn. In addition, P4P programmes are often introduced together with other policies, making it even harder to attribute any change in practice solely to these incentives.

P4P programmes vary across many different parameters, all of which can influence how effective they are at meeting their objectives (Table 9.2).

The level at which the financial reward is directed – individual, group or system – will be important in determining the strength of the incentive. Payment at these different

Table 9.2   Stylised facts from existing literature

Design parameter	Evidence from literature
Unit of assessment	• Incentives at the individual level are most effective (Armour et al., 2001) • Group- and system-level incentives run the risk of being ineffective if there is no clear distribution of the incentive among the individual members, thus creating weakened individual incentives (Petersen et al., 2006) • System-level incentives are good for changing the administration and management of organisations (Berthiaume et al., 2006; Cameron et al., 1999; Norton, 1992)
Type of service targeted	• Initial P4P programmes focused on preventive and primary care, such as immunisations • Many P4P programmes are targeted at primary care areas that are known to affect patient outcomes in the longer term • The last five years have seen P4P programmes extended to emergency care and acute services
Magnitude and type of payment	• Rewards that make up a small percentage of physicians' salaries will draw little attention (Rosenthal et al., 2005) • Rewards should not be too large, as they may 'crowd out' providers' intrinsic motivation (McDonald et al., 2007; Young and Conrad, 2007) • Complex reward systems that are poorly communicated and do not provide feedback to providers are likely to be less successful
Data and measurement system	• Performance measures used in incentive programmes should be carefully constructed and consult physicians in order to avoid backlash, ineffectual policy and unintended effects • P4P policies improve administration and documentation in practices, which in turn improves quality of care • While rare, P4P can result in adverse selection, gaming and fraud if not carefully designed

levels creates different incentives: individual rewards will provide stronger incentives, whereas group- and system-level incentives are important in encouraging teamwork. Evidence from the literature shows that physicians are most likely to respond to individual-level incentives; however, group- or system-level incentives will differ according to how the incentive itself is distributed among the individuals within the groups or departments within the organisations (Petersen et al., 2006). Group- or system-level incentives are better at inducing group work or managerial and administrative changes. Ideally, the level at which payment is made should correspond to the entity responsible for the service so that the optimal behaviour is incentivised. Many of the studies reviewed in these areas did not provide details of the internal distribution of a group- or system-level financial reward. The distribution of the rewards will determine how effective it is in inducing different members of the team to try to meet the objectives targeted.

All incentives will be ineffectual if the tasks required to receive the reward are not clearly communicated to the individuals whose behaviour is being targeted. This is especially relevant to the group- and system-level incentives, where obtaining the reward may depend on group work, or the efforts of many individuals. In such cases it is important to provide clear instructions, indicators and feedback. While this seems obvious, many P4P programmes have been unsuccessful due to the complexity of the incentive design or lack of knowledge of its existence (Felt-Lisk et al., 2007; Hillman et al., 1998; Hillman et al., 1999).

While the unit of reimbursement is fundamental in defining the design of the payment system, the amount of reimbursement is also important. Research has shown that relative as well as absolute payment levels have substantial incentive effects on providers (Conrad and Christianson, 2004). Generally, low payment levels will reduce quality incentives in almost any payment design. However, incentives will tend to create some change in behaviour as long as they are large enough to cover any transaction and opportunity costs (Conrad, 2009; Young and Conrad, 2007). Incentives should not be too large, as this may crowd out the intrinsic incentives of providers and may also lead them to neglect other untargeted areas. However, more research is needed in this area to determine the extent of this problem.

Payment design is also crucial to determining how powerful an incentive will be; if a payment is constructed in such a way that providers feel it may be very difficult to obtain, such as a high benchmark or relative payment, they may be less likely to attempt it. However, if payments are fixed, providers who are already meeting targets will not have to change their behaviour at all, and this may be a waste of resources. The selection indicators to which rewards are tied will also be important in order to ensure the cooperation of physicians. For this reason, physicians are often consulted during the selection or construction of indicators to ensure that they correspond to best clinical practice and established norms.

7.   CONCLUSIONS

This chapter has examined some of the existing literature on P4P programmes, focusing on four key areas of their design in order to draw some conclusions as to how these can influence the overall effectiveness of these programmes. While much more work is still necessary to tease out the optimal design, certain conclusions as to what constitutes an effective P4P can be drawn. An effective P4P programme should have:

1. clear communication of the incentive to all stakeholders involved;
2. an incentive that is proportionate to the initial costs of service area targeted, as well as further transaction and opportunity costs;
3. incentives directed to the correct level for the type of service being incentivised (so that it reaches all parties necessary in the correct implementation of the service);
4. adequate risk adjustment or exemption mechanisms to ensure that providers will not be penalised for treating riskier patients;
5. performance indicators that have been constructed with the consultation of physicians and policy in order to ensure their clinical relevance.

Finally, there are still many areas where further research would be beneficial. More work should be done on the distribution of financial incentives within groups or systems, and how this impacts effectiveness. Little to no work has reviewed the effectiveness of using process or outcome indicators to reward performance. Furthermore, better understanding of the degree to which intrinsic motivation may be influenced by directed payments is important in understanding the full effects of these policies.

REFERENCES

Achat, H., McIntyre, P. and Burgess, M. (1999), 'Health care incentives in immunization', *Australian and New Zealand Journal of Public Health*, **23**, 205–0.

Amundson, G., Solberg, L.I., Reed, M., Martini, E.M. and Carlson, R. (2003), 'Paying for quality improvement: compliance with tobacco cessation guidelines', *Joint Commission Journal on Quality and Safety*, **29**, 59–65.

Armour, B.S., Pitts, M.M., Maclean, R., Cangialose, C., Kishel, M., Imai, H. and Etchason, J. (2001), 'The effect of explicit financial incentives on physician behaviour', *Archives of Internal Medicine*, **161**, 1261–6.

Ashworth, M., Armstrong, D., de Freitas, J., Boullier, G., Garforth, J. and Virji, A. (2005), 'The relationship between income and performance indicators in general practice: a cross-sectional study', *Health Services Management Research*, **18**, 258–64.

Baker, G. and Delbanco, S. (2007), *Pay for Performance: National Perspective. 2006 Longitudinal Survey Results with 2007 Market Updates*, San Francisco, CA: MedVantage.

Banker, R.D., Lee, S. and Potter, G. (1996), 'A field study of the impact of a performance-based incentive plan', *Journal of Accounting and Economics*, **21**, 195–226.

Beaulieu, N.D. and Horrigan, D.R. (2005), 'Organizational processes and quality', *Health Services Research*, **40**, 1318–34.

Berthiaume, J.T., Chung, R.S., Ryskina, K.L., Walsh, J. and Legoratta, A. (2006), 'Aligning financial incentives with quality of care in the hospital setting', *Journal for Health Care Quality*, **28**, 36–50.

Berwick, D.M. (1995), 'The toxicity of pay for performance', *Quality Management in Health Care*, **4**, 27–33.

Bodenheimer, T. (1999), 'The American health care system: the movement from improved quality in health care', *The New England Journal of Medicine*, **340**, 488–92.

Bokhour, B.G., Burgess, J.F., Hook, J.M., White, B., Berlowitz, D., Guilden, M.R., Meterko, M. and Young, G.J. (2006), 'Incentive implementation in physician practices: a qualitative study of practice executive perspectives on pay for performance', *Medical Care Research and Review*, **63**, 73S–95S.

Cameron, P.A., Kennedy, M.P. and McNeil, J.J. (1999), 'The effects of bonus payments on emergency service performance in Victoria', *Medical Journal of Australia*, **171**, 243–6.

Casalino, L.P., Elster, A., Eistenberg, A. et al. (2007), 'Will pay-for-performance and quality reporting affect health care disparities?', *Health Affairs*, **26**, 465–14.

Centers for Medicare and Medicaid Services (CMS) (2004), *CMS HQI Demonstration Project:*

Composite Quality Score Methodology Overview, 26 March available at https://www.cms.hhs.gov/ HospitalQualityInits/downloads/HospitalCompositeQualityScoreMethodologyOverview.pdf. (accessed 14 April 2009).

Christianson, J.B., Leatherman, S. and Sutherland, K. (2007a), 'Paying for quality: understanding and assessing physician pay-for-performance initiatives', Robert Wood Johnson Foundation: Research Synthesis Report, no. 13.

Christianson, J.B., Leatherman, S. and Sutherland, K. (2007b), *Financial Incentives, Healthcare Providers and Quality Improvements: A Review of the Evidence*, London: The Health Foundation.

Conrad, D. (2009), 'Incentives for performance measurement improvement', in P.C. Smith, E. Mossialos, S. Leatherman and I. Papanicolas (2009), *Performance Measurement for Health System Improvement: Experiences, Challenges and Prospects*, Cambridge: Cambridge University Press, pp. 582–611.

Conrad, D.A. and Cristianson, J.B. (2004), 'Penetrating the "black box": financial incentives for enhancing the quality of physician services', *Medical Care Research and Review*, **61**, 37S–68S.

Damberg, C.L., Raube, K., Williams, T. and Shortell, S.M. (2005), 'Paying for performance: implementing a statewide project in California', *Quality Management in Health Care*, **14**, 66–79.

Davies, H. (2005), 'Measuring and reporting the quality of health care: issues and evidence from the international research literature', NH Quality Improvement Scotland.

Deci, E.L. (1971), 'Effects of externally mediated rewards on intrinsic motivation', *Journal of Personality and Social Psychology*, **18**, 105–15.

Department of Health (DOH) (2004), *Investing in General Practice: The New General Medical Services Contract*, London: Department of Health.

Donabedian, A. (1966), 'Evaluating the quality of medical care', *The Milbank Memorial Fund Quarterly*, **44** (3), 166–206.

Doran, T., Fullwood, C., Gravelle, H., Reeves, D., Konotopantelis, E., Hiroeh, U. and Roland, M. (2006), 'Pay-for-performance programs in family practices in the United Kingdom', *The New England Journal of Medicine*, **355**, 375–84.

Doran, T., Kontopantelies, E. and Valderas, J.M. (2011), 'Effect of financial incentives on incentivised and non-incentivised clinical activities: longitudinal analysis of data from the UK Quality and Outcomes Framework', *British Medical Journal*, **324**, d3590.

Duckett, S., Daniels, S., Kamp, M. et al. (2008), 'Pay for performance in Australia: Queensland's new clinical practice improvement payment', *Journal of Health Services Research and Policy*, **13**, 174–7.

Engels, Y., van den Hombergh, P., Mokkink, H. et al. (2006), 'The effects of a team-based continuous quality improvement intervention on the management of primary care: a randomised controlled trial', *British Journal of General Practice*, **56**, 781–7.

Ettner, S.L., Thompson, T.L., Stevens, M.R., Mangione, C.M., Kim, C. and Steers, W.N. (2006), 'Are physician reimbursement strategies associated with processes of care and patient satisfaction for patients with diabetes in managed care?', *Health Services Research*, **41**, 1221–41.

Fairbrother, G., Hanson, K.L., Friedman, S. and Butts, G.C (1999), 'The impact of physician bonuses, enhanced fees, and feedback on childhood immunization coverage rates', *American Journal of Public Health*, **89**, 171–5.

Fairbrother, G., Siegel, M.J., Friedman, S., Kory, P.D. and Butts, G.C. (2001), 'Impact of financial incentives on documented immunization rates in the inner city: results of a randomized controlled trial', *Ambulatory Pediatrics*, **1**, 206–12.

Felt-Lisk, S., Gimm, G. and Peterson, S. (2007), 'Making pay-for-performance work in Medicaid', *Health Affairs*, **26**, 516–27.

Glickman, S.W., Ou, F.S., DeLong, E.R., Roe, M.T., Lytle, B.L., Mulgund, J., Rumsfeld, J.S., Gilber, E., Ohman, M., Schulman, K.A. and Peterson, E.D. (2007), 'Pay for performance, quality of care, and outcome in acute myocardial infarction', *Journal of the American Medical Association*, **297**, 2373–80.

Grady, K.E., Parr Lemkau, J., Lee, N.R. and Caddell, C. (1997), 'Enhancing mammography referral in primary care', *Preventative Medicine*, **26**, 791–800.

Grossbart, S.R. (2006), 'What's the return? Assessing the effect of "pay-for-performance" initiatives on the quality of care delivery', *Medical Care Research and Review*, **63**, 29S–48S.

Gulliford, M.C., Ashworth, M., Robotham, D. and Mohiddin, A. (2007), 'Achievement of metabolic targets for diabetes by English primary care practices under a new system of incentives', *Diabetic Medicine*, **24**, 505–11.

Health Departments of Great Britain (1989), *General Practice in the National Service: The 1990 Contract*, London: Department of Health and Social Security.

Hillman, A.L., Ripley, K., Goldfarb, N., Nuamah, I., Weiner, J. and Lusk, E. (1998), 'Physician financial incentives and feedback: failure to increase cancer screening in Medicaid managed care', *American Journal of Public Health*, **88**, 1699–701.

Hillman, A.L., Ripley, K., Goldfarb, N., Nuamah, I., Weiner, J., Nuamah, I. and Lusk, E. (1999), 'The use of physician financial incentives and feedback to improve pediatric preventative care in Medicaid managed care', *Pediatrics*, **104**, 931–5.

Holmstrom, B. and Milgrom, P. (1991), 'Multitask principal agent analyses: incentive contracts asset ownership and job design', *Journal of Law, Economics and Organization*, **7**, 24–52.

Iezzoni, L. (2009), 'Risk adjustment', in P.C. Smith, E. Mossialos, S. Leatherman and I. Papanicolas (2009), *Performance Measurement for Health System Improvement: Experiences, Challenges and Prospects*, Cambridge: Cambridge University Press, pp. 251–85.

Kouides, R.W., Bennett, N.M., Lewis, B., Cappuccio, J.D., Barker, W.H., LaForce, M. and the primary-care physicians of Monroe County (1998), 'Performance-based physician reimbursement and influenza immunization rates in the elderly', *American Journal of Preventive Medicine*, **14**, 89–95.

Larsen, D.L., Cannon, W. and Towner, S. (2003), 'Longitudinal assessment of a diabetes care management system in an integrated health network', *Journal of Managed Care Pharmacy*, **9**, 552–8.

Levin-Scherz, J., DeVita, N. and Timbie, J. (2006), 'Impact of pay-for-performance contracts and network registry on diabetes and asthma HEDIS measures in an integrated delivery network', *Medical Care Research and Review*, **63**, 14S–28S.

Lindenauer, P.K., Remus, D., Roman, S. et al. (2007), 'Public reporting and pay for performance in hospital quality improvement', *The New England Journal of Medicine*, **356**, 486–96.

Mant, J. (2001), 'Process versus outcome indicators in the assessment of quality of health care', *International Journal for Quality in Health Care*, **13**, 475–80.

Marshall, M.N., Shekelle, P.G., Hue, T.O. and Smith, P.C. (2003), 'Public reporting on quality in the United States and the United Kingdom', *Health Affairs*, **22**, 134–48.

McDonald, R., Harrison, S., Checkland, K. et al. (2007), 'Impact of financial incentives on clinical autonomy and internal motivation in primary care: ethnographic study', *British Medical Journal*, **334**, 1357–62.

McLean, G., Sutton, M. and Gurthrie, B. (2006), 'Deprivation and quality of primary care services: evidence for persistence of the inverse care law from the UK Quality and Outcomes Framework', *Journal of Epidemiology and Community Health*, **60**, 917–22.

McMahon, L.F., Hofer, T.P. and Hayward, R. (2007), 'Physician-level P4P – DOA? Can quality-based payment be resuscitated?', *The American Journal of Managed Care*, **13**, 233–6.

Meterko, M., Young, G.J., White, B., Bokhour, B., Burgess, H., Berlowitz, D., Guldin, M.R. and Nealon Seibert, M. (2006), 'Provider attitudes toward pay-for-performance programs: development and validation of a measurement instrument', *Health Services Research*, **41**, 1959–78.

Norton, E.C. (1992), 'Incentive regulation of nursing homes', *Journal of Health Economics*, **11**, 105–28.

Petersen, L.A., Woodard, L.D., Uroeh, T., Daw, C. and Sookanan, S. (2006), 'Does pay-for-performance improve the quality of health care?', *Annals of Internal Medicine*, **145**, 265–72.

Rosenthal, M.B. and Adams Dudley, R. (2007), 'Pay-for-performance: will the latest payment trend improve care?', *Journal of the American Medical Association*, **297**, 740–44.

Rosenthal, M.B. and Frank, R.G. (2006), 'What is the empirical basis for paying for quality in health care?', *Medical Care Research and Review*, **63**, 135–57.

Rosenthal, M.B., Frank, R.G., Zhonghe, L. and Epstein, A.M. (2005), 'Early experience with pay-for-performance: from concept to practice', *Journal of the American Medical Association*, **294**, 1788–93.

Rosenthal, M.B., Landon, B.E., Normand S.L.T., Frank, R.G. and Epstein, A.M. (2006), 'Pay for performance in commercial HMOs', *The New England Journal of Medicine*, **355**, 1895–902.

Rosenthal, M.B., Landon, B.E., Howitt, K., Song, H.R. and Epstein, A.M. (2007), 'Climbing up the pay-for-performance learning curve: where are the early adopters now?', *Health Affairs*, **26**, 1674–82.

Roski, J., Jeddeloh, R., An, L., Lando, H., Hannan, P., Hall, C. and Zhu, S. (2003), 'The impact of financial incentives and a patient registry on preventive care quality: increasing provider adherence to evidence-based smoking cessation practice guidelines', *Preventive Medicine*, **36**, 291–9.

Rothstein, R. (2008), 'Holding accountability to account: how scholarship and experience in other fields inform exploration of performance incentives in education', National Center on Performance Incentives, Working Paper 2008-04.

Scheider, E.C. and Epstein, A. (1996), 'Influence of cardiac-surgery performance reports on referral practices and access to care', *The New England Journal of Medicine*, **335**, 251–6.

Scott, I.A. (2007), 'Pay for performance in health care: strategic issues for Australian experiments', *The Medical Journal of Australia*, **187**, 31–5.

Shen, Y. (2003), 'Selection incentives in a performance-based contracting system', *Health Services Research*, **38**, 535–52.

Shohet, C., Yelloly, J., Bingham, P. and Lyratzoponlos, G. (2007), 'The association between the quality of epilepsy management in primary care, general practice population deprivation status and epilepsy-related emergency hospitalizations', *Seizure*, **16**, 351–5.

Sikka, R. (2007), 'Pay for performance in emergency medicine', *Annals of Emergency Medicine*, **49**, 756–61.

Smith, P.C. and York, N. (2004), 'Quality incentives: the case of U.K. general practitioners', *Health Affairs*, **23**, 112–18.

Smith, P.C., Mossialos, E., Leatherman, S. and Papanicolas, I. (2009), *Performance Measurement for Health System Improvement: Experiences, Challenges and Prospects*, Cambridge: Cambridge University Press.

Srirangalingam, U., Sahatheran, S.K., Lasker, S.S. and Chowdhury, T. (2006), 'Changing pattern of referral to a diabetes clinic following implementation of the new UK GP Contract', *British Journal of General Practice*, **56** (529), 624–6.

Steel, N., Melzer, D., Wenger, N.S. et al. (2004), 'Developing quality indicators for older adults: transfer from the USA to the UK is feasible', *Quality and Safety in Health Care*, **13**, 260–64.

Steel, N., Maisey, S., Clark, A. et al. (2007), 'Quality of clinical primary care and targeted incentive payments: an observational study', *British Journal of General Practice*, **57**, 449–54.

Town, R., Douglas, W.R., Kralewski, J. and Bowd, B. (2004), 'Assessing the influence of incentives on physicians and medical groups', *Medical Care Research and Review*, **61**, 80S–118S.

Town, R., Kane, R., Johnson, P. and Butler, M. (2005), 'Economic incentives and physicians' delivery of preventative care: a systematic review', *American Journal of Preventative Medicine*, **28**, 234–40.

Young, G.J. and Conrad, D. (2007), 'Practical issues in the design and implementation of pay-for-quality programs', *Journal of Healthcare Management*, **51**, 10–19.

Young, G.J., White, B., Burgess, J.F., Berlowitz, D., Meterko, M., Guldin, M.R. and Bokhour, B.G. (2005), 'Conceptual issues in the design and implementation of pay-for-quality programs', *American Journal of Medical Quality*, **24**, 144–50.

Young, G.J., Meterko, M., Beckman, H., Baker, E., White, B., Sautter, K.M., Greene, R., Curtin, K., Bokhour, B., Berlowitz, D. and Burgess, J.F. (2007a), 'Effects of paying physicians based on their relative performance for quality', *Health Policy*, **22**, 872–6.

Young, G.J., Meterko, M., Beckman, H., White, B., Bokhour, B., Sautter, K.M., Berlowitz, D. and Burgess, J.F. (2007b), 'Physician attitudes toward pay-for-quality programs: perspectives from the front line', *Medical Care Research and Review*, **64**, 331–4.

10 Social health protection: policy options for low- and middle-income countries
Philipa Mladovsky

1. INTRODUCTION

Financing health care has become an increasingly central policy issue in national and international efforts to improve health and health care in low- and middle-income countries (LMIC). The increased attention can partly be explained by the realisation that high levels of out-of-pocket expenditure on health reduce access to health care, especially among the poorest (Hjortsberg, 2003, Pieker et al., 2002, Lagarde and Palmer, 2008), and increase the financial risks of ill health to households due to selling of assets, indebtedness, impoverishment and reduction of essential expenditure on food, education and so on, in addition to the costs of being unable to carry out normal income-generating activities due to ill health (van Doorslaer et al., 2006; Xu et al., 2003; Wagstaff, 2009; McIntyre et al., 2006). Another driving factor for the focus on health financing is the further realisation that international development mechanisms aiming to support public health, such as aid, loans, debt reduction and global health initiatives, are unlikely to succeed without the presence of strong health, including health-financing, systems (Travis et al., 2004).

Before commencing an overview of the various policy options for financing health care available to LMIC, it is important to understand what the objectives of such policies might be. WHO outlined a set of objectives for health financing policy in the resolution on 'Sustainable health financing, universal coverage and social health insurance' (World Health Assembly, 2005), as well as in two world health reports (WHO, 2000, 2010) and other policy documents (Kutzin, 2008; Carrin et al., 2008). According to WHO, universal coverage is a key goal for any health system and is defined as securing access for all to appropriate promotive, preventive, curative and rehabilitative services at an affordable cost. National health-financing policies aiming for universal coverage need to incorporate three complementary dimensions of financial protection (i.e. protection against the financial risk of ill health): breadth of coverage (universality or the extent of the population covered); scope of coverage (i.e. the range of benefits); and depth of coverage (the share of service cost covered by the third party, i.e. user charges). The further goal of social health protection is related to and includes the goal of universal coverage, but more explicitly defines the values that a health-financing system should embody, namely equity, solidarity and social justice (International Labour Office, 2007).

The broad goals of universal coverage and social health protection incorporate a series of specific objectives that are commonly accepted as fundamental to the development and reform of health financing policy (Carrin et al., 2008; WHO, 2000). These are:

- sufficient, equitable and efficient revenue collection;
- risk pooling in order to ensure equitable financial access to health care; and
- efficiency and equity in the purchasing and provision of good-quality health care.

The strengths and weaknesses of specific health-financing mechanisms discussed in this report will be analysed in relation to these objectives.

It is recognised that the goals of universal coverage and social health protection can be, and usually are, met through a mix of health-financing mechanisms (International Labour Office, 2007; World Health Assembly, 2005). These may include:

- tax-funded national health insurance;
- contribution-based mandatory regulated social health insurance (SHI) financed by employers and workers;
- mandated or regulated private (non-profit in the case of the goals of social health protection) health insurance (PHI) schemes;
- mutual and community non-profit health-financing schemes such as community-based health insurance or subsidised vouchers.

The following discussion will take each of these financing mechanisms in turn and analyse the extent to which they have the potential to meet the above-mentioned objectives, including in terms of their effect on the rest of the health system. Each mechanism's strengths and weaknesses will be outlined from a theoretical perspective, and where possible also in terms of specific contexts and country experiences. At the same time, it is recognised that in practice each mechanism may adopt collection, pooling and purchasing features classically associated with another mechanism. For example, in many countries contribution-based mandatory SHI financed by employers and workers does include significant non-payroll tax revenue (such as in the form of government subsidies); or in countries such as England, tax financing is associated with contracting autonomous or private sector health care providers. Nevertheless, we retain categorisation by financing mechanism for ease of reference.

2.   SOCIAL HEALTH PROTECTION POLICY OPTIONS

2.1   Tax-funded National Health Insurance

Tax-funded NHI systems are characterised by three main features: funding comes from general revenues; the entire population is entitled to medical coverage; and health care is usually delivered through a network of public providers (Gottret and Schieber, 2006), although the last feature is gradually becoming less prominent as countries experiment with different provider systems.

Revenue collection
In high-income countries, tax-based NHI systems have the advantage over SHI systems in that they rely on a much broader revenue base. Rather than relying on formal sector employers and employees, as well as income tax, other taxes such as value-added tax

(VAT), sales tax and import tax may be drawn upon for health care funding, spreading the financial burden over a larger segment of the population (Gottret and Schieber, 2006) and lowering labour costs. However, in LMIC there is typically a much lower tax base than in high-income countries (Gottret and Schieber, 2006), and this has been proposed as one of the main reasons for LMIC to promote SHI instead of/in addition to a tax-based health financing system. For example, in 2003 Ghana decided to introduce a national SHI scheme in order to supplement tax revenue for the health system. However, introducing SHI is also associated with numerous problems in LMIC, discussed below. On the other hand, it has been argued that a low tax base need not remain a permanent obstacle: in several LMIC tax bases have been widened through reforms such as simplifying taxes, limiting incentives and exemptions, as well as changing tax rates to encourage tax compliance and reduce the informalising of the economy (Wagstaff, 2007). Such reforms have been used to expand government health financing in Bolivia, for example, where government health spending as a share of GDP grew at an annual rate of nearly 10 per cent during the 1990s (Wagstaff, 2007).

While it may be possible to increase the tax base, it should be noted that there is no guarantee that the health system will benefit. Another perceived weakness of tax-based financing systems is that the source of funding is vulnerable to changes in political priorities, with the MoH having to compete with other sectors for the same resources – a situation that does not arise in SHI systems (Gottret and Schieber, 2006). However, conceptually there is no reason why taxes cannot be earmarked for health.

Risk pooling

A pure tax-based NHI system is a universal pooling arrangement, preventing risk selection and potentially making this the most equitable form of health financing (Gottret and Schieber, 2006). However, in practice pooling may not necessarily be at the national level (there may be pooling at a regional level, for example), and many LMIC combine tax-based NHI systems with other financing mechanisms, such as user charges, which are often characterised by wide socioeconomic inequalities. It is challenging to include diverse populations in one risk pool; if there is a relatively small budget, as in most LMIC, one national risk pool may be equitable in that it may allow for the provision of a basic level of care for all, but it may not be politically feasible since it may not respond to the demands for more sophisticated health care among the wealthy and middle classes. African and former Soviet Union countries with tax-based health-financing systems have responded to this problem by allowing these groups access to expensive care at the taxpayer's expense in elite urban facilities that are inaccessible to large segments of the population (Wagstaff, 2007). If government-funded primary care is not sufficiently resourced and is of low quality (often the case in LMIC), this approach typically results in the highly inequitable situation where the rich receive a greater proportion of the public subsidy than the poor (Gottret and Schieber, 2006).

One response to this situation evident in high-income countries as well as LMIC such as Brazil, Malaysia and Sri Lanka is to develop private health insurance to cover the wealthier segments of the population (Wagstaff, 2007), although this may not improve equitable risk pooling (see below). This may be especially so if private health insurance benefits from tax relief, as in Brazil, India and South Africa. In addition to PHI, countries such as Egypt have additionally introduced SHI as a third parallel health-financing system to cover the formal sector. Such fragmentation typically erodes the benefits of tax-based systems by increasing administrative costs and limiting the equity and efficiency of pooling arrangements.

Purchasing and provision of health care

Typically in tax-based systems the Ministry of Health (MoH) delivers health care through its own network of providers that are paid through a mixture of budgets and salaries. The hierarchical command-and-control structure can be more efficient than less integrated systems such as SHI, due to lower transaction costs and the greater ability to control health expenditure. Such structures have helped MoHs in many LMIC implement successful public health programmes (Gottret and Schieber, 2006). However, overly bureaucratic civil service systems with poor incentive structures for efficiency and quality of care along with government corruption have often resulted in an inefficient and poor-quality state-run national health service in LMIC. This has led to health sector reforms that sought to reduce the role of central government in direct health care provision, introducing decentralisation of provision, increased provider autonomy and contracting out to private providers in many LMIC. It is unclear whether these reforms have resulted in efficiency gains, since the same lack of institutional capacity and poor governance that hindered pre-reform health systems often continues to hinder the reform process (Mills, 1998; Bennett et al., 1997).

2.2   Social Health Insurance

SHI systems are characterised by mandatory earmarked payments legally required from certain population groups, often in the form of employee payroll deductions and employer contributions. Independent or quasi-independent non-profit insurance funds (or a single fund) typically provide access to a defined benefit package that is available only to those who make contributions or are covered by the insurance.

Revenue collection

A strength of SHI is said to be its capacity to raise greater and more predictable revenues for health care than tax-funded systems, particularly in LMIC where the ability to collect taxes is said to be weak (see above). SHI may be preferred by governments in countries where the informal sector is large because it may encourage people to declare their earnings, assuming they are willing to trade off lost tax revenue for access to health benefits. Formal sector employees may also be more willing to finance health care via SHI than under a tax-based system since under the former, contributions are more clearly linked to benefits. Other causes of comparatively greater willingness to pay are thought to be increased solidarity within a clearly defined risk pool (this idea derives from the European experience where it has been argued that SHI institutions embody a set of social values deeply rooted in civil society (Saltman, 2004)) and a lack of trust in government health systems.

However, in countries such as China and Vietnam, 50 per cent or more formal sector employees evaded enrolment in SHI. SHI schemes in Eastern Europe and the former Soviet Union have not resulted in additional revenues for health care, in part because of problems in collecting revenues (Wagstaff, 2007). In addition, SHI may incur higher administrative costs resulting from a revenue collection system that runs parallel to existing tax collection systems. Furthermore, more could be done to increase the tax base in LMIC (see above). Finally, as in Europe (Normand and Busse, 2002; Thomson et al., 2009), in LMIC with SHI it is likely that the health system will also rely on tax-based financing of health care, for example in order to fund subsidies and preventive health. It is important that the introduction of SHI does not erode the commitment of the Ministry of Finance to fund such activities (Wagstaff, 2007).

In terms of the increased predictability of funds under SHI, it is not necessarily clear that this is an advantage to the more negotiable and flexible flow of funds in a tax-based system. Under SHI, funds are protected from cuts made by the Ministry of Finance, but just as this can prevent underinvestment, it can also lead to overinvestment, as has arguably been the case in France and Germany (Wagstaff, 2007; Thomson et al., 2009). Furthermore, relying almost exclusively on employment-based contributions is called into question by rising unemployment, growing informal economies, concerns about international competitiveness and changing dependency ratios (Thomson et al., 2009), although whether tax-based health-financing systems have a more favourable effect on unemployment rates is not clear (Wagstaff, 2007).

Finally, an important point to consider is the degree of equity in the financing system. Studies have found that payroll contributions are often regressive, due to contribution ceilings (Wagstaff, 2007). The degree of progressiveness of a tax-based financing system depends on the tax structure in the particular national context. Income tax is often designed to be proportional if not progressive. Indirect taxes are normally considered to be regressive, although in LMIC where poorer households rely on subsistence farming and luxury goods are taxed at high rates, even VAT can be progressive (Wagstaff, 2007).

Risk pooling
Due to its mandatory nature, SHI implies income and risk cross-subsidies, whereby individuals contribute to the insurance according to their ability to pay (or their income) and benefit from coverage according to their need for health care. However, if the SHI system is limited to the formal sector and benefits are linked only to contributions, there will be little risk pooling between the formal and informal sectors. This is the case in many Latin American countries, where parallel, often inferior quality and underfunded tax-financed systems operated by the MoH serve the informal sector (Wagstaff, 2007; Lloyd-Sherlock, 2006). This violates the core values of social health protection and suggests that in LMIC many of the advantages of SHI may benefit only those enrolled in SHI, while negatively affecting the rest of the health system as a result of fragmentation of the risk pool. Another potentially negative effect of mandating coverage only among the formal sector that has been of concern in Latin America is that this may create a perverse incentive for people to leave formal employment and opt instead for subsidised state health care or private health insurance, resulting in the increased informalisation of the economy (Wagstaff, 2007).

If SHI is intended to cover the whole population, contributions from the formal sector may be used to subsidise the informal sector, but to achieve this the contribution rate would need to be (probably unsustainably) high in LMIC, where the formal sector is typically in the minority. One solution to this is state subsidies for contributions to cover poor segments of the population. However, in practice this has been difficult to implement. For example, in countries such as Vietnam and Colombia less than 50 per cent of the eligible population has actually applied for subsidised enrolment; Colombia and Mexico also experience the reverse problem whereby high numbers of eligible people have fraudulently applied for subsidised coverage (Wagstaff, 2007). Another problem with subsidies is that they may create a perverse incentive to poor households not to increase their income above the subsidy threshold. Raising contributions from the non-poor informal sector is another option, but this has also been associated with low enrolment rates in countries such as Vietnam, Philippines, Tanzania and Ghana (Wagstaff, 2007). The reasons for non-enrolment are varied but may typically include high co-payments and under-the-table payments, low quality of care and lack of information.

Purchasing and provision of health care
The configuration of purchasers and providers in SHI systems typically involves either autonomous health care provision in cases where there is a dedicated SHI delivery system, as in some Latin American countries, or a purchaser–provider split where the insurer has the role of purchaser while the delivery of health care is the responsibility of the MoH, as in Vietnam, for example, or is contracted out to the private sector, as in Argentina (Wagstaff, 2007). If purchasers create appropriate incentives, this configuration may enhance efficiency, reduce health care costs and improve quality of care (Normand and Busse, 2002). The autonomy of providers can be contrasted with some tax-based systems, which entail the state taking the role of both purchaser and provider (see above), an integrated structure that is said to create relatively few incentives for improved efficiency and quality of care. It may also be the case that providers in SHI systems are more accountable to the public due to the clearer link between contributions and benefits than in the tax-based system (Wagstaff, 2007). If there are several SHI funds, then efficiency may also be increased through competition, although this also introduces the potential for risk selection (Normand and Busse, 2002).

However, it has been argued that evidence from Europe does not support the arguments in favour of SHI, with tax-based systems often performing better in certain aspects of accountability, quality and costs (Wagstaff, 2007), and with SHI systems in LMIC such as Armenia, Kazakhstan, Kenya (Gottret and Schieber, 2006), Argentina and Mexico (Lloyd-Sherlock, 2006) often performing poorly on these criteria. Furthermore, tax-based systems can be (re)structured to incorporate the advantages of the SHI model without actually adopting SHI, through the separation of purchasers from providers, as in Canada, England and most EU countries financed predominantly through taxation (Wagstaff, 2007; Thomson et al., 2009).

2.3   Private Health Insurance

While public insurance is funded through taxes, either general or social security taxes, private insurance is provided through the direct payment of premiums to insurers. Private health insurance (PHI) arrangements in LMIC are highly varied and can include voluntary insurance and mandatory insurance if it is not in the direct control of government; for-profit insurers, non-profit and community-based insurers (Sekhri and Savedoff, 2006). Community-based insurance is discussed separately in the next section. Furthermore, PHI can have a supplementary, substitutive or complementary role (Mossialos and Thomson, 2002).

Revenue collection

PHI is proposed as an alternative or complement to public health-financing mechanisms such as taxation and social health insurance (SHI) and private mechanisms in the form of user charges, both of which are argued to have largely failed to raise sufficient revenues for health care in LMIC (Pauly et al., 2006; Drechsler and Jutting, 2005; Preker, 2007; Sekhri and Savedoff, 2005, 2006), due to the problems discussed above.

However, voluntary health insurance currently represents a minimal source of revenue for health care in low-income countries, representing less than 5 per cent of total expenditure on health, although in some LMIC, such as Brazil, Chile, Namibia, South Africa and Zimbabwe, this rises to more than 20 per cent (Gottret and Schieber, 2006; Sekhri and Savedoff, 2006). The importance of PHI is probably set to increase, though: measured in terms of premium volume, the insurance industry in LMIC grew more than twice as fast as in industrialised economies during the past ten years (Drechsler and Jutting, 2007).

Three possible causes of small or non-existent markets for private insurance in LMIC have been proposed: inadequate demand because of low risk aversion or misperception; restrictions on supply because of regulation; and high administrative costs (Pauly et al., 2006). Regulation may restrict supply because of the high minimum capital requirement needed to obtain a licence to operate PHI in many countries (Sekhri and Savedoff, 2006). Other regulatory issues are addressed in the next sub-sections. Low risk aversion is argued to be related to the third problem, administrative costs. The main problem associated with risk aversion is argued to exist in insurance markets mainly in a relative sense, in relation to the price of the premium (Pauly, 2007). Due to loading to cover administrative and other costs, premiums are normally priced higher than the 'fair' price, unless they are subsidised. Assuming that a consumer's amount of risk aversion is equal to the maximum loading they are willing to pay for, in order to increase demand, private insurers in LMIC must keep administrative costs low enough to maintain the prices of premiums at an acceptable level. Another important cause of escalation of the price of premiums is the desire of PHI providers to increase profit. In Latin American and other LMIC this may have contributed to the dramatic rise in the price of premiums (Drechsler and Jutting, 2007). It has therefore been argued that either for-profit PHI providers must be regulated, or policy makers should concentrate their efforts on the development of non-profit PHI schemes (Drechsler and Jutting, 2005). Group insurance might be preferable since it reduces administrative costs and the need for information for individual risk rating, which may not be available in LMIC contexts (Drechsler and Jutting, 2005). However, policies to make PHI premiums more affordable are unlikely to improve enrolment among much of the poor population in many LMIC.

Risk pooling

The benefits of pooling risks of losses from high levels of out-of-pocket medical spending among the poor is one of the main arguments proposed for the promotion of voluntary health insurance (mutual or community insurance, non-profit private insurance, and for-profit private insurance) in LMIC (Pauly et al., 2006; Drechsler and Jutting, 2005; Preker, 2007; Sekhri and Savedoff, 2005, 2006).

There are three main risk-pooling options for governments aiming to promote PHI. The first option entails introducing voluntary supplementary or substitutive PHI for formal sector employees only, among whom demand (determined by willingness to pay and risk aversion) may be higher than among the general population. Indigents and informal sector workers would continue to be covered by subsidised public sector health care. It is argued that this arrangement is not only efficient but also in line with equity objectives since it allows indirect targeting of limited government resources to those who cannot afford to pay for themselves. However, while market segmentation for formal sector or wealthier groups may relieve pressure on the public system, it may lead to a differentiation of insurance pools with increased, rather than reduced, pressure on the public system due to overloading and underfunding (Sekhri and Savedoff, 2006). If, as in the case of substitutive PHI, these groups, representing good risks, are permitted to opt out of the public system, it has been argued that the public system should be compensated through financial transfers or a clear separation of each domain of coverage; otherwise PHI is likely to jeopardise the goal of universal coverage (Drechsler and Jutting, 2005).

The second option is to introduce substitutive PHI to a broader segment of the population by providing government subsidy for the premiums of those lacking the resources to pay for themselves. It is argued that this approach is preferable to the first since it allows more direct targeting of the poor by focusing subsidies on the demand, rather than supply, side, and it reduces the fragmentation of the risk pool (Preker, 2007). However, if PHI is to be a primary alternative to other forms of health financing, the coverage offered must be comprehensive and must include low-cost/high-frequency events. In reality, in most countries, most people covered by PHI are covered by supplementary coverage for high-cost/low-frequency events such as hospitalisation (Drechsler and Jutting, 2005).

It has been argued that a lack of regulation has prevented PHI from improving equitable access to financial protection in LMIC, illustrated by many Latin American countries such as Chile, Argentina, Colombia and Brazil, where there were delays in establishing regulatory agencies for PHI (Drechsler and Jutting, 2007; Sekhri and Savedoff, 2006). Different types of regulation can be considered. Mandating or standardising benefit packages is considered to have both merits and disadvantages, increasing the potential to prevent cream skimming but also possibly resulting in increased cost of premiums and limited innovation. The effect of mandating or standardising prices for the premium, for example through community rating, is also seen as having mixed results, increasing solidarity but also increasing risk selection and reducing the attractiveness of the scheme to low-risk individuals (adverse selection). Regulating the benefits to include a basic package of care and to address limited coverage of pre-existing conditions, contract exclusions and waiting periods would also be needed to introduce financial protection for the conditions for which insurance is most needed in LMIC.

However, it has been argued that, while regulation is needed to mitigate the risk of insolvency of insurance schemes, regulation of the premium and benefit package should be kept to a minimum and grading premiums according to risk should be permitted (Zweifel et al., 2007). These conditions are argued to preserve efficiency and prevent risk selection and cream skimming. From this free-market perspective, equity aims, expressed through the *ex ante* redistribution of resources through the regulation of the premium and benefit package, for example, are wholly inappropriate for PHI in LMIC (Zweifel and Pauly, 2007). These aims, it is argued, harm consumer choice and competition, and threaten the viability of the scheme. Risk adjustment could control some of the negative effects of regulation, but this is seen as probably too complicated for many LMIC (Zweifel et al., 2007).

Purchasing and provision of health care

One argument, discussed above, explaining the development of PHI in many Latin American and other countries is that economic growth has led to diversified consumer demand that might not be met by public services (Drechsler and Jutting, 2005, 2007). In addition, due to its association with private health care provision, PHI may be more trusted than public entities; also, since PHI does not require a strong service infrastructure it may be able to develop despite institutional weaknesses (Drechsler and Jutting, 2005). However, in many LMIC PHI has not led to high-quality care and it has been argued that improved regulation of insurer–provider integration, contracting and provider payment is needed in order to maintain access and quality of care, to reduce provider-induced demand and to help control price inflation and prevent it from increasing prices in the public sector (Sekhri and Savedoff, 2006). However, the institutional capacity to regulate PHI in this way is lacking in many LMIC (Sekhri and Savedoff, 2006).

An alternative perspective views vertical integration as primarily driven by insurers and/or providers themselves (Zweifel et al., 2007), with government playing a regulatory role only in terms of guaranteeing the rule of law so that contracts are honoured, something that is acknowledged to be challenging in many LMIC where there is relatively high corruption.

2.4   Community Health Financing

Community health financing schemes have three main features: prepayment for health services covers; community control; and voluntary membership (Hsiao, 2001). This section covers three types of community health financing. The first involves schemes involving direct government subsidy to the individuals (such as the Thai Health Card). The second and third types can be classified as community-based health insurance (CBHI) and involve either community-sponsored third-party insurance or provider-sponsored prepayment (free access to specific providers in exchange for monthly premiums).

Data on community financing is scarce (Ekman, 2004; Jakab and Krishnan, 2001), but it has been of increasing interest to international funders who have encouraged the rapid growth of schemes in LMIC. For example, it is estimated that in West Africa there was more than a twofold increase in the number of CBHI schemes in just three years, from 199 schemes in 2000 to 585 in 2003 (Bennett et al., 2004). However, it should be noted that in most contexts levels of population coverage continue to remain low.

Revenue collection

In theory, prepayment by community members is the main source of revenue for community health financing schemes, but in reality most schemes cannot raise sufficient resources through this method alone and also rely on co-payments, government subsidies and donor support (Jakab and Krishnan, 2001). A review of 26 studies reporting the contribution of community financing schemes to the operational revenues of local providers found a large variation, with some schemes achieving full financing of the recurrent costs of their local health centre, including some drug and referral expenditures. Others, particularly hospital-based schemes, had a modest contribution to the resources of the facility (Jakab and Krishnan, 2001). The main reason for a lack of resource mobilisation is poverty of the target population, which limits the degree of redistribution taking place within the limited risk pool.

Risk pooling
International development agencies construe CBHI as a transitional pooling mechanism to achieving universal coverage for health care in low-income countries (Arhin-Tenkorang, 2001; Davies and Carrin, 2001; WHO, 2000, 2005). The current international policy model linking CBHI and universal coverage is implicitly informed by the history of health service financing in nineteenth-century Europe and Japan, where CBHI schemes covering small risk pools eventually merged to form a national pool (Criel and Van Dormael, 1999). However, it is too early to tell whether CBHI schemes in their current form will develop into forms of national health financing according to the historical precedent.

Community health financing is mainly considered to be a method of increasing risk pooling among the informal sector. If schemes are successful in enrolling poorer segments of the population, they may increase equity in health financing. A review of 13 studies that report evidence regarding the socioeconomic composition of scheme members (Jakab and Krishnan, 2001) found that while community health financing extends coverage to a large number of people who would otherwise not have financial protection, the poorest of the poor are often not included in the benefits of community-based health financing. The Gonosasthya Kendra and Grameen Bank (GB) schemes in Bangladesh and the Thai Health Card scheme are among those that have managed to enrol relatively high rates of poor households, compared to non-poor households, in the target population. Mutual health insurance schemes in the Thies region in Senegal and the Nkoranza scheme in Ghana are among those that have enrolled relatively wealthier (although still poor by international standards) households and not the poorest of the poor in the target population. Where data are available, lack of affordability and distance to scheme hospital appear to be the main factors affecting the decision to enrol (Jakab and Krishnan, 2001).

In order to increase equity through risk pooling, community schemes also need to reduce catastrophic expenditures. Evidence from India suggests that community financing has been successful in this to a degree: the SEWA and ACCORD schemes halved the number of households that would have experienced catastrophic health expenditure (spending >10 per cent of annual household income) by covering hospital costs. However, 4 per cent and 23 per cent of households with admissions still experienced catastrophic expenditure at ACCORD and SEWA, respectively due to high co-payments (Devadasan et al., 2006).

The typically small size of risk pools in community health financing may threaten the viability of schemes by reducing the potential to spread risk, actuarially correctly assess the probability of the loss occurring and therefore maintain solvency, to cross-subsidise and lower transaction costs (Schieber and Maeda, 1997). However, on the positive side, it is also thought that problems associated with voluntary health insurance such as adverse selection, moral hazard and low demand may in part be counteracted by the smallness of community financing schemes, through informal safeguards such as full information, social sanctions, increased social capital and increased solidarity (Davies and Carrin, 2001; Zweifel, 2004; Pauly, 2007; Zhang et al., 2006). However, in some contexts such as Vietnam, strong intra-community ties may have favoured informal financial networks such as borrowing money that have prevented more formal and institutionalised types of mechanisms such as CBHI from emerging (Jowett, 2003). Evidence from Senegal (Bennett et al., 2004), India (Devadasan et al., 2006) and elsewhere suggests that links with NGOs, umbrella organisations or local government (within and beyond the health sector) could be used to foster scheme mergers, a more generalised sense of trust and more formalised community networks, which might increase willingness to participate in CBHI and enlarged risk pools (Mladovsky and Mossialos, 2008).

Purchasing and provision of health care
A major obstacle to community health financing is the poor quality of health services (Criel and Waelkens, 2003). Some types of community financing such as CBHI can potentially contribute to improving quality, efficiency and sustainability of health services through strategic purchasing (WHO, 2000; Hsiao, 2001) if the provider is separate from the purchaser. However, for strategic purchasing there must be an enabling environment: information about the quality and quantity of services must be provided; there needs to be investment in new skills in contracting on the part of both the purchaser and provider (Bennett et al., 1997); and a revision of the balance of power between purchaser and provider must be accepted (Desmet et al., 1999, Meessen et al., 2002, Carrin et al., 2005; Criel et al., 2005). In light of these numerous preconditions, it is not surprising that in a study of 258 CBHI schemes in low-income countries only 16 per cent conducted strategic purchasing (ILO, 2002).

One method of creating these conditions is for government to provide the function of monitoring, regulating and/or accrediting providers, so that schemes do not need to develop the technical skills to conduct these activities themselves. China's rural cooperative medical system (RCMS) provides an example of this (Bloom and Shenglan, 1999).

Another possible avenue for improving quality of care in LMIC is demand-side financing such as subsidised voucher schemes. Demand-side financing allows patients to choose the provider, assuming there are sufficient providers to choose from (often not the case in poor rural areas). This potentially creates competition among providers and consequently incentives for improved quality and responsiveness (Sandiford et al., 2002), although whether patients are well informed enough to choose providers on the basis of clinical quality (rather than factors such as waiting times and responsiveness of staff) is not clear.

While many schemes may not achieve the goal of quality improvement, by removing the cost of health care at the point of use community health financing has been found to increase health care utilisation rates (Jakab and Krishnan, 2001). In addition to co-payments, high indirect costs such as transport costs and opportunity costs of time away from income-generating activities mean that this is unlikely to represent moral hazard in most poor, rural contexts.

3. SUMMARY AND DISCUSSION

High rates of out-of-pocket and catastrophic expenditure on health care, combined with low total rates of health expenditure and high rates of mortality from easily and cheaply treatable diseases, make improving health care financing an urgent priority in many LMIC. However, the experience of high-income countries suggests that reaching the goal of universal coverage takes time (50 years in many cases) and requires nationally specific and relevant solutions. This review of the four principal mechanisms for financing health care in LMIC, tax-based NHI systems, SHI, PHI and community financing, suggests that no single model is likely to provide all the answers. Each mechanism is associated with strengths, but also serious weaknesses that limit the likelihood of its achieving successful social health protection in many country contexts.

While tax-based financing may in theory be the most equitable system, in practice governments have been unable to raise sufficient resources to provide health care that meets the diverse demands of both rural poor populations and wealthier and politically more powerful groups. This is particularly a problem in countries that have high socio-economic inequalities. SHI and PHI, on the other hand, do have the potential to serve wealthier, formal sector populations. However, in many countries these mechanisms have had a negative impact on the rest of the health system by fragmenting the risk pool and creating increased inequity. In addition, successfully enrolling the informal sector is extremely difficult in economically underdeveloped countries. PHI has the additional drawback of being highly unregulated in many LMIC, leading to expensive and poor-quality care even for those covered. Community financing does have the potential to cover poorer population groups, and countries such as the Philippines have used it in combination with SHI in an effort to move towards universal coverage. While such a mixed approach could successfully draw on different strengths of different financing mechanisms, the high levels of complexity and fragmentation of risk pools also make it likely to be associated with high transaction costs.

ACKNOWLEDGEMENTS

The author would like to thank Sarah Thomson for her comments on a previous draft of this chapter.

REFERENCES

Arhin-Tenkorang, D. (2001), 'Health insurance for the informal sector in Africa: design features, risk protection, and resource mobilization', CMH Working Paper Series, No. WG3: 1.
Bennett, S., Kelley, A.G. and Silvers, B. (2004), *21 Questions on CBHF: An Overview of Community-Based Health Financing*, Bethesda, MD: The Partners for Health Reformplus Project, Abt Associates Inc.
Bennett, S., McPake, B. and Mills, A. (1997), *Private Health Providers in Developing Countries: Serving the Public Interest?*, London and Princeton, NJ: Zed Books.
Bloom, G. and Shenglan, T. (1999), 'Rural health prepayment schemes in China: towards a more active role for government', *Social Science and Medicine*, **48**, 951–60.
Carrin, G., Mathauer, I., Xu, K. and Evans, D.B. (2008), 'Universal coverage of health services: tailoring its implementation', *Bulletin of World Health Organization*, **86**, 857–63.

Carrin, G., Waelkens, M.P. and Criel, B. (2005), 'Community-based health insurance in developing countries: a study of its contribution to the performance of health financing systems', *Tropical Medicine and International Health*, **10**, 799–811.

Criel, B. and Van Dormael, M. (1999), 'Mutual health organizations in Africa and social health insurance systems: will European history repeat itself?', *Tropical Medicine and International Health*, **4**, 155–9.

Criel, B. and Waelkens, M.P. (2003), 'Declining subscriptions to the Maliando Mutual Health Organisation in Guinea-Conakry (West Africa): what is going wrong?', *Social Science and Medicine*, **57**, 1205–19.

Criel, B., Diallo, A.A., Van Der Vennet, J., Waelkens, M.P. and Wiegandt, A. (2005), 'Difficulties in partnerships between health professionals and Mutual Health Organisations: the case of Maliando in Guinea-Conakry', *Tropical Medicine and International Health*, **10**, 450–63.

Davies, P. and Carrin, G. (2001), 'Risk-pooling – necessary but not sufficient?', *Bulletin of the World Health Organization*, **79**, 587.

Desmet, M., Chowdhury, A.Q. and Islam, M.K. (1999), 'The potential for social mobilisation in Bangladesh: the organisation and functioning of two health insurance schemes', *Social Science and Medicine*, **48**, 925–38.

Devadasan, N., Ranson, K., Van Damme, W., Acharya, A. and Criel, B. (2006), 'The landscape of community health insurance in India: an overview based on 10 case studies', *Health Policy*, **78**, 224–34.

Drechsler, D. and Jutting, J. (2005), *Private Health Insurance in Low- and Middle-income Countries. Scope, Limitations, and Policy Responses*, Paris: OECD.

Drechsler, D. and Jutting, J. (2007), 'Different countries, different needs: the role of private health insurance in developing countries', *Journal of Health Politics, Policy and Law*, **32**, 497–534.

Ekman, B. (2004), 'Community-based health insurance in low-income countries: a systematic review of the evidence', *Health Policy Planning*, **19**, 249–70.

Gottret, P.E. and Schieber, G. (2006), *Health Financing Revisited: A Practitioner's Guide*, Washington, DC: The World Bank.

Hjortsberg, C. (2003), 'Why do the sick not utilise health care? The case of Zambia', *Health Economics*, **12**, 755–70.

Hsiao, W.C. (2001), 'Unmet health needs of two billion: is community financing a solution?', HNP Discussion Paper, Washington, DC: The World Bank.

ILO (2002), 'Extending social protection in health through community based health organizations. Evidence and challenges', Discussion Paper, Geneva: International Labour Organization.

ILO (2007), 'Social health protection: an ILO strategy towards universal access to health care. Draft for consultation. Issues in Social Protection', Discussion Paper 19, Geneva: International Labour Organization.

Jakab, M. and Krishnan, C. (2001), *Community Involvement in Health Care Financing: Impact, Strengths and Weaknesses: A Synthesis of the Literature*, Washington, DC: The World Bank.

Jowett, M. (2003), 'Do informal risk sharing networks crowd out public voluntary health insurance? Evidence from Vietnam', *Applied Economics*, **35**, 1153–61.

Kutzin, J. (2008), *Health Financing Policy: A Guide for Decision-makers*, Copenhagen: WHO.

Lagarde, M. and Palmer, N. (2008), 'The impact of user fees on health service utilization in low- and middle-income countries: how strong is the evidence?', *Bulletin of the World Health Organization*, **86**, 839–48.

Lloyd-Sherlock, P. (2006), 'When social health insurance goes wrong. Lessons from Argentina and Mexico', *Social Policy and Administration*, **40**, 353–68.

McIntyre, D., Thiede, M., Dahlgren, G. and Whitehead, M. (2006), 'What are the economic consequences for households of illness and of paying for health care in low- and middle-income country contexts?', *Social Science and Medicine*, **62**, 858–65.

Meessen, B., Criel, B. and Kegels, G. (2002), 'Formal pooling of health risks in sub-Saharan Africa: reflections on the obstacles encountered', *International Social Security Review*, **55**(2), 71–93.

Mills, A. (1998), 'To contract or not to contract? Issues for low and middle income countries', *Health Policy Planning*, **13**, 32–40.

Mladovsky, P. and Mossialos, E. (2008), 'A conceptual framework for community-based health insurance in low-income countries: social capital and economic development', *World Development*, **36**, 590–607.

Mossialos, E. and Thomson, S. (2002), 'Voluntary health insurance in the European Union', in E. Mossialos, A. Dixon, J. Figueras and J. Kutzin (eds), *Funding Health Care Options for Europe*, Buckingham: Open University Press, pp. 128–60.

Normand, C. and Busse, R. (2002), 'Social health insurance financing', in E. Mossialos, A. Dixon, J. Figueras and J. Kutzin (eds), *Funding Health Care: Options for Europe*, Buckingham: Open University Press, pp. 59–79.

Pauly, M.V. (2007), 'Insights on demand for private voluntary health insurance in less developed countries', in A.S. Preker, R.M. Scheffler and M. Bassett (eds), *Private Voluntary Health Insurance in Development. Friend or Foe?*, Washington, DC: The World Bank, pp. 25–54.

Pauly, M.V., Zweifel, P., Scheffler, R.M., Preker, A.S. and Bassett, M. (2006), 'Private health insurance in developing countries', *Health Affairs (Millwood)*, **25**, 369–79.

Preker, A., Langenbrunner, J. and M. Jakab (2002), 'Rich–poor differences in health care financing', in D. Dror and A. Preker (eds), *Social Re-insurance: A New Approach to Sustainable Community Health Care Financing*, Washington, DC: The World Bank, pp. 21–36.

Preker, A.S. (2007), 'The evolution of health insurance in developing countries', in A.S. Preker, R.M. Scheffler and M. Bassett (eds), *Private Voluntary Health Insurance in Development. Friend or Foe?*, Washington, DC: The World Bank, pp. 1–22.

Saltman, R.B. (2004), 'Social health insurance in perspective: the challenge of sustaining stability', in R.B. Saltman, R. Busse and J. Figueras (eds), *Social Health Insurance Systems in Western Europe*, Maidenhead: Open University Press, pp. 3–20.

Sandiford, P., Gorter, A. and Salvetto, M. (2002), 'Vouchers for Health. Using voucher schemes for output-based aid', *Public Policy for the Private Sector*, World Bank, Note no. 243.

Schieber, G. and Maeda, A. (1997), 'A curmudgeon's guide to financing health care in developing countries', in G. Schieber (ed.), *Innovations in Health Care Financing: Proceedings of a World Bank Conference, March 10–11, 1997*, Washington DC: The World Bank, pp. 1–38.

Sekhri, N. and Savedoff, W. (2005), 'Private health insurance: implications for developing countries', *Bulletin of the World Health Organization*, **83**, 127–34.

Sekhri, N. and Savedoff, W. (2006), 'Regulating private health insurance to serve the public interest: policy issues for developing countries', *International Journal of Health Planning and Management*, **21**, 357–92.

Thomson, S., Foubister, T. and Mossialos, E. (2009), *Financing Health Care in the European Union. Challenges and Policy Responses*, Copenhagen. WHO on behalf of the European Observatory on Health Systems and Policies.

Travis, P., Bennett, S., Haines, A., Pang, T., Bhutta, Z., Hyder, A.A., Pielemeier, N.R., Mills, A. and Evans, T. (2004), 'Overcoming health-systems constraints to achieve the Millennium Development Goals', *Lancet*, **364**, 900–906.

Van Doorslaer, E., O'Donnell, O., Rannan-Eliya, R.P., Somanathan, A. et al. (2006), 'Effect of payments for health care on poverty estimates in 11 countries in Asia: an analysis of household survey data', *Lancet*, **368**, 1357–64.

Wagstaff, A. (2007), 'Social health insurance reexamined', World Bank Policy Research Working Paper 4111, Washington DC: The World Bank.

Wagstaff, A. (2009), 'Measuring financial protection in health', in Peter C. Smith, Elias Mossialos, Irene Papanicolas and Sheila Leatherman (eds), *Performance Measurement for Health System Improvement: Challenges and Prospects*, Cambridge: Cambridge University Press, pp. 114–37.

World Health Assembly (2005), Resolution 58.33. Geneva: World Health Organization. Available at http://www.who.int/gb/ebwha/pdf_files/WHA58/WHA58_33-en.pdf.

WHO (2000), *World Health Report, 2000: Health Systems: Improving Performance*, Geneva: World Health Organization.

WHO (2005), 'Achieving universal health coverage: developing the health financing system', Technical briefs for policy-makers. Number 1. Geneva: World Health Organization.

WHO (2010), *The World Health Report. Health Systems Financing: The Path to Universal Coverage*, Geneva: WHO.

Xu, K., Evans, D.B., Kawabata, K., Zeramdini, R., Klavus, J. and Murray, C.J. (2003), 'Household catastrophic health expenditure: a multicountry analysis', *Lancet*, **362**, 111–17.

Zhang, L., Wang, H., Wang, L. and Hsiao, W. (2006), 'Social capital and farmer's willingness-to-join a newly established community-based health insurance in rural China', *Health Policy*, **76**, 233–42.

Zweifel, P. (2004), 'Private health insurance in developing countries: supply. Report submitted to the World Bank', Background paper presented at Wharton Impact Conference on Voluntary Health Insurance in Developing Countries, 15–16 March, University of Pennsylvania, USA. http://hc.wharton.upenn.edu/impactconference/index.html, accessed 3 March 2006.

Zweifel, P. and Pauly, M.V. (2007), 'Market outcomes, regulation, and policy recommendations', in A.S. Preker, R.M. Scheffler and M. Bassett (eds), *Private Voluntary Health Insurance in Development. Friend or Foe?*, Washington, DC: World Bank, pp. 115–46.

Zweifel, P., Krey, B.B. and Tagli, M. (2007), 'Supply of private voluntary health insurance in low-income countries', in A.S. Preker, R.M. Scheffler and M. Bassett (eds), *Private Voluntary Health Insurance in Development. Friend or Foe?*, Washington, DC: World Bank, pp. 55–114.

PART IV

PHARMACEUTICALS AND NEW TECHNOLOGIES

11 Technology diffusion in health care: conceptual aspects and evidence
Victoria Serra-Sastre and Alistair McGuire

1. INTRODUCTION

The relevance of technological change in the health care sector has received attention recently as it has become commonly accepted that this is the main component driving the increasing growth in health care expenditure. Technological change in the health care market over the past decades has been rapid, broadening the capacity of patient treatment. One manifestation of this technological change is the actual number of drugs, surgical procedures and medical devices that are introduced every year in the global health care market. However, the introduction of such innovations does not necessarily lead to instantaneous widespread diffusion and there is usually a lapse between an innovation introduction and its extensive use. The diffusion process plays a key role in that it delineates a change in preferences expected to modify the provision of health care services. Despite the significance of the diffusion process as the aspect of technological change that places the innovation into use, diffusion analysis in health care has not received much economic attention.

The aim of this chapter is to provide a follow-up of the analysis of technology diffusion starting from the stylised facts that motivated the interest in technology diffusion. First, the chapter examines technology diffusion in the health care market, providing an overview of those aspects that characterise this context and presenting competing analytical structures. The conceptual and definitional aspects considered in this chapter refer to the different approaches that can be used to examine diffusion and the different types of innovations. The diffusion process plays a key role in that it represents a change in preferences that will then modify the provision of health care services. This discussion will therefore consider the conceptual underpinnings of how diffusion affects the health production function. Second, this chapter presents a review of the literature on the theoretical and empirical sides of technology diffusion in health markets. The objective is to identify those elements of market structure, institutional aspects and technology characteristics that shape diffusion in health care. Given the limited research in this topic, the theoretical and empirical literature review will allow the identification of potential areas of research in diffusion analysis that remain unexplored.

The chapter is structured as follows. The next section discusses the relationship between medical technology and expenditure, and how this motivates diffusion analysis. Section 3 presents and discusses different approaches to the analysis of diffusion as well as presenting the different types of innovations available in health markets. The following two sections refer to the evidence provided in the literature and what can be inferred from this evidence. In particular, the fourth section discusses the different theoretical approaches to the factors that push technology uptake in the health care sector. The fifth section includes a summary of the results found in empirical studies. Section 6 presents the concluding remarks and some policy implications.

2.   MEDICAL TECHNOLOGY AND EXPENDITURE

In a general economic context, technological change brings economic growth through lower input resource usage to produce certain goods with the specific goal of achieving both technical and allocative efficiency. However, the health care market faces medical innovation in a different manner given that new technologies are generally accompanied by a greater new technology input use. Thus the reduction in input and costs expected in the standard production function in other markets is not applicable to the health production function. On the contrary, it is generally the case that new technologies bring along input increases that expand the cost of health production. This effect can be partly explained by an expansive effect whereby the new technology will be used for treating a greater range of patients given that it increases the number of patients eligible for treatment. The cost implications are translated into higher expenditure on the production of health that at an aggregate level implies a large contribution to growing national health care expenditure.

The increasing trend in medical expenditure has been a common pattern observed in developed countries. As pointed out in Chapter 8, health care expenditure per capita growth has outpaced the growth of GDP per capita generally over the past 30 years. Initially, the responsibility for expenditure increase relied on population ageing, higher income or higher insurance generosity. However, it was later recognised that technological change had the highest influence on this trend (Aaron, 1991; Newhouse, 1992, 1993; Fuchs, 1996). Why thus is technology diffusion important? Having a good understanding of the mechanisms that drive diffusion will provide an insight into how innovations are introduced into the market. The relevance of diffusion will thus stem from its link to the changes in the production of health and its relationship with expenditure.

Given the recognised importance of medical technology in health care expenditure growth, the question arising concerns the contribution of technology to this increase. Some empirical studies have quantified this relationship using one of the following two approaches. The first is the residual approach,[1] which measures the technology impact on the average annual growth rate as a residual after accounting for other confounding factors. Among the confounders considered to affect the annual growth rate are population ageing, income levels and changes in insurance demand. Some of the studies using the residual approach report that technology accounts for more than 50 per cent of health care expenditure (Newhouse, 1992; Oxley and MacFarlan, 1994). More recent estimates by Smith et al. (2009) show that technology is responsible for 27 per cent to 48 per cent of annual growth in per capita health spending. An alternative method to the residual approach is the so-called direct approach, which quantifies the relationship between expenditure and the factors considered to determine expenditure using proxies to quantify the technological change factor.[2] Recently, a report by the Australian government's Productivity Commission (2005) linked the contribution of technology to expenditure not only at the aggregated level but also at the level of the individual contribution of particular technologies to expenditure. In all cases new technologies were considered an important contributory factor in increasing health care expenditure.

In the UK, the Wanless report (Wanless, 2001) estimated that in the future the contribution of medical technology to health care expenditure growth would be between two and three percentage points. This seems to contrast with the evidence of the impact of technology on expenditure growth observed in other countries. However, international comparisons may not be appropriate as the UK appears not to have a leading position with respect to technology uptake. Evidence from the Technological Change in Health Care (TECH) research network shows differences across countries in their adoption and diffusion speed (TECH, 2001). The UK is among a group of countries (together with Finland and Norway) that not only has delays in adoption of new technologies but also shows a slow uptake.

Once it has been recognised that technology and expenditure growth are intertwined, the important issue is to identify those elements of technology through which the increase in expenditure may be channelled. Total expenditure on specific treatments that involve the use of new technology follows the standard decomposition in prices and quantities. It has been observed elsewhere (Chapter 8) that increases in expenditure can be attributed to increases in quantities rather than increasing prices. Thus the introduction of medical innovations leads to a more intensive use of the technology explained by an increase in the production possibilities frontier in the production of health. Cutler and McClellan (1998) and Cutler et al. (1998) also find that the vast majority of the growth in expenditure in the treatment for heart attack is derived from the use of new technologies or increasing quantity of existing technologies. In fact, they show that prices are fairly stable for some of the treatments. As such, the key issue is to understand the factors explaining more intensive demand (quantities) of technologies that leads to a diffusion process of medical innovations. Before discussing the factors found in the literature relating to responsibility for diffusion, there are some definitional aspects of diffusion and several types of technology that are worth examining in order to define a framework that contextualises the diffusion analysis.

3. ASPECTS OF TECHNOLOGY DIFFUSION

3.1 Definition of Diffusion

Diffusion of new technologies has been extensively studied in neoclassical economics. It is defined as the spread of the use of the technology across the relevant market in which prospective users (firms) operate. As pointed out by Stoneman (2002, p. 9),

> diffusion concerns issues that are among the more difficult to analyse adequately. Time is involved. Uncertainty is inherent. Change is the main topic. Imperfect markets abound. All such characteristics mean that the analysis of diffusion stands apart from much of the economic textbooks where perfect competition, full information, static models tend to hold sway.

By definition, diffusion is hence inherently dynamic not only in terms of the time path but also in terms of likely modifications to the technology and changes in the market/

industry. In order to understand the nature of diffusion in itself, it is important first to define the concept.

Following the definition given by Stoneman (1983), diffusion is the process by which the new technology is converging towards a threshold. Let x^* be the post-diffusion technology level and x_t the technology usage in period t; thus diffusion is the process and elements that drive this process whereby x_t tends to x^*. If $x_t = x^*$ for any period t, the diffusion is instantaneous. Diffusion can be seen as the accumulation of goods or as the population that owns the technology. If diffusion refers to goods, y^* is the convergence stock of technology and diffusion considers the process by which the stock of technology products y_t moves towards the convergence level. If diffusion is seen as the rate at which individuals purchase the new technology, n^* is the maximum number of individuals in the pool of potential adopters and n_t is the number of individuals owning the technology at period t, the diffusion is the process by which n_t converges to n^*.

This definition of diffusion serves as the basis to differentiate between diffusion as the number of potential adopters that purchase the technology and diffusion as the degree to which the new technology is being used over time by each individual. The first case can be considered as the number of firms adopting the technology in a given market; that is, it represents the first contact of the user with the technology, defining the process as 'inter-firm' diffusion. Using the terminology above the inter-firm level captures the proportion of firms or individuals that have adopted the technology over the total pool of adopters, n_t/n^*. This is equivalent to measuring diffusion as the first contact with the innovation by the pool of potential adopters. Embedded in the definition of inter-firm diffusion is the notion of acceptance across the market. Nevertheless, adoption itself does not necessarily explain how usage evolves after adopters have purchased the new technology. In such an analysis of inter-firm diffusion, the speed of diffusion might not provide an accurate picture of the process itself. Thus, as an alternative, the second case refers to the 'intra-firm' diffusion, which measures the intensity of new technology use. Intra-firm diffusion refers to the rates at which different firms produce goods using the new technology, y_t/y^*.[3] Intra-firm diffusion looks at the individual acceptance of the technology as the proportion of output produced with the new technology. The definition of intra-firm diffusion characterises the diffusion analysis as a process undertaken by the firm and its individual acceptance.[4]

The definition of diffusion in both cases is intrinsically linked to a time dimension; however, there are differences with respect to their location on the timeline.[5] The inter-firm concept is related to the time elapsed between technology availability and time to adoption. Sequentially, after the technology is adopted, intra-firm diffusion is related to the factors that foster an increasing acceptance over time until the technology is well established as input in the production function. The terms adoption and diffusion are generally used interchangeably not only in the health care market but also in other sectors. Nevertheless, the concepts include definitional aspects of measurement that characterise them as separate aspects of the same research area. Thus adoption is closely linked to the inter-firm aspect whereas diffusion would strictly refer to the intra-firm element of the analysis. The distinction between adoption and diffusion is of special relevance within the health care sector. Little attention has been paid to the possibility of firms or hospitals suspending the use of a new innovation. For example, as noted by Sloan et al. (1986), some hospitals disrupted technology use after adoption. As they argue, situations that involve changes in demand may also reflect changes in competitive advantage from superior innovations or changes in the overall market structure.

The diffusion process can be therefore defined as a two-stage process in which first adoption (inter-level) is the initial step and diffusion (intra-level) comprises the second stage. Adoption has been represented above as the number of potential adopters acquiring the innovation over the pool of adopters, n_t/n^*. In practical terms, this has been seen as the decision by the provider to adopt and the factors that induce this decision or as the time to adoption by the provider. The common representation has been seen as the hazard of acquiring the technology depicted by a hazard function of the type $\lambda_i(t) = \lambda_0(t) \cdot \exp(x_i(t) \cdot \beta)$, where the vector $x_i(t)$ represents a number of co-variates assumed to affect the decision. Intra-level diffusion is an indicator of the degree of acceptance of the new technology and can be measured as the speed at which the new technology penetrates the production process. Assuming that the health production function is given by

$$H_t = f(M_t, T_t), \text{ where } T_t = T_{ot} + T_{nt}$$

where H_t is health, M_t refers to medical inputs and T_t refers to specific total stock of technology comprised by T_{ot}, the old technology capital used, and T_{nt}, the new technology capital stock. A measure of intra-firm diffusion is the growth rate of the proportion of new capital over the total capital used in the production function,[6]

$$T_{nt}/T_t = T_{nt}/(T_{ot} + T_{nt})$$

Depending on the nature of the innovation, the intra-firm diffusion will be automatic or progressive.[7] The equation above is expressed as a function of several factors thought to lead this process that account for the increasing proportion of output produced with the innovation. This is the common approach for intra-firm diffusion in non-health markets. However, an alternative to this definition more commonly used in health markets is the representation of the intra-level diffusion analysis as the demand for the new technology in terms of technology volume.

Despite the definitional differences, inter- and intra-firm diffusion have common features. The sigmoid-shaped (S-shaped) curve that commonly represents inter-firm diffusion may also be representative of the intra-firm diffusion path. There is an initial time span where diffusion happens at a slow rate and only a reduced number of early adopters use the technology. The next stage is characterised by quick general adoption, with the number of adopters increasing gradually and a final levelling phase. These stylised facts have been observed in different industries such as engineering, transport and agriculture.[8] The S-shaped curve obtained when plotting time against diffusion shows an inflexion point from a concave to a convex function that captures a slow initial path followed by a faster process, as seen in Figure 11.1. The sigmoid diffusion curve represents the increase in the number of adopters over time when the inter-firm diffusion is under consideration. If the diffusion relates to the intra-firm aspect, the sigmoid curve shows the proportion of output produced with the new technology.

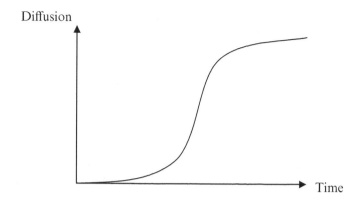

Diffusion

Time

Figure 11.1   S-shaped diffusion curve

3.2   Health Care Technologies

Technologies are generally differentiated according to the nature of the innovation and whether the production function is modified under input change. An innovation is classified as process innovation if the technology introduces a change in the production process. Stoneman (2002) refers to process innovation as any change in equipment, factory structure, inputs used or management methods. It generally involves lower costs. A product innovation is a technology that is a new product in itself. Zweifel and Breyer (1997) distinguish this classification for technologies in the health care market. In addition, they explicitly differentiate the case in which technology refers to an organisational innovation. Stoneman's (1981) definition of process innovations included any management methods. Zweifel and Breyer (1997) separate this out as an additional category of technology. According to them, technology can be classified as process, product or organisation innovation. The last refers to the restructuring of the firm, for example the generation of health maintenance organisations (HMOs) or the separation of two types of specialised care within a hospital. Organisational innovations share the characteristic with process innovation of being technologies that entail a lower cost of production. Drugs and clinical procedures are examples of product innovations. New product innovations in health care have generally higher costs than the alternative existing ones.[9]

Medical technologies also differ in the process they follow in their development, technology evaluation and degree of regulation during the introductory stage. Chang and Luft (1991) sum up the differences in several aspects for three different types of product and process innovations: drugs, devices and procedures. They argue that the cost of development is high for the development of drugs, whereas surgical procedures are associated with low cost as they are generally developed in an academic environment. Drugs and surgical devices are patentable products generally required to go through an approval process, in which the safety of the product is assessed. Medical device innovation is characterised by the diversity of devices produced (Foote, 1991). R&D in the device market is mainly carried out in small companies, where the innovator is typically the decision maker (Kahn, 1991). Chang and Luft (1991) also point out that the diffusion of drugs and devices is at the corporate level whereas the diffusion of surgical procedures is professional.[10] Drugs are more costly to develop than the other technologies and also have a strongly regulated approval process, but patentability provides them with the opportunities to obtain high return rates to investment. The market for pharmaceuticals is based on a strong patent system and characterised by restrictive regulatory policies regarding pre-marketing approval and reimbursement systems (Grabowski, 1991). Finally, surgical procedure innovation is carried out in a context not driven by profit-maximising purposes and regulation is scarce or inexistent; it has a low cost of development and is not patentable (Chang and Luft, 1991).

4.   MODELLING TECHNOLOGY DIFFUSION

As mentioned above, technology diffusion analysis has been motivated by the increasing expenditure growth experienced by developed countries over recent decades. The diffusion process is crucial in order to place technologies in the market. The definitional aspects defined above were set with the objective of offering a framework in which technology diffusion can be considered according to the diffusion stage of interest and the type of technology under consideration. Still, formal considerations of the channels through which diffusion is happening have not been examined in detail. Rather than dealing explicitly with technology diffusion, the conceptual literature is mainly focused on the interaction between health insurance, technological change and adoption of medical innovations. Generally, the models available in the literature adopt the inter-level diffusion approach and examine technological change as a decision process based on the profits and costs of adopting.

There are several agents involved in the diffusion process, namely, patients, providers (physicians and hospitals) and insurance companies. The perspective adopted when analysing their behaviour will differ on the basis of the incentives in favour of technological change that each individual is facing. As a first approach, it is interesting to examine the position of patients in relation to technological change. This has been mainly examined in terms of the influence of third-party reimbursement schemes on patients' behaviour. In particular, the relationship between technological change and welfare under different forms of insurance contracts has been explored (Goddeeris, 1984a, 1984b; Baumgardner, 1991). These approaches consider individual patient behaviour under the standard economic utility function representation. The optimal choice is the result of a maximisation problem given the health production function. Technology (technological change) enters the maximisation problem through the changes that innovation introduces in the production function to induce improvements in the individual's health. In these models the presence of insurance induces moral hazard, which distorts demand for technical advances. These models, however, consider the effect of insurance on the patient's demand for new technology generally and do not specify the technology type under consideration. In a framework in which there is no specific insurance contract arrangement, the patient's allocation of spending among process, product and organisational innovations has been examined (Zweifel and Breyer, 1997). The optimal allocation requires that the marginal health improvement brought by the technology to be larger than the utility loss from reduced income derived from purchasing medical technology.

Although representative of the individual optimal distribution of resources to medical innovations, the models presented above do not consider the decision to adopt a new technology from the perspective of the provider. These are approaches more representative of health markets dominated by private insurance contracts rather than markets highly represented by public insurance coverage. Nevertheless, one of the characteristics of health markets is the presence of asymmetric information that leads to the doctor–patient relationship. Eventually, it is the physician as agent who decides about possible treatments and technologies available, and thus the physician perspective becomes relevant. Along the same lines, it is also important to examine diffusion from the hospital point of view, as it is the organisational unit responsible for technology availability.

Turning to the perspective of diffusion as seen by the health provider, the analysis approached from the physician and hospital side is not very well documented. The process of adoption by physicians can be modelled as a dynamic investment problem. The existence of an existing technology alternative to the new technology implies that there is a process whereby physicians weight the benefits and costs of using the new technology. Factors such as increased income gained from technology adoption, potential gains of extensive technology use in a great number of consultations and reimbursement schemes that are not restrictive in technology are ideal environments with a large scope for adoption (Klausen et al., 1992).[11] There is an important element of technology diffusion that has been at the centre of the attention in diffusion analysis: the uncertainty related to the innovation. Before seeing the potential benefits of adopting the technology, physicians need to invest their effort in an information-seeking process that will provide information on the attributes of the new technology. There is a body of literature that examines diffusion of experience goods of the type of new drugs as a Bayesian learning process (Coscelli and Shum, 2004; Crawford and Shum, 2005). In these models, beliefs in technology quality are updated over time such that experimentation with the innovations brings familiarity with the product and its benefits. In addition, if individual experimentation influences other physicians' technology choices, there might be alternative ways to propagate diffusion of technologies based on colleagues' information derived from self-experimentation such that there is a convergence towards treatment choice (Bikchandani et al., 2001). Physicians learn about colleagues' choice among dosage decisions that can be weighted to converge to a routine practice through the constant learning by physicians.

If physicians are thought to be part of an integrated health care provision system, their decisions for adoption and diffusion are likely to be highly conditioned by the interaction of physicians and the organisation (hospital) for which they are working. In this context, Zweifel (1995) examined differences in hospital adoption of product and process innovations as a joint decision by hospitals and physicians with an integrated approach of the health care system that dominates the diffusion context. Two different settings are examined, the USA, in which there is a maximisation goal in the provision of health care services, and the Western European context, in which hospitals operate under a not-for-profit setting although they receive subsidies from the government. In both types of setting, the adoption of product innovations will be more profitable than the adoption of process innovations. Other types of model look at the behaviour strictly from the hospital side. A strategic timing, game-theoretic approach is used in Schmidt-Dengler (forthcoming) to model the diffusion of magnetic resonance imaging (MRI) with respect to the degree of competition existing in the market.[12] This model suggests that the return to adoption is higher, the smaller the number of adopters. On the other hand, the reduction in costs over time may enhance longer adoption waiting time. In a more general context, Miraldo (2007) looks at the relationship between incentives provided by different hospital reimbursement schemes and diffusion, and the influence that this exerts over the R&D process. The model proposes a mixed or prospective scheme as the optimal reimbursement system in order to enhance the development and adoption of quality-increasing and cost-reducing technologies.

5.   EVIDENCE ON MEDICAL TECHNOLOGY DIFFUSION

The health care sector is constantly undergoing rapid technological change. Newhouse (2002, p. 18) argues that 'rapid change makes knowledge quickly obsolete and places a heavy burden on mechanisms that enable physicians and other health professionals to keep up'. In addition to the rapid technological change, new medical technology is characterised by uncertainty. Usually this uncertainty has been linked to the early stage of adoption; however, this uncertainty may persist after initial adoption as new technologies may experience incremental improvements along their paths of diffusion. Hence technological change cannot be considered as a static issue but as an evolutionary process of learning (Gelijns and Rosenberg, 1994; Gelijns et al., 2001). Different factors have been identified that affect the dissemination of medical innovations. Cutler and McClellan (1996) find six categories to explain technological diffusion: organisational factors, insurance generosity, technology regulations, malpractice pressure, provider interactions and demographic factors. In addition to these factors, Berwick (2003) also identifies the perception of the innovation by the potential adopter as a driver of diffusion. Thus, apart from the contextual factors outlined above, the degree of innovativeness of the technology may also be a key factor in diffusion.

The empirical literature has been largely devoted to the diffusion analysis of product and process innovations rather than organisational innovations. In general, the literature has been devoted to the analysis of physical capital,[13] surgical procedures and new drugs. Most of the research on physical capital and surgical innovations has been approached as a hospital decision process. The diffusion of drugs is either examined at the market level or from the perspective of the individual physician. Variables such as socioeconomic factors of patients, insurance variables or hospital characteristics are frequent in diffusion analysis.

5.1   Main Factors Explaining Diffusion of Physical Capital

The majority of the studies presented here examine the diffusion process as an inter-level process. The different types of physical capital technologies have been generally categorised according to their acquisition costs and classified as 'little-ticket' or 'big-ticket' technologies. The early work by Russell (1977) examined the diffusion rate of five little-ticket technologies using epidemic models.[14] Diffusion of physical capital has been primarily devoted to big-ticket technologies of the type represented by computed tomography (CT) and magnetic resonance imaging (MRI).[15] The diffusion of these types of costly technologies has been shown to be faster for larger hospitals (Baker, 1979; Banta,

1980; Globerman, 1982). Technological value, safety and efficacy, incremental profitability gained from adoption, communication channels and the structure of the medical system account for the bulk of factors explaining MRI diffusion (Hillman et al., 1984). Differences in technology costs and regulatory environments have been identified as factors leading to a slower diffusion path (Hillman and Schwartz, 1985).

The role of the third-party payer in the adoption and diffusion of new medical technologies has focused most of the attention in the research addressing capital-embodied technologies. In general, the generosity of the insurance coverage is positively associated with adoption (Chou et al., 2004). Some evidence suggests that prospective systems restrict technology adoption; however, this also depends on the characteristics of the innovations (Romeo et al., 1984; Lee and Waldman, 1985).[16] The restrictions introduced by prospective systems may change the type of technologies that hospitals will adopt. Lee and Waldman (1985) find stronger evidence about prospective reimbursement making cost-reducing innovations more attractive. Along the same lines, some research has been particularly interested in the effect of managed care on adoption. Managed care refers to schemes designed to reduce utilisation and high costs associated with fee-for-service plans (Baker and Phibbs, 2002). Empirical evidence has shown a consistent and systematic negative relationship between managed care and new capital-embodied technologies (Hill and Wolfe, 1997; Baker and Wheeler, 1998; Baker and Phibbs, 2002; Baker, 2001).[17] Managed care has been shown to achieve the cost-containment objective and to reduce the level of health care expenditure. Nevertheless, evidence on the effect of managed care on health care cost growth is mixed (Chernew et al., 1997; Cutler and Sheiner, 1997).

5.2   Evidence on New Pharmaceuticals Diffusion

Pharmaceuticals represent a large share of the health expenditure bill in most developed countries. In the UK, total expenditure on pharmaceuticals accounted for 12 per cent of total expenditure on health in 2008 (OECD, 2010). In addition, the pharmaceutical market is characterised as highly dynamic in regard to R&D activities and the number of new products launched. According to the Association of the British Pharmaceutical Industry (ABPI), in the UK the market share of medicines that were launched in the previous five years to 2007 accounted for 11 per cent of the market and the R&D activities for the UK industry were 26 per cent of the industry gross output. Despite the relevance of pharmaceuticals in the health care market, drug diffusion analysis has been fairly restricted, partly due to the higher complexity of this market and also partly due to data constraints. Pharmaceutical spending has come with benefits for patients as new drugs have been shown to bring significant improvements in their health outcomes (Lichtenberg, 1996, 2003; Duggan and Evans, 2005). This may lessen demand for further health care services, although results on that front are inconclusive (Lichtenberg, 2001; Duggan, 2005).[18]

In the case of drugs, there is a general concern about the role that product uncertainty has in the diffusion process. This has been the starting point for the analysis of drug diffusion in a number of papers that have approached diffusion analysis emphasizing rather different aspects. In general, information has been accepted as the key to overcoming product uncertainty that leads to drug diffusion. The publication of scientific evidence regarding new drugs has acted as a channel to propagate information, and this has led to increasing sales. Consumption externalities have also been identified as an influential mechanism that mirrors market behaviour, giving information on overall prescription patterns (Azoulay, 2002; Berndt et al., 2003).

A third information channel has been identified, namely, physician self-experience. As part of the learning process in which physicians engage in order to familiarise themselves with the new product, feedback received from actual drug prescription to patients will confer first-hand information. These models have used a Bayesian learning approach as the framework to examine the role of uncertainty and information from self-experience. Informational spillovers from prescription experience define the learning process at the same time that uncertainty is reduced (Coscelli and Shum, 2004; Crawford and Shum, 2005; Chintagunta et al., 2009; Ching, 2010). Any learning process may imply that physicians' investment in product familiarisation will establish persistence in drug prescription that generates a barrier when new products are introduced (Johannesson and Lundin, 2001).[19] Pharmaceuticals are product innovations entailing higher unit cost as compared to alternative existing treatment options. Drug prices have been generally dismissed by physicians, facilitated by the presence of third-party reimbursement and empirical evidence (Hellerstein, 1998; Lundin, 2000). In accordance to that, additional evidence has shown that prices of new pharmaceuticals do not influence prescription behaviour (Johannesson and Lundin, 2001).

5.3   Perspectives on Diffusion of Surgical Procedures

The part of the literature devoted to the analysis of surgical procedures is mainly focused on the hospital decision to adopt (inter-firm-level approach). The exception to that is a study by Sloan et al. (1986), which also looked at the intra-firm level of analysis. Few studies have examined technology adoption decision by the surgeon, despite the shared importance of diffusion analysis examining both hospital and surgeon determinants (Lewit, 1986). From the surgeon's perspective, economic incentives lead to earlier adoption of technologies (Escarce et al., 1995; Escarce, 1996). However, additional factors may enhance the individual adoption of technologies. As such, individuals may learn from peers, inducing the presence of herd behaviour through informational spillovers such that early adopters induce faster adoption by surgeons in the same hospital (Escarce, 1996). When the unit of interest in adoption analysis changes to the hospital level, the variables examined refer more to organisational and regulatory factors of the type of arrangement the hospital has with third-party payers.[20] Diffusion has been shown to be greater the more commercially oriented the insurance market; larger hospitals tend to adopt faster; location or university affiliation has been shown to have a positive impact on adoption and more competitive markets tend to slow diffusion (Sloan et al., 1986; Fendrick et al., 1994).

The case of surgery to treat heart attack has been largely analysed with the aim to identify the source of its expenditure growth, the factors of diffusion and the impact on health outcomes. Diffusion of angioplasty (PTCA) is mainly analysed as an alternative to coronary artery bypass graft (CABG), the former being a less invasive and costly procedure than the latter. Expenditure growth in heart attack care has been attributed to an increase in the number of intensive procedures rather than to an increase in treatment costs (Cutler and McClellan, 1996; Cutler and McClellan, 1998). At the same time, increases in quantities have been articulated to operate at two levels: treatment substitution, referring to the substitution of CABG by PTCA; and expansion effect, which concerns PTCA treatment for a segment of the population not suitable for surgical treatment prior to technological change (Cutler and McClellan, 2001; Cutler and Huckman, 2003).[21] Cutler and McClellan (1996) identify insurance variables, technology regulation and provider interactions as the factors influencing the diffusion of PTCA. The introduction of PTCA has brought improvements in mortality and morbidity rates, offsetting overall expenditure (Cutler et al., 1998; Cutler et al., 1999).

Cross-national comparison of the determinants of technological change for the case of heart attacks is being carried out by the Technological Change in Health Care (TECH) research network.[22] The objective is to study the effect of payment systems, technology regulation, competition and physician supply on the adoption of high-tech (surgical procedures) and low-tech treatments (drugs), and how this affects health outcomes and medical expenditure growth (McClellan and Kessler, 1999; McClellan and Kessler, 2002; TECH, 2001). Three different patterns of diffusion have been identified. The first defines early adoption and fast growth, as represented by the USA and Japan. The second group covers those countries with late adoption and fast growth (Canada, France, Italy, Singapore and Taiwan). The third group comprises those countries with late adoption and slow growth. The UK, Scandinavian countries and Ontario are among the countries in the third group. In the USA, the use of high-tech procedures is the cause of expenditure growth and the effect of regulatory and financial incentives on uptake seems to be minimal (McClellan et al., 2002; Robinson et al., 2002).

6.   CONCLUDING REMARKS AND POLICY IMPLICATIONS

This chapter aimed to present the motivation of the importance of new medical technology diffusion analysis. Two different aspects were presented. The first one refers to the different conceptual aspects regarding technology diffusion to be considered when setting the framework for analysis. The second aspect is related to the evidence presented in the literature on diffusion of several types of medical technologies. The common ground between these two aspects is that they present different available perspectives for analysis and potential areas for future research in this area. Analysis on technology diffusion is fairly limited, given the relevance of technological change on health care expenditure. In general, the evidence presented here is technology specific and generalisations can only be made if there are supporting results that verify general statements on technology. Further research is required into the analysis of diffusion of different innovation types and diffusion in health markets defined by different regulatory environments. With additional analysis, results obtained would contribute to make strong recommendations for policy making.

In general, there is evidence on the benefits derived from the use of new medical technologies. This implies that new technologies may imply higher costs but that this translates into benefits in the form of improved health outcomes. However, for this to happen the crucial stage of technological change is the diffusion stage. Several variables are relevant to diffusion, and their importance should be weighted when designing health policies that will affect the approach taken by providers with regard to new technologies.

Similarly, by, common elements have been identified across technologies to affect largely the adoption (inter-level diffusion) of new technologies. Factors such as structure of health insurance, hospital size or market competition have been shown to hasten technology uptake. As a result, policies that have occupied the agendas of health policy makers in attempts to increase efficiency and reduce costs should consider the role of new technologies and the factors that boost their demand. For instance, policies designed for cost containment may have collateral effects on technology uptake, and this might translate into lower health outcomes as compared to the scenario in which the innovation had diffused more quickly and widely. In the long term this may induce higher costs as the non-use of the medical innovation will not prevent further development of specific health conditions.

NOTES

1. Fuchs (1972) pointed out the role of the 'technology imperative' in the increased demand for health care services using the residual approach to explain demand growth.
2. A description of the two methods can be found in the Productivity Commission report (2005), where the advantages of each method are discussed. The report also offers a summary of the empirical evidence found in studies using these methods.
3. In addition to these two concepts of diffusion, there is also a concept of economy-wide diffusion that involves the analysis as an aggregation of all the industries that could adopt the technology.
4. Note that the inter- and intra-level definitions of diffusion analysis may refer to both individuals and firms.
5. Inter-firm and intra-firm diffusion have been shown to have different importance levels at different stages of the process (Battisti and Stoneman, 2003, 2005).
6. An example in the health sector would be the process by which PTCA is introduced as a treatment for heart attack as opposed to the old technology CABG. Cutler and Huckman (2003) examine the process by which PTCA is replacing CABG.
7. In the first case, the use of the innovation requires immediate substitution of the old by the new technology and output being produced uniquely with the new technology. In this case, the new technology capital will replace the total technology stock and $T_t = T_{nt}$. The majority of technologies will involve a gradual process of substitution in which the new technology will progressively replace the old capital input in the production function. The share of the old technology might grow towards a convergence level in which the new technology completely replaces the old technological capital. In this case the following relation holds: $T_{nt}/(T_{ot} + T_{nt}) = 1$ in $t = t^*$, where t^* represents the terminal date for the substitution process. Alternatively, the new technology might not be designed to fully substitute old-type capital and a certain proportion of the old technology might be required for the production process to take place. If this is the case, there will be growth over time in the share of the new capital in total capital and at the end of the intra-diffusion period: $T_{nt}/(T_{ot} + T_{nt})$ is bounded such that $T_{nt}/T_t \in [0, 1]$.
8. The seminal work by Griliches (1957) on the diffusion of hybrid corn in the USA and the research by Mansfield (1961, 1968) on the diffusion of several industrial technologies first noted the S-shaped diffusion pattern. Griliches (1957) and Mansfield (1961) highlight the significant impact that economic incentives and innovation profitability on technology adoption; however, over time other factors, such as the role of marketing, barriers and regulatory constraints, have been incorporated.
9. Technological change experienced in the health care sector implies that, depending on the type of innovation, the impact on the production function will be defined as embodied or disembodied technological change. Technological change is said to be embodied when the new technology defines a new input set and the production process is transformed. On the contrary, when the production function remains unaltered in the input vector, technological change is said to be disembodied. The analytical computation of embodied technological change is complicated and the analysis in standard production theory is mainly devoted to disembodied technological change. In the disembodied technological change case there is no major change in the production function such that there are no changes in inputs or in the production process (Chambers, 1988). It is important to understand how the new technology might influence the production function. Health technologies differ in their nature, but, as an input in the production process, the effect of the technology might not be quantitative in terms of the amount of inputs required

to produce health but to introduce qualitative differences. If the aim is to achieve a specific level of output (health outcome) using a specific input bundle, the introduction of a new technology that improves the health outcome by being more effective does not change the amount of inputs used. The variation is in the input quality. As such, studying technological change in health care as disembodied technological change does not represent a deviation from reality. Nevertheless, this will depend on the type of technology. Whereas this might be true for product innovations, it may not hold for process and organisational innovations.

10. The diffusion of drugs is corporate when it is considered to occur within a specific sector such as the primary care market. However, drug diffusion is also professional (individual) if the diffusion is assumed to be the result of a number of prescription choices by the individual physician.

11. They consider the process of adoption of dry chemical laboratory equipment by Norwegian physicians within the primary health care sector.

12. In each period, firms decide whether or not to adopt, and they move sequentially. The hospital faces a trade-off between adoption and waiting.

13. Physical capital technology refers to capital-embodied innovations.

14. These models were initially developed to study how infectious diseases spread across populations (Karshenas and Stoneman, 1995). Epidemic models are based on the contact that users have with non-users within a pool of potential users. Over time there is a declining number of non-users and an increasing growth of users. The underlying assumption is that the diffusion process is the result of the distribution of information.

15. International comparisons have also been undertaken regarding the diffusion of big-ticket technologies in the OECD countries (Lázaro and Fitch, 1995). Technologies included in the analysis are CTs, MRIs, extracorporal shock wave lithotripters (ESWLs), cobalt units (CU) and linear accelerators (LAs). Their findings suggest that countries with similar national income and health expenditure have different distribution of technologies and there are within-country differences across technologies.

16. Romeo et al. (1984) consider the effect of prospective reimbursement systems on technology adoption in a context of intra-firm analysis.

17. The effect of managed care may have indirect costs to patients not enrolled in this type of insurance arrangements. Markets with high proportions of HMO share may slow down adoption by health care providers with different financing systems (Baker, 1999).

18. Differences between Duggan (2005) and Lichtenberg (2001) are on whether their studies are drug-specific or cover a wider range of new drugs, respectively. This may be the origin of the disparity in their results. Duggan (2005) argues there is no lower demand for other health care services derived from new drug consumption.

19. Persistence in adoption pattern has been confirmed at more aggregated levels. In the USA, Skinner and Staiger (2005a, 2005b) showed the same adoption patterns at state level for four different types of technologies (new drugs among them) compared to those observed in a much earlier work by Griliches (1957).

20. The regulatory environment and the reimbursement system have been shown to influence diffusion in several directions. Under prospective payment systems there may be incentives to invest in less invasive procedures in order to increase the margin between the payment per procedure and the actual hospital cost (Greenberg et al., 2001). There are other restrictions imposed by the regulator that may affect the adoption and diffusion. Some US states have Certificate of Need (CON) legislation whereby new investments in hospitals need approval from a review board. CON legislation has been shown to change hospital investment composition but not lead to a reduction in technology spending (Salkever and Bice, 1976). CON legislation has been shown to slow diffusion (Caudill et al., 1995); however, this type of regulation does not seem to change technology diffusion in those US states in which this type of legislation has been removed (Conover and Sloan, 1998).

21. Cutler and Huckman (2003) estimate the degree of treatment expansion and substitution of PTCA in New York State for the period 1992–2000. There is a growth in PTCA in the 1980s interpreted as treatment expansion while during the 1990s there is an improvement in PTCA performance that leads to treatment substitution. Increases in PTCA volume implied better health outcomes. Cost-wise, they find that cost increases arise due to higher PTCA volume but that was partly offset by the cost reduction due to the substitution of CABG for PTCA. McGuire et al. (2010) extend Cutler and Huckman's (2003) work to examine the UK case. Two improvements are introduced: the use of medical management to control for the potential bias due to the correlation of unobserved factors with CABG and PTCA; and the hospital as the unit of analysis under consideration. Their findings suggest that the UK has had lower treatment substitution and higher expansion than the USA.

22. Nystedt and Lyttkens (2003) also undertake an international comparison across countries to compare the diffusion trends of carotid endarterectomy use among the elderly. They compare the Swedish system with the USA and Canada. Overall patterns show similar procedure rates, suggesting that differences in health care systems do not affect the pattern of procedure rates.

REFERENCES

Aaron, H.J. (1991), *Serious and Unstable Condition: Financing America's Health Care*, Washington, DC: Brookings Institution.

Azoulay, P. (2002), 'Do pharmaceutical sales respond to scientific evidence?', *Journal of Economics & Management Strategy*, 11, 551–94.

Baker, L.C. (1999), 'Association of managed care market share and health expenditures for fee-for-service medicare patients', *Journal of the American Medical Association*, 281, 432–7.

Baker, L.C. (2001), 'Managed care and technology adoption in health care: evidence from magnetic resonance imaging', *Journal of Health Economics*, 20, 395–421.

Baker, L.C. and C.S. Phibbs (2002), 'Managed care, technology adoption, and health care: the adoption of neonatal intensive care', *The RAND Journal of Economics*, 33, 524–48.

Baker, L.C. and S.K. Wheeler (1998), 'Managed care and technology diffusion: the case of MRI', *Health Affairs*, 17, 195–207.

Baker, S.R. (1979), 'The diffusion of high technology medical innovation: the computed tomography scanner example', *Social Science & Medicine*, 13D, 155–62.

Banta, H.D. (1980), 'The diffusion of the computed tomography (CT) scanner in the United States', *International Journal of Health Services*, 10, 251–69.

Battisti, G. and P. Stoneman (2003), 'Inter- and intra-firm effects in the diffusion of new process technology', *Research Policy*, 32, 1641–55.

Battisti, G. and P. Stoneman (2005), 'The intra-firm diffusion of new process technologies', *International Journal of Industrial Organization*, 23, 1–22.

Baumgardner, J.R. (1991), 'The interaction between forms of insurance contract and types of technical change in medical care', *The RAND Journal of Economics*, 22, 36–53.

Berndt, E.R., R.S. Pindyck and P. Azoulay (2003), 'Consumption externalities and diffusion in pharmaceutical markets: antiulcer drugs', *The Journal of Industrial Economics*, 51(2), 243–70.

Berwick, D.M. (2003), 'Disseminating innovations in health care', *Journal of the American Medical Association*, 289, 1969–75.

Bikhchandani, S., A. Chandra, D. Goldman and I. Welch (2001), 'The economics of iatroepidemics and quakeries: physician learning, informational cascades and geographic variation in medical practice', Paper prepared for the 2001 NBER Summer Institute.

Caudill, S.B., J.M. Ford and D.L. Kaserman (1995), 'Certificate-of-need regulation and the diffusion of innovations: a random coefficient model', *Journal of Applied Econometrics*, 10, 73–8.

Chambers, R.G. (1988), *Applied Production Analysis: A Dual Approach*, Cambridge: Cambridge University Press.

Chang, S.W. and H.S. Luft (1991), 'Reimbursement and the dynamics of surgical procedure innovation', in A.C. Gelijns and E.A. Halm (eds), *The Changing Economics of Medical Technology*, Washington, DC: National Academy Press, pp. 96–162.

Chernew, M., A.M. Fendrick and R.A. Hirth (1997), 'Managed care and medical technology: implications for cost growth', *Health Affairs*, 16, 196–206.

Ching, A.T. (2010), 'Consumer learning and heterogeneity: dynamics of demand for prescription drugs after patent expiration', *International Journal of Industrial Organization*, 28, 619–38.

Chintagunta, P., R. Jiang and G. Jin (2009), 'Information, learning, and drug diffusion: the case of cox-2 inhibitors', *Quantitative Marketing and Economics*, 7, 399–443.

Chou, S.-Y., J.-T. Liu and J.K. Hammitt (2004), 'National health insurance and technology adoption: evidence from Taiwan', *Contemporary Economic Policy*, 22, 26–38.

Conover, C.J. and F.A. Sloan (1998), 'Does removing certificate-of-need regulations lead to a surge in health care spending?', *Journal of Health Politics, Policy and Law*, 23, 455–81.

Coscelli, A. and M. Shum (2004), 'An empirical model of learning and patient spillovers in new drug entry', *Journal of Econometrics*, 122, 213–46.

Crawford, G.S. and M. Shum (2005), 'Uncertainty and learning in pharmaceutical demand', *Econometrica*, 73, 1137–73.

Cutler, D.M. and R.S. Huckman (2003), 'Technological development and medical productivity: the diffusion of angioplasty in New York state', *Journal of Health Economics*, 22, 187–217.

Cutler, D.M. and M. McClellan (1996), 'The determinants of technological change in heart attack treatment', National Bureau of Economic Research WP 5751.

Cutler, D.M. and M.B. McClellan (1998), 'What is technological change?', in D.A. Wise (ed.), *Inquiries in the Economics of Aging. A National Bureau of Economic Research Project Report*, Chicago, IL: University of Chicago Press, ch. 2.

Cutler, D.M. and M.B. McClellan (2001), 'Is technological change in medicine worth it?', *Health Affairs*, 20, 11–29.

Cutler, D.M. and L. Sheiner (1997), 'Managed care and the growth of medical expenditures', National Bureau of Economics Research, WP 6140.

Cutler, D.M., M. McClellan and J.P. Newhouse (1998), 'What has increased medical-care spending bought?', *American Economic Review*, **88**, 132–6.

Cutler, D.M., M. McClellan and J.P. Newhouse (1999), 'The costs and benefits of intensive treatment for cardiovascular disease', in J.E. Triplett (ed.), *Measuring the Prices of Medical Treatments*, Washington, DC: Brookings Institution Press, pp. 34–71.

Duggan, M. (2005), 'Do new prescription drugs pay for themselves?: The case of second-generation antipsychotics', *Journal of Health Economics*, **24**, 1–31.

Duggan, M.G. and W.N. Evans (2005), 'Estimating the impact of medical innovation: the case of HIV antiretroviral treatments', NBER, WP 11109.

Escarce, J. (1996), 'Externalities in hospitals and physician adoption of a new surgical technology: an exploratory analysis', *Journal of Health Economics*, **15**, 715–34.

Escarce, J.J., B.S. Bloom, A.L. Hillman, J.A. Shea and J.S. Schwartz (1995), 'Diffusion of laparoscopic cholecystectomy among general surgeons in the United States', *Medical Care*, **33**, 256–71.

Fendrick, A.M., J.J. Escarce, C. McLane, J.A. Shea and J.S. Schwartz (1994), 'Hospital adoption of laparoscopic cholecystectomy', *Medical Care*, **32**, 1058–63.

Foote, S.B. (1991), 'The impact of public policy on medical device innovation: a case of polyintervention', in A. Gelijns and E. Halm (eds), *The Changing Economics of Medical Technology*, Washington, DC: National Academy Press, pp. 69–88.

Fuchs, V.R. (1972), *Essays in the Economics of Health and Medical Care*, New York: NBER; Columbia University Press.

Fuchs, V.R. (1996), 'Economics, values, and health care reform', *The American Economic Review*, **86**, 1–24.

Gelijns, A. and N. Rosenberg (1994), 'The dynamics of technological change in medicine', *Health Affairs*, **13**, 28–46.

Gelijns, A.C., J.G. Zivin and R.R. Nelson (2001), 'Uncertainty and technological change in medicine', *Journal of Health Politics, Policy and Law*, **26**, 913–24.

Globerman, S. (1982), 'The adoption of computer technology in hospitals', *Journal of Behavioral Economics*, **11**, 67–95.

Goddeeris, J.H. (1984a), 'Insurance and incentives for innovation in medical care', *Southern Economic Journal*, **51**, 530–39.

Goddeeris, J.H. (1984b), 'Medical insurance, technological change, and welfare', *Economic Inquiry*, **22**, 56–67.

Grabowski, H. (1991), 'The changing economics of pharmaceutical research and development', in A. Gelijns and E. Halm (eds), *The Changing Economics of Medical Technology*, Washington, DC: National Academy Press, pp. 35–52.

Greenberg, D., J.G. Peiser, Y. Peterburg and J.S. Pliskin (2001), 'Reimbursement policies, incentives and disincentives to perform laparoscopic surgery in Israel', *Health Policy*, **56**, 49–63.

Griliches, Z. (1957), 'Hybrid corn: an exploration in the economics of technological change', *Econometrica*, **25**, 501–22.

Hellerstein, J.K. (1998), 'The importance of the physician in the generic versus trade-name prescription decision', *The RAND Journal of Economics*, **29**, 108–36.

Hill, S.C. and B.L. Wolfe (1997), 'Testing the Hmo competitive strategy: an analysis of its impact on medical care resources', *Journal of Health Economics*, **16**, 261–86.

Hillman, A.L. and J.S. Schwartz (1985), 'The adoption and diffusion of CT and MRI in the United States. A comparative analysis', *Medical Care*, **23**, 1283–94.

Hillman, B.J., J.D. Winkler, C.E. Phelps, J. Aroesty and A.P. Williams (1984), 'Adoption and diffusion of a new imaging technology: a magnetic resonance imaging prospective', *American Journal of Roentgenology*, **143**, 913–17.

Johannesson, M. and D. Lundin (2001), 'The impact of physician preferences and patient habits on the diffusion of new drugs', Stockholm School of Economics, Working Paper Series in Economics and Finance No. 2001.

Kahn, A. (1991), 'The dynamics of medical device innovation: an innovator's perspective', in A. Gelijns and E. Halm (eds), *The Changing Economics of Medical Technology*, Washington, DC: National Academy Press, pp. 89–95.

Karshenas, M. and P.L. Stoneman (1995), 'Technological diffusion', in P. Stoneman (ed.), *Handbook of the Economics of Innovation and Technological Change*, Oxford: Blackwell, pp. 265–97.

Klausen, L.M., T.E. Olsen and A.E. Risa (1992), 'Technological diffusion in primary health care', *Journal of Health Economics*, **11**, 439–52.

Lázaro, P. and K. Fitch (1995), 'The distribution of "big ticket" medical technologies in OECD countries', *International Journal of Technology Assessment in Health Care*, **11**, 552–70.

Lee, R.H. and D.M. Waldman (1985), 'The diffusion of innovations in hospitals: some econometric considerations', *Journal of Health Economics*, **4**, 373–80.

Lewit, E.M. (1986), 'The diffusion of surgical technology: who's on first?', *Journal of Health Economics*, **5**, 99–102.

Lichtenberg, F.R. (1996), 'Do (more and better) drugs keep people out of hospitals?', *The American Economic Review*, **86**, 384–8.

Lichtenberg, F.R. (2001), 'Are the benefits of newer drugs worth their cost? Evidence from the 1996 MEPS', *Health Affairs*, **20**, 241–51.

Lichtenberg, F.R. (2003), 'Pharmaceutical innovation, mortality reduction, and economic growth', in K.M. Murphy and R.H. Topel (eds), *Measuring the Gains from Medical Research: An Economic Approach*, Chicago, IL and London: The University of Chicago Press, 74–108.

Lundin, D. (2000), 'Moral hazard in physician prescription behavior', *Journal of Health Economics*, **19**, 639–62.

Mansfield, E. (1961), 'Technical change and the rate of imitation', *Econometrica: Journal of the Econometric Society*, **29**, 741–66.

Mansfield, E. (1968), *Industrial Research and Technological Innovation: An Econometric Analysis*, New York: Norton.

McClellan, M. and D. Kessler for the TECH Investigators (1999), 'A global analysis of technological change in health care: the case of heart attacks', *Health Affairs*, **18**, 250–55.

McClellan, M.B. and D.P. Kessler (2002), 'Introduction: a global analysis of technological change in health care, with a focus on heart attacks', in their *Technological Change in Health Care: A Global Analysis of Heart Attack*, Ann Arbor, MI: University of Michigan Press, pp. 1–20.

McClellan, M.B., N. Every, A.M. Garber, P. Heidenreich, M. Hlatky, D.P. Kessler, J.P. Newhouse and O. Saynina (2002), 'Technological change in heart attack care in the United States', in M.B. McClellan and D.P. Kessler (eds), *Technological Change in Health Care: A Global Analysis of Heart Attack*, Ann Arbor, MI: University of Michigan Press, pp. 21–54.

McGuire, A., M. Raikou, F. Windmeijer and V. Serra-Sastre (2010), 'Technology diffusion and health care productivity: angiolpasty in the UK', LSE Health Working Paper Series in Health Policy and Economics.

Miraldo, M. (2007), 'Hospital financing and the development and adoption of new technologies', Centre for Health Economics, University of York, Research Paper 26.

Newhouse, J.P. (1992), 'Medical care costs: how much welfare loss?', *The Journal of Economic Perspectives*, **6**, 3–21.

Newhouse, J.P. (1993), 'An iconoclastic view of health cost containment', *Health Affairs*, **12** (Supplement), 152–71.

Newhouse, J.P. (2002), 'Why is there a quality chasm?', *Health Affairs*, **21**, 13–25.

Nystedt, P. and C.H. Lyttkens (2003), 'Age diffusion never stops? Carotid endarterectomy among the elderly', *Applied Health Economics and Health Policy*, **2**, 3–7.

OECD (2010), Health Data, Paris: OECD.

Oxley, H. and M. MacFarlan (1994), 'Health care reform: controlling spending and increasing efficiency', OECD Economics Depament Working Papers no. 149.

Productivity Commision (2005), 'Impacts of advances in medical technology in Australia', Research Report, Melbourne.

Robinson, M.B., R. Manning, M. Pettigrew, N. Rice, M. Sculpher and T. Sheldon (2002), 'Technological change in heart attack care in England', in M.B. McClellan and D.P. Kessler (eds), *Technological Change in Health Care: A Global Analysis of Heart Attack*, Ann Arbor, MI: University of Michigan Press, pp. 268–88.

Romeo, A.A., J.L. Wagner and R.H. Lee (1984), 'Prospective reimbursement and the diffusion of new technologies in hospitals', *Journal of Health Economics*, **3**, 1–24.

Russell, L.B. (1977), 'The diffusion of hospital practices: some econometric evidence', *Journal of Human Resources*, **12**, 482–502.

Salkever, D.S. and T.W. Bice (1976), 'The impact of certificate-of-need controls on hospital investment', *Milbank Memorial Fund Quarterly Health & Society*, **54**, 185–214.

Schmidt-Dengler, P. (forthcoming), 'The timing of new technology adoption: the case of MRI'.

Skinner, J. and D. Staiger (2005a), 'The diffusion of health care technology', *Mimeo*, Dartmouth College.

Skinner, J. and D. Staiger (2005b), 'Technology adoption from hybrid corn to beta blockers', NBER, WP 11251.

Sloan, F.A., J. Valvona, J.M. Perrin and K.W. Adamache (1986), 'Diffusion of surgical technology: an exploratory study', *Journal of Health Economics*, **5**, 31–61.

Smith, S., J.P. Newhouse and M.S. Freeland (2009), 'Income, insurance, and technology: why does health spending outpace economic growth?', *Health Affairs*, **28**, 1276–84.

Stoneman, P. (1981), 'Intra-firm diffusion, Bayesian learning and profitability', *The Economic Journal*, **91**, 375–88.

Stoneman, P. (1983), *The Economic Analysis of Technological Change*, Oxford: Oxford University Press.

Stoneman, P. (2002), *The Economics of Technological Diffusion*, Oxford: Blackwell Publishers.
Stoneman, P. and N.J. Ireland (1983), 'The role of supply factors in the diffusion of new process technology', *The Economic Journal*, **93**, 66–78.
TECH (2001), 'Technological change around the world: evidence from heart attack care', *Health Affairs*, **20**, 25–42.
Wanless, D. (2001), 'Securing our future health: taking a long-term view', Interim Report, HM Treasury, London.
Zweifel, P. (1995), 'Diffusion of hospital innovations in different institutional settings', *International Journal of the Economics of Business*, **2**, 465–83.
Zweifel, P. and F. Breyer (1997), *Health Economics*, New York: Oxford University Press.

12 Do international launch strategies of pharmaceutical corporations respond to changes in the regulatory environment?

Nebibe Varol, Joan Costa-Font and Alistair McGuire

1. INTRODUCTION

The purpose of this chapter is to investigate how the regulatory environment impinged on the launch strategies of pharmaceutical corporations across the main OECD markets during 1960–2008. How regulation affects adoption of innovation is a question open to empirical scrutiny, especially in highly regulated industries such as the pharmaceutical industry where products and processes are protected by intellectual property rights. Although several studies have been carried out, the existing evidence in the pharmaceutical context is limited. Particularly important is the role of the timing of a new drug launch, which is typically carried out by international companies following some corporate strategy. Paradoxically, the impact of regulation on generic products within a therapeutic group has received even less attention. Expected proliferation of bioequivalent products in the near future, rising concerns over cost containment and the resulting push for genericisation makes timing of generic launch a question of interest for both the pharmaceutical industry and the policy makers.

Normally, firms facing a competitive environment would ideally like to launch new chemical entities (NCE) as quickly as possible into several markets while the product is still under patent protection to amortise the substantial R&D outlays. However, there are at least two regulatory hurdles that firms have to overcome before commercialising a new drug product. The first hurdle is that manufacturers have to prove the threefold requirement of quality, safety and efficacy of new molecules, which is estimated to take around ten years of pre-clinical and clinical research (Permanand, 2006). The second hurdle typically includes the review of the new product dossier by the regulatory authority (FDA,[1] EMEA[2] or any national authority) and approval of marketing authorisation (MA). Finally, the third hurdle following marketing approval is pricing and reimbursement (P&R), which involves negotiations between manufacturers and P&R authorities regarding the price of the new product and its reimbursement status. Price regulation can arguably delay launch through the negotiation processes alongside the resulting firm strategies of delaying or forgoing launch in low-priced markets[3] (Danzon et al., 2005; Kyle, 2007a). Non-homogeneity in these hurdles across markets results in launch delays, with welfare implications for the consumer and the pharmaceutical producer.

Lags in adoption of new pharmaceutical innovations may affect consumer welfare through impaired access to new drug products, in particular cost-effective products. Empirical evidence shows that lack of access to new drugs leads to compromises in health outcomes (Schöffski, 2002), shifts volume to older molecules of lower therapeutic value (Danzon and Ketcham, 2004) and results in higher expenditures on other forms of medical care and compromises in quality of health care (Kessler, 2004; Wertheimer and Santella, 2004). Innovative medications offer economic benefits through fewer work days missed and lives saved (Lichtenberg, 1996; Hassett, 2004; Lichtenberg, 2005). Delays in the launch of new molecules could be costly to the pharmaceutical industry through reduced market exclusivity periods, lower returns to R&D and eventually fewer innovations.[4]

Generic products are by definition bioequivalent, and therefore perfect substitutes (on objective quality grounds) to their branded counterparts that usually claim substantial price mark-ups over the marginal cost of production.[5] Generic entry following patent expiry is argued to enhance efficiency and competition in the drug market; however, the main hurdle before generic entry is the cost of bioequivalence tests which have been estimated to be significantly cheaper than the average costs of safety and clinical evaluation.[6] Generic imitations largely free-ride on the R&D efforts of originator firms, which enables them to compete based solely on price. Timely adoption of generic products, therefore, carries significant importance to improve allocative efficiency and stimulate competition (DG Competition, 2009).

The analysis here draws upon an extensive database on the timing and entry of new pharmaceutical molecules along with the entry of bioequivalent competitors. The chapter makes several contributions to the literature on regulation and changes in corporate behaviour. First, previous studies do not use such an extensive database, so that results are likely to be limited to a specific, small time period. Second, one of the most important dimensions of market dynamics, the timing dimension of new and old products, has traditionally been left out of the analysis of drugs. Finally, the chapter assesses corporate behaviour with respect to two main regulatory changes that substantially reshaped the barriers to entry: (1) the US Hatch Waxman Act in 1984;[7] (2) the establishment of the European Medicines Agency (EMEA) in 1995 along with the adoption of the centralised procedure that grants a Community marketing authorisation.

This chapter is organised as follows: Section 2 describes the data and methods used in the analysis; Section 3 discusses the results of the analysis along with corresponding regulatory triggers; and finally Section 4 concludes.

2.   DATA AND METHODS

2.1   Data

The IMS data used in the analysis contain quarterly sales in dollars and standard units for molecules from 14 different ATC groups and 20 countries.[8, 9] Additional data fields include global and local launch date of drug products, pharmaceutical form, anatomic therapeutic class of the product, the distribution channel of sales (hospital versus retail) and patent protection status of the drug. The markets in the data set comprise the majority of the global pharmaceutical sales and are all based in the OECD except for South Africa. Results are reported for the main seven pharmaceutical markets comprising of the USA, Japan and the EU-5 (namely the UK, Germany, France, Italy and Spain).

Multi-country drug lag studies apply several criteria to identify significant NCEs. Some consider molecules that have launched in the USA and/or the UK as an indication

Table 12.1   Number of molecules by period of global launch

	US & UK (all)	US & UK (generic)
1960–84	385	214
1984–95	194	90
1995–2008	266	46
Total	845	350

of therapeutic significance and potential for global launch (Parker, 1984; Danzon et al., 2005). Several studies find a direct relationship between the therapeutic contribution of a new drug and its likelihood of achieving widespread introduction (Parker, 1984; Barral, 1985). This finding suggests that most one-market NCEs do not simply disperse among countries more slowly than others, but will never be widely available due to their marginal therapeutic advantages. Molecules that have not launched in the USA and the UK are excluded to avoid any potential bias due to one-market molecules and to ensure that molecules with potential global importance are considered. Hereafter, this potentially global set of molecules is referred as US & UK molecules.

In addition, a global molecule set comprising molecules that have diffused to all 20 markets on the database is defined. These two sets provide a means to compare relative drug lags for molecules with different levels of international spread and to assess whether there is a systematic difference between the two. For brevity, the results for US & UK molecules only are reported. Findings for global molecules are broadly in line with the estimates for US & UK molecules.

Table 12.1 presents the breakdown of molecules by the period of global launch. The majority of the molecules had their global launch during 1960–84. In total, 845 molecules were launched in the USA and the UK since 1960, 200 of which diffused to all markets. Only 350 of the molecules had a generic launch in both the USA and the UK. The USA, the UK, Germany, France, Canada and Switzerland are among countries that had the greatest number of launches, whereas Portugal, Japan, Spain, Belgium, Sweden and Turkey had the least number of launches. The highest number of generic molecule launches occurred in the USA, the UK, Germany, Canada, Poland, Australia and the Netherlands.

2.2   Definitions

Launch times are the most important information to feed a non-parametric survival analysis. The advantage of non-parametric approaches lies in that it provides a good fit for any distribution without any prior assumptions about the functional form of the failure time. The analysis takes place at the molecule level, whereby subjects are defined as potential molecule-country launches. The failure event is interpreted as the launch of a given molecule in the destination market. The failure indicator is set to one if the molecule launches in the given market and to zero if the molecule is censored (i.e. does not launch by the end of the observation period, 2008).[10]

The time-to-failure event is defined as the time lapse from the first global launch date of the molecule (the onset of risk) to the date of launch in a particular country (the failure). The global launch date is the first date the molecule launched in any country in the IMS database. Since drug products may differ with respect to the local launching corporation, dosage and form, the local launch date of each molecule is defined as the minimum launch date among drug products of the same molecule in individual countries. Missing global launch dates are proxied by the minimum local launch date across all 20 markets. Relative launch lags are defined as the difference between the global launch date and the country-specific local launch date.[11] Differential timing of launch could be due to variations in market authorisation dates or delays in pricing and reimbursement procedures as well as strategic firm delays to avoid threats of price spillovers across markets (Danzon et al., 2005). The global launch date is used to define the onset of risk for molecule launches due to unavailability of data to isolate the delays due to these components.

The risk onset in the case of pharmaceutical imitation is defined as the date when the first generic product of a given molecule launched in any of the 20 markets. It would have been informative to carry out the analysis by considering generic delays following the local protection expiry dates. This approach was not followed because expiry date is available only in 3 per cent of the data, and in 56 per cent of these cases expiry date exceeds local launch by more than a year, which could be due to the presence of copy products in some markets, launch of pseudogenerics[12] (also known as authorised generics) or errors in reporting the expiry dates.

Kaplan–Meier (KM) estimates of the survivor function $S(t)$ at time t are obtained using STATA 10. Due to the significant right-skewed nature of failure time distributions, inferences are based primarily on the median delays. The median survival times are estimated in each market for molecules by period of entry into the risk set, that is, first global launch during 1960–84, 1984–95 and 1995–2008. This framework allows the comparison of the evolution of relative launch lags both across countries and over time. Since the cut-off points of 1984 and 1995 correspond to two major regulatory changes in the USA and Europe, their impact on timing of launch can be assessed comparatively using medians before and after these cut-off values.

3. RESULTS

3.1 Trends in the Adoption of Pharmaceutical Innovation

3.1.1 Evolution of median delays over decades
Figure 12.1 shows the trend in overall median delays for US & UK molecules across the 20 markets from 1960 to 2008. A marked acceleration in the international diffusion speed of pharmaceuticals is observed. While the overall median is 11 years for molecules with a global launch in 1960–85, the median drops to 4 and 2 years for molecules that launched in 1984–95 and 1995–2008 respectively (see Table 12A.1 in the Appendix for the medians in individual countries over time). The significance of this trend is tested by a Cox proportional hazard model that controls for the period of global launch. Coefficients are estimated both by a Cox model with country fixed effects and a random effects Cox model with shared frailties for the same country launches. Both the fixed effects and the random effects indicate that hazard of launch[13] is significantly higher for molecules that

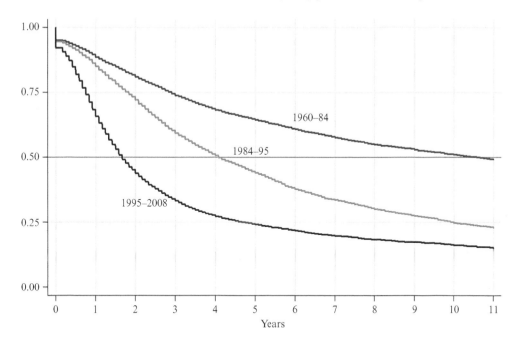

Figure 12.1   Kaplan–Meier (KM) survival estimates by period of first launch, US & UK molecules

first launched during 1995–2008 compared to 1984–95. Similarly, the hazard is higher for molecules that launched in 1984–95 compared to 1960–84. The Hausman test that compares the fixed and random effects specifications indicates that the fixed effects model is the correct specification (p-value: 0.0135). Based on the fixed effects specification, launch in 1960–84 reduces the hazard by 48 per cent and launch in 1995–2008 increases the hazard by 82 per cent, both compared to launch in 1984–95.

The acceleration of the international diffusion of pharmaceutical products may be attributed to the evolution in barriers to entry as a result of changes in the regulatory environment and an increasingly global and interdependent market environment. The increasing international reach of pharmaceutical corporations as evidenced by the spread of the manufacturing, marketing and innovative R&D activities to different countries has overcome prior geographical barriers. Harmonisation of safety and efficacy and marketing authorisation requirements across markets has contributed to a reduction in regulatory costs (Busfield, 2003). The following sections present the survival estimates for individual markets in the biggest seven pharmaceutical markets and describe in more detail the regulatory changes that may explain the evolutionary trend in the lags.

3.1.2   1960–84: stringency in MA regulations and the US drug lag
The Thalidomide tragedy in the late 1950s, which caused congenital anomalies in babies and a degenerative nerve disorder in pregnant women, marked the beginning of a new era in modern medicine regulation. Until the early 1960s most countries except the Nordic countries and the USA had no independent safety and efficacy protocols for

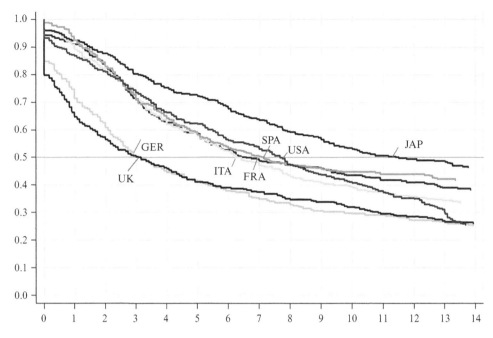

Figure 12.2   Kaplan–Meier (KM) survival estimates in years, molecules with global launch during 1960–84

new drugs. The USA had a regulatory office for pharmaceuticals, the FDA, which was empowered to license medicines subject to certain safety standards. US drug companies had to show only the safety of their new products before 1960. However, in 1962 the US Kefauver Harris Amendments introduced an additional proof-of-efficacy requirement as a response to the Thalidomide disaster. Other countries in Europe aligned their marketing, authorising procedures for increased safety and efficacy only in the late 1960s and early 1970s (Permanand, 2006).

The debate about launch delays extends back to the 1960s, when the main concern was the significant US drug lag compared to the main EU markets, mainly as a result of the more stringent US regulations. Wardell, a pharmacologist, coined the term 'drug lag' and increased awareness of the unavailability of new drugs in the USA, and stressed that the delay affected therapeutically important drugs as well (Wardell, 1973, 1974, 1978). Later studies by Grabowski (1980), Berlin and Jonsson (1986) and Kaitin et al. (1989) confirmed the findings of Wardell.

The survival estimates in this study for molecules that first launched during 1960–84 confirm findings of the early literature that the US market was relatively disadvantaged for the timely adoption of pharmaceutical innovations as a result of much stricter requirements for regulatory approval. The survival graph in Figure 12.2 shows $S(t)$, the probability that molecule launch in a given country occurs after t years following global launch, conditional on the fact that the molecule has not launched in that country up to time t. Hence it takes longer for countries with a higher survival curve to adopt new pharmaceutical innovations. The median survival time, the time point at which half of the molecule candidates have launched, is given by the *t*-value where the survival probability is 0.5.

During 1960–84, Europe is found to be leading in the introduction of pharmaceutical innovation. As expected, free price countries such as the UK and Germany are leading markets, with a median delay of three years, followed by Italy, France and Spain with a corresponding lag of 3.5–4 years. The US lags behind the slowest European market by about half a year. Japan has the most dramatic delay of 12 years, which can be attributed to geographical barriers and the predominantly domestic nature of the market, especially in a period when the global expansion of pharmaceutical corporations was relatively limited.

3.1.3   1984–95: the US Hatch–Waxman Act and stimulus for innovation

The Hatch–Waxman Act, also known as the Drug Price Competition and Patent Term Restoration Act of 1984, was enacted to compensate for the loss in effective patent life during drug development. The Act extended pharmaceutical patents for the time lost in clinical testing and regulatory review, but the entire patent term restored was restricted to five years and the term of the restored patent following FDA approval was restricted to 14 years. In addition, the Act introduced a five-year market exclusivity period for new molecular entities (NMEs) such that once an NME is approved a generic manufacturer cannot submit an application until five years after the approval of the pioneer and thus cannot enter the market for at least five years. These amendments enabled pharmaceutical innovators to recoup some of the revenue losses due to regulatory delay after 1962. The main aim of the Act, however, was to maintain incentives for innovation while ensuring quick generic entry. Although the impact on the brand-name drugs is somewhat contentious, data from the literature suggest that the stimulation for innovation resulted in increased R&D funding and R&D intensity (Branes, 2007).

Survival estimates in this study indicate a stark improvement in the USA for the timing of new product launches *vis-à-vis* Europe (Figure 12.3). The median delay in the USA decreased from about eight years to three years following the enactment of the Act, whereas the corresponding decrease in the leading markets of UK and Germany was on the order of one year only. While the USA was the second-slowest market to adopt new pharmaceutical molecules in 1960–84, after the 1984 Act the USA becomes one of the leading markets, along with the UK and Germany. The estimates present a clear indication that the 1984 Act has generated a more favourable environment for market entry in the USA and suggests an increase in overall R&D activity in the US pharmaceutical industry.

The remaining markets in Europe also experience faster introductions after 1984. In particular, the medians in France and Italy decrease by three years (to about 3.5 years). The one-year reduction in the Spanish median delay is more modest and can be partially attributed to the lack of product patent protection for new pharmaceuticals before ratification of the Agreement on Trade Related Aspects of Intellectual Property Rights (TRIPS) in 1995. Overall, Spain and Japan emerge as the slowest adopters following the 1984 Act. Local clinical trial requirements are the core factor for the Japanese drug lag and the exclusion of foreign corporations from the Japanese market. According to a study that analyses the Japanese lag during 1981–93, the second influential factor is the

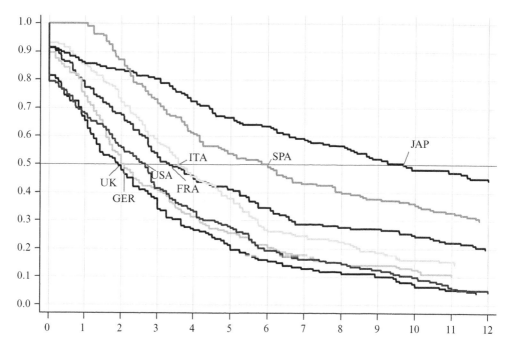

Figure 12.3   Kaplan–Meier (KM) survival estimates in years, molecules with global launch during 1984–95

price regulations since 1981 that sharply lowered launch prices and the life-cycle sales of drugs launched into Japan (Thomas, 2001).

Patent term restoration in Europe was enacted only eight years following the 1984 Act in the USA. In 1992, the Supplementary Protection Certificate (SPC) extended the protection period of pharmaceutical products in the European Community (EC) by five years following patent expiry or 15 years of protection from the date of first market authorisation in the EC, instead of 20 years after patent application, as under the European Patent Convention.[14] This prolonged the profit life of products as drug sales are generally highest during the period of market exclusivity. In addition, the SPC prevented generic companies from engaging in R&D prior to patent expiry, which essentially ensured a longer shelf-life for branded products and provided stimulus for innovation. The relative delay in providing financial stimulus for innovation through patent term restoration in the EU could be an additional factor that explains the drastic improvement in the timing of new product launches in the USA *vis-à-vis* Europe during 1984–95.

3.1.4   1995–2008: EMEA and harmonisation across the globe

The set-up of a single market in 1993 and a common currency in 1999 (when exchange rates were pegged) ensured free movement of people, goods and services within the EU. Since then, market authorisation has been streamlined by the establishment of the European Medicines Agency (EMEA) in 1995, although a complete harmonisation of the pharmaceutical market has not taken place. This was a significant step to speed up approval times across Europe, which had begun to suffer from an increasing number

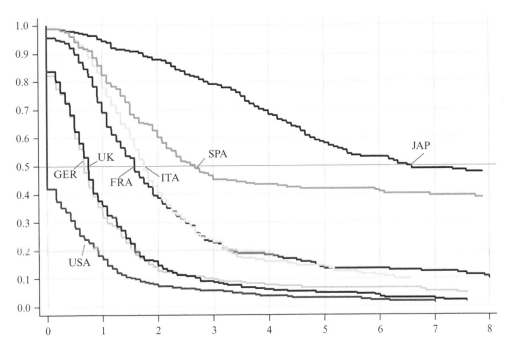

Figure 12.4   Kaplan–Meier (KM) survival estimates in years, molecules with global launch during 1995–2008

of applications as the industry grew and technical and scientific issues became more complex. In addition, EU Directive 2004/27/EC introduced a uniform level of data protection for ten years across the EU and precluded the launch of the generic copy until the expiry of the ten-year period.

A centralised approval procedure, which grants a Community-wide authorisation valid in all member states, would increase efficiency by obviating the duplication of effort through a single market authorisation process and reducing the annual expenditure of drug firms to get separate approvals from individual member countries. The centralised procedure, however, does not apply to all products. It is mandatory for all biotechnology processes and optional for innovative chemical drugs provided the product offers a significant therapeutic, scientific or technical innovation.[15]

After 1990, the pharmaceutical industry witnessed further harmonisation efforts. The TRIPS Agreement in 1994 strengthened intellectual property rights and provided significant financial incentives for companies by blocking generic competition until the expiry of the 20 years' patent life and by extending the scope of patent protection to both products and processes (WTO OMC, 2003). Similarly, the International Conference on Harmonisation of Technical Requirements for Registration of Pharmaceuticals for Human Use (ICH) has aimed to achieve greater harmonisation in the application of technical guidelines and requirements for product registration across the EU, the USA and Japan to reduce or obviate the need of duplicative testing in the R&D stage.[16]

Figure 12.4 shows that the median delays continued to decrease throughout 1995–2008 as a response to the harmonisation efforts across the biggest seven pharmaceutical

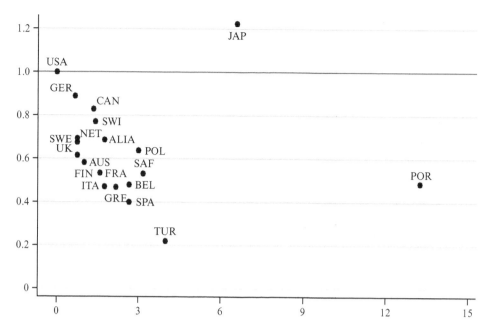

Figure 12.5   2004 price index (US = 1) vs median delay (yrs), US & UK molecules
            during 1995–2008

markets, yet the differential delays have not been eliminated totally.[17] Most of the molecules launch immediately in the USA followed by launch in the free-priced European markets of Germany and the UK within one year. The USA emerges as the most favourable market because of high profit potentials. This is because the USA has the largest market size and a more liberal pricing environment compared to other OECD markets that employ some form of price control, either in the form of statutory pricing whereby the price is set on a regulatory basis or through price negotiations (Vogler, 2008). Stringent price controls have been criticised for having negative implications on the extent and timing of launch via knock-on effects on foreign markets through external referencing and parallel trade within the EU; however, the available evidence is limited (Danzon and Epstein, 2005; Kyle, 2007a; Danzon and Epstein, 2008).

The relative launch delays in Europe suggest an ordering with respect to price levels of pharmaceutical products. Figure 12.5 illustrates the correlation between median delays and the bilateral price indexes with respect to US prices for 2004.[18] The correlation is −0.47 and is significant at the 0.01 level. France and Italy seem to have a comparable speed of launch, with a median delay of around two years. The median lag in Spain has decreased compared to 1984–95 but it still lags about a year behind France and Italy. The lack of product patent protection for new pharmaceuticals before EU membership contributes to launch delays in Spain. EU accession in 1986 required Spain to comply with the European Patent Convention (EPC), which allowed the patentability of both products and processes. Spain enacted a new patent law in 1986 that introduced patent protection for pharmaceuticals. However, effective patentability was delayed until 7 October 1992 through Reservation under Article 167 of the EPC, which essentially meant that pharmaceutical and chemical products could not be patented in Spain before 7 October 1992. In 1995, Spain ratified the TRIPS Agreement, which substantially changed the patent protection landscape.[19] In addition, Spain is one of the major parallel exporters in the EU due to its relatively lower drug prices, which are further pushed downwards by unilateral price cuts imposed on pharmaceutical prices. The delay in Spain, therefore, is consistent with pharmaceutical firm strategies to avoid parallel trade as suggested by Kyle (2007b).

The Japanese drug lag extends to this period as well, although the median Japanese delay decreases by two years with respect to the previous period. This is paradoxical given the international competitiveness of numerous Japanese high-tech industries including electronics and automobiles during the 1990s. The Japanese pharmaceutical market is the second-largest market in the world and offers a great profit potential because of a large market size and relatively high drug prices (see Figure 12.5). Nevertheless, the Japanese pharmaceutical industry remains predominantly domestic and uncompetitive.

Japanese regulations for new drug approval have required Japanese clinical data for evaluating the efficacy and safety of the drug even if foreign clinical data are available due to racial and ethnic variations in responses to medicines. In the past, all three phases of clinical trials had to be carried out on the Japanese population, which has driven launch delays in addition to other factors such as language barriers and longer times for patient enrolment in clinical trials. In 1998, Japan adopted the ICH E5 guideline entitled 'Ethnic Factors in the Acceptability of Foreign Clinical Data', which recommends the use of foreign clinical data for new drug approval if there is one additional bridging study[20] showing that the drug will behave similarly in the Japanese population. According to Uyama et al. (2005), new drug approvals based on a bridging strategy in Japan have increased from 3.2 per cent in 1999 to 25 per cent in 2003. Tabata and Albani (2008) report that companies are increasingly trying to leverage their operations globally in order to take advantage of the Japanese efforts to comply with the trend for globalising clinical trials (Tabata and Albani, 2008). These developments suggest that the drug lag in Japan may decrease over the next years (Uyama et al., 2005).

Ranking countries by median lags, countries may be characterised as leaders (the USA, the UK, Germany, Sweden, the Netherlands, Finland, Austria and Switzerland) and laggards (Belgium, Greece, South Africa, Poland, Portugal and Turkey). The remaining countries (France, Canada, Italy, Australia and Spain) rank as intermediaries, with the rank dependent on the period and extent of global launch. The laggards and leaders, as defined by countries with median lags above and below the overall delays, are similar for the global and the US & UK molecules; however, the extent of the relative lag is shorter for the truly global molecules, as is expected because global molecules have diffused to all markets and have non-censored survival times. Similarly, launch in all markets may indicate higher therapeutic or commercial importance at the product level.

3.1.5   EMEA sub-analysis
Differences in the survival behaviour among the EU markets in Figure 12.4 indicate that pharmaceutical firms have adopted different launch strategies across markets in the EU and that efforts of harmonisation in market authorisation procedures have not eliminated the differentials in timing of launch across European countries. Sub-analysis for the EU countries[21] is carried out to further investigate the impact of the establishment of a centralised regulatory procedure in the EU. In order to compare relative delays for

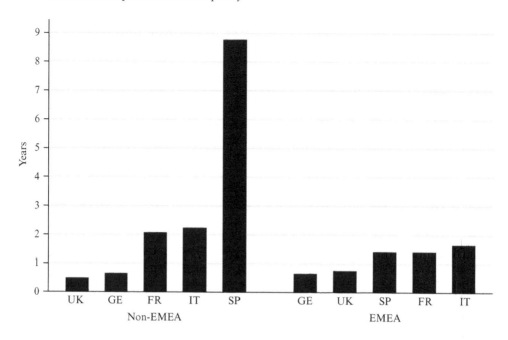

Figure 12.6   Median delays for central vs non-central molecules in EU-5

molecules that obtained centralised approval (central molecules) with those that did not (non-central molecules), data were collected for all centrally approved molecules from the EMEA website (the EMEA publishes information following the grant of a Marketing Authorisation as a European Public Assessment Report[22]). This information was combined with the IMS database to estimate delays within the EU for molecules with a first global launch post-1995 (see Figure 12.6[23]).

There is a statistically significant difference in launch behaviours between the central and non-central molecules (*p*-value: 0.000 for the test of the null hypothesis that the survival behaviours of EMEA and non-EMEA molecules are identical). The effectiveness of a more streamlined authorisation is demonstrated by the lower variation in launch timing for EMEA molecules compared to molecules that did not go through the centralised procedure. The median delay for non-central molecules is greater by more than two years compared to the median delay of central molecules, which is on the order of one year. The faster diffusion of centrally approved molecules can be attributed to the elimination of differentials in regulatory approval times as well as a potentially higher therapeutic/commercial value of the centrally approved drugs.

Central approval speeds up the introduction of molecules in laggard countries such as France, Italy and Spain. Spain exhibits the most dramatic reduction in median delays – a reduction from 5 years to 1.5 years – among the five main European pharmaceutical markets due to central approval. For France and Italy the reduction is on the order of half a year only. The centralised EU procedure is compulsory for all medicinal products derived from biotechnology and other high-technology processes. If the product does not belong to the designated disease categories[24] for central approval, companies can

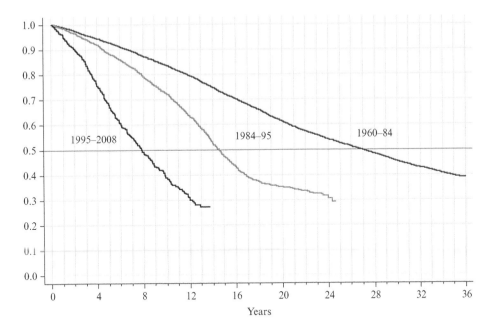

Figure 12.7   Kaplan–Meier (KM) survival estimates by first launch period, generic molecules

submit an application for a centralised marketing authorisation, provided the product offers a significant therapeutic, scientific or technical innovation.[25] A more homogeneous cross-country launch for central molecules across the EU indicates that on average European patients have more equitable access to drugs that have priority from a health policy perspective – at least to the extent that these drugs are diffused at comparable times (the take-up and access post-launch may introduce further differentials in access due to differences in reimbursement policies as well as cultural factors).

3.2   Trends in the Adoption of Generic Products

The lags in generic entry across countries depend on differentials in patent expiry dates or market exclusivity as well as originator firm strategies to block or delay generic competition. Due to unavailability of data to control for patent expiry dates or originator firm actions, the estimates provide generic lags as the time elapsed between the first global generic product launch and local generic launch for a given molecule–country pair. This measure therefore provides only a relative measure of differentials in the timing of generic availability across countries.

3.2.1   Evolution of median delays over decades
The trend in overall median delays for generic molecules that launched in both the USA and the UK from 1960 to 2008 is similar to the case in the cross-country diffusion of pharmaceutical innovation; the diffusion of imitative pharmaceutical has accelerated over time (see Figure 12.7). In each period, medians are reduced by half compared to

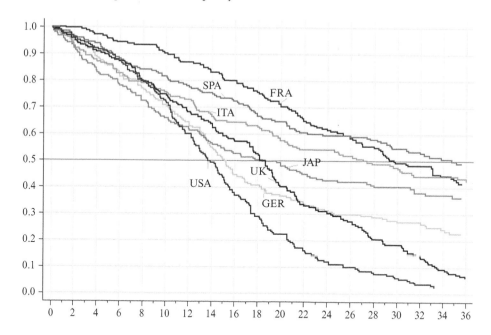

*Figure 12.8   Kaplan–Meier (KM) survival estimates in years, US & UK generic
molecules with first launch during 1960–84*

the previous period. The overall median delay has decreased from 26 to 14.5 years from
1960–84 to 1984–95 and to eight years during 1995–2008.

In parallel with the case with innovative molecules, fixed and random effect Cox
estimates for the impact of the period of first launch indicate that generics launched
significantly faster after 1984. The Hausman test comparing fixed and random effects
indicates that the shared frailty specification is correct (p-value 0.154). First launch
during 1984–95 is associated with a 2.5 times faster hazard rate compared to first launch
during 1960–84, and first launch during 1995–2008 is associated with a 6.5 times faster
hazard rate compared to first launch during 1960–84. The significance of the difference in the median delays across decades can also be inferred from the non-intersecting
confidence intervals of medians estimated by STATA (see Appendix Table 12A.2). The
acceleration in generic adoption over time can be mainly attributed to new regulations
in the USA and EU that have enabled generic drug development before patent expiry
and reduced capital requirements by obviating the need to reproduce data from clinical
trials.

3.2.2   1960–84: stringency in MA regulations and the US drug lag

In the previous sections, significant lags in the USA were observed for innovative
products (i.e. new molecules launching for the first time). As Figure 12.8 shows, the
USA exhibits no lag with respect to the adoption of pharmaceutical imitation. Based
on a cross-country perspective, Italy, Spain and France adopt generics latest, and are
surpassed by Germany and the UK. This pattern in Europe is broadly in line with the
case for innovative pharmaceutical diffusion, except for the fact that the UK lags behind

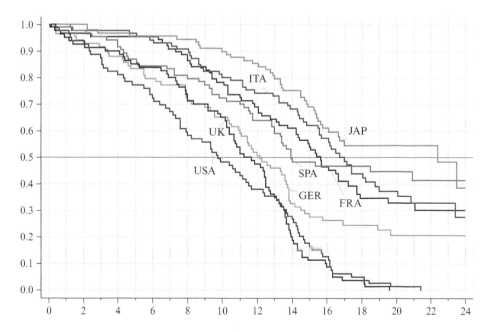

Figure 12.9   Kaplan–Meier (KM) survival estimates in years, US & UK generic molecules with first launch during 1984–95

Germany during this period by about three years (see Appendix Table 12A.3 for the exact figures). Also, generics reach Japan relatively quickly during this period compared to the relative adoption speed of innovative molecules in Japan.

3.2.3   1984–95: the Hatch–Waxman Act and improved generic access in the USA

The Hatch–Waxman Act of 1984 aimed to facilitate generic entry by elimi- nating the entry barrier of duplicative testing required for generic substitutes while ensuring adequate return for innovator firms through patent restoration (Wittner, 2004). As the most immediate benefit, the 1984 Act allowed generic manu- facturers to develop generic drugs before patent expiry of the originator product (often referred as the 'Bolar' clause).[26] Generic producers were allowed to reference the originator's safety and efficacy data, obviating the need to repeat the same tests, which reduced development costs substantially and therefore alleviated barriers to generic entry. The Act introduced 180 days of market exclusivity period to the first company to file a new generic application (known as ANDA, Abridged New Drug Application).

Figure 12.9 shows the pattern of differential lags during 1984–95. Compared to 1960–84, three main differences emerge. First, following the provisions for quicker generic entry in the Hatch–Waxman Act, the median delay in the USA is reduced by four years (from 14 years to about ten years). Second, the Japanese lag for generics increases by four years. Third, the UK and Germany show equally fast generic adoption with a median lag on the order of 11–12 years. Finally, France, Italy and Spain follow with a median delay of 14–17 years.

3.2.4   1995–2008: EMEA and new generic legislation in Europe

The period from 1995 to 2008 witnessed important regulatory changes in generic legislations in both the USA and Europe. Europe followed the USA in providing incentives for generic development and timely market access in Europe. The USA, on the other hand, focused mainly on the prevention of originator firm strategies to delay or block generic competition.

3.2.5   Changes in the US generic legislation

Two revisions (McCain–Schumer legislation in 2002, Gregg–Schumer Act in 2003) to the Hatch–Waxman Act in the USA sought to improve the balance between the needs of the branded companies and those of the generic companies. First, the new revisions set up a new mechanism to prevent the inclusion of frivolous patents or those filed at the last moment as a blocking mechanism. Second, the new legislation addressed the use of an 180-day exclusivity period by generic companies for special arrangements with originators as a means to prevent market entry of other generics.[27] The Gregg–Schumer revisions included 'forfeiture' provisions, which put the generics company under risk of losing the exclusivity if found to have made such an arrangement.

3.2.6   Changes in the European generic legislation

Europe's fragmented market structure has presented a major barrier to generic growth compared to the US market where federal law applies uniformly across different states. Directive 2004/27/EC has aimed to remove some of these barriers by updating Directive 2001/83. As with the US Hatch–Waxman Act, the legislation was intended to balance the needs of the branded pharmaceutical companies and generics companies. Directive 2001/83, the overall body of EU law governing the manufacture and trade in pharmaceuticals, had flaws such as the lack of a generic-product definition and allowed branded companies to withdraw reference products before generic entry.

The new laws introduced a specific 'generic' definition. One of the most important aspects for generics companies was the 'Bolar' clause permitting generic companies to do their own development work within the EU during the period of patent protection for the original molecule. The practical impact of the clause on the timing of product launches may be minimal because wherever the development is carried out, generics cannot be launched prior to patent expiry. The main benefit, however, is that companies could maintain generic drug development in the EU.[28] Under the new legislation, the same product can be used as a reference product for generics everywhere in the EU, even if not registered in particular countries. This is a small step towards unification of European generic legislation. An additional benefit of the new legislation is that if originator companies withdraw a brand before any generic versions are marketed, the generics can still use it as a reference product. Finally, the establishment of the EMEA in 1995 had little direct impact on generics companies. However, the centralised procedure is open to generics provided that the original is approved through the centralised system (Wittner, 2004).

3.2.7   Generic lags across markets follow the pattern of non-generic lags

Figure 12.10 demonstrates that the pattern of launch for the first imitative generic product is quite similar to the pattern for innovative molecules (Figure 12.4).[29] New

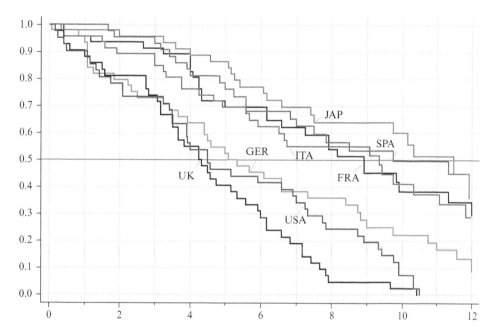

Figure 12.10   Kaplan–Meier (KM) survival estimates in years, US & UK generic molecules with first launch during 1995–2008

generic legislations have proven effective in the EU in further reducing the generic lag. The fastest adopters are as usual markets with relatively high originator prices (the USA, the UK and Germany) that offer higher profit prospects for imitative products. The median delay for the leaders is on the order of four–five years, with a reduction of five–six years compared to 1984–95. More regulated markets (Italy, Spain and France) lag by about five years behind the leaders, with a median delay of nine–ten years (which is a significant reduction from 14–17 years in 1984–95).

The Japanese lag for the adoption of imitative products is not as dramatic as for innovative molecules; however, Japan is still the slowest market among the biggest seven markets, with a median delay of 11 years. Generic drugs have been regarded in Japan as inferior. Similarly, physicians have had financial incentives for prescribing non-generic drugs. However, the government has recently initiated educational and advertising campaigns to improve generic use as well as changes on the provider side, including elimination of the link between prescribing practices and physician salaries (Business Insights, 2009).

The similar survival profiles for new molecules and generic products indicate that the negative impact of price controls on the launch timing of pharmaceutical innovation translates into the adoption of imitative pharmaceutical products. The launch patterns show that regulated markets access innovation later but also face temporal disadvantage in terms of their access to cost-saving generic products. To what extent this is balanced by lower branded prices remains an open question for further exploration.

4.   CONCLUSIONS

This chapter has sought to provide an overview of the evolution of the drug lag for pharmaceutical innovation (new molecules) as well as generic copies across the main OECD markets with regard to changes in the regulatory environment during 1960–2008 using non-parametric methods. This is the first study to provide a descriptive evolution of relative lags across a number of markets over a lengthy period of time and a comprehensive set of molecules, for both innovative products and generic copies.

Lower transaction costs due to reductions in geographical barriers and lower regulatory costs (harmonised market authorisation procedures, strengthened IP rights, patent term restorations) have exerted a downward pressure over time on median delays in individual countries as well as overall delays across the main OECD markets. All markets experience a decreasing trend over time for median delays following global launch. With the wider use of the centralised procedure over the coming years, the delays in the diffusion of pharmaceutical innovation across the EU may be further smoothed out. However, the relative lags across countries remain significant for both new molecules and generic products due to the variety in pricing and reimbursement regulations. In fact, an important finding is that the negative impact of price controls on new molecules translates into a later generic availability, which suggests that regulation delays patient access to new pharmaceutical technologies but also creates opportunity costs for governments through forgone savings due to later generic availability compared to free markets. Assessing the impact on overall welfare, however, would require a comparison of savings from lower branded product prices and savings forgone due to late generic launch and possibly lower generic penetration. Relative delays in the diffusion of generics are expected to reduce further due to the impact of the new European legislation in 2004 and the push for genericisation as a cost-containment mechanism in regulated markets that have been further challenged by the recent economic downturn.

Globally, the relative lags exhibit a change in the geographical pattern of lags over time. The US lag back in the 1960s has switched to more price-stringent European markets throughout 1960–2008. Relatively free-priced European markets of Germany and the UK,[30] which also have strong local pharmaceutical industries, led in the EU as the fastest adopters of pharmaceutical innovation (and imitation). Product launch strategically takes place first in higher-priced EU markets as a result of threat of arbitrage and price dependence across the member states, which puts European markets with low prices and/or small market sizes such as Spain and Portugal at a disadvantage. Paradoxically, the Japanese market with its large market size and relatively high prices remains a laggard throughout 1960–2008. The idiosyncratic nature of clinical trial requirements in Japan has been the major driver of asymmetric costs for foreign pharmaceutical firms. Harmonisation efforts on foreign clinical data use seem to be taking effect slowly, and expected future rise in the use of the bridging strategy may further reduce the Japanese drug lag in coming years.

The R&D activity of leading pharmaceutical companies is largely carried out in the major OECD markets. Reducing delays in these markets will offer higher returns to R&D and stimulate further innovation, contributing to dynamic efficiency over the long run. On the other hand, new pharmaceutical technologies impose additional pressure on the tight health care budgets, and quick diffusion of new technologies with uncertain benefits could lead to inefficiencies in the provision of health care (Garber and Skinner, 2008). The introduction of new drugs in individual markets, therefore, should be balanced by the expansion of drug expenditure and the evidence of cost-effectiveness. From a cross-country perspective, reducing the differential delays for globally important molecules will enable more equitable access to new and possibly more effective treatment alternatives.

ACKNOWLEDGEMENTS

We are grateful for the financial support provided by Merck Foundation Trust, and to Tim Williams and Elizabeth Finch from MSD, UK for their help during the data collection process.

NOTES

1. Food and Drug Administration.
2. European Medicines Agency.
3. The USA, the UK and Germany do not require price approval; however, in the UK, Germany and several other markets, cost-effectiveness evaluation may further delay the adoption of new pharmaceutical innovation as the fourth hurdle.
4. Both profit expectations and lagged cash flows have been shown to have significantly positive impacts on pharmaceutical firms' R&D investment intensity (Vernon, 2005).
5. A generic is defined by the European Directive 2004/27/EC as 'a medicinal product which has the same qualitative and quantitative composition in active substances and the same pharmaceutical form as the reference medicinal product, and whose bioequivalence with the reference medicinal product has been demonstrated by appropriate bioavailability studies'.
6. Eighteen times cheaper, according to the Pharmaceutical Manufacturers' Association (1993).
7. The cut-off value of 1984 has been suggested as a pivotal year in the history of drug introduction patterns between the USA and the UK (Coppinger et al., 1989).
8. IMS (Intercontinental Medical Services) MIDAS data were collected at Merck Sharp and Dome Limited (MSD) premises in Hoddesdon, UK.
9. Australia (ALIA), Austria (AUS), Belgium (BEL), Canada (CAN), Finland (FIN), France (FRA), Germany (GER), Greece (GRE), Italy (ITA), Japan (JAP), Netherlands (NET), Poland (POL), Portugal (POR), South Africa (SAF), Spain (SPA), Sweden (SWE), Switzerland (SWI), Turkey (TUR), the UK, and the USA.
10. For global molecules right-censoring is not an issue since the exact launch time of every molecule is known in all countries.
11. Spain, Turkey, Belgium, Greece, Portugal, Spain and South Africa have only retail channel data; therefore, the first local launches in these countries represents launch in the retail sector.
12. Pseudogenerics are generics marketed by brand-name companies to compete against independent generics.
13. The instantaneous probability of launch conditional on not launching before.
14. The SPC became effective in January 1993 and applied to drugs granted market authorisation in the EU after January 1985.
15. http://www.emea.europa.eu/.
16. http://www.ich.org.
17. Log-rank test for equality of survivor functions indicate that the difference in median delays between countries is significant (p-value: 0.0000). In addition, significant heterogeneity exists with respect to the ATC group (p-value: 0.0021), which implies that the relative delays vary across ATC groups.
18. Bilateral price indexes are calculated by considering common molecules in the USA and the respective country; prices are weighted by the US volume.
19. https://www.eversheds.com/uk/Home/Articles/index1.page?ArticleID=templatedata\Eversheds\articles\

data\en\Healthcare\BioBrief_Stop_press_Direct_applicability_in_Spain_of_patent_provisions_of_the_
TRIPS_Agreement.

20. A bridging study aims to confirm that the efficacy, safety and dose–response relationships of the drug in the new population are similar to those in the population evaluated in the foreign studies.

21. Austria, Belgium, Finland, France, Germany, Italy, the Netherlands, Poland, Portugal, Spain, Sweden and the UK.

22. http://www.emea.europa.eu/htms/human/epar/a.htm.

23. Kaplan–Meier estimate for Spain not available, the restricted mean which provides a lower bound for the median is reported.

24. These categories include all human medicines intended for the treatment of HIV/AIDS, cancer, diabetes, neurodegenerative diseases, auto-immune and other immune dysfunctions, and viral diseases, and all designated orphan medicines intended for the treatment of rare diseases.

25. http://www.emea.europa.eu/.

26. The name is derived from a landmark case between Roche and the generic companies Bolar. Bolar won the right to start developing the generic copy of Roche's patented compound Flurazepam Hydrochloride prior to its patent expiry, which was incorporated into the 1984 Act.

27. According to the 1984 Act, if the first generic company chose not to market the generic copy, all other generic competitors from the market would be excluded and all competition would be blocked for a period of 180 days. Authorised generics, copies made under licence from the innovator companies, were introduced whereby the originator receives royalties on sales in return. For example, Par Pharma's generic version of Glaxo's Paxil (Paroxetine) was launched with Glaxo's approval even though Apotex had obtained six-month exclusivity for its own generic.

28. As mentioned before, the SPC had prevented generic companies from engaging in R&D prior to patent expiry.

29. Similar to the non-generic case, equality by country, atc1, form1 and first launch period rejected (p-value < 0.001 for all).

30. However, prices may be indirectly affected through regulations in other parts of the market. In the UK, profits are regulated through the PPRS (Pharmaceutical Price Regulation Scheme) and products are subject to NICE appraisals for cost-effectiveness ('the fourth hurdle'). The flexible pricing scheme and risk sharing agreements introduced in the 2009 PPRS will further emphasise value for money in NHS purchases of medicinal products. In Germany, reimbursement regulation through reference pricing includes patented pharmaceuticals in reference groups unless novelty and therapeutic improvement are demonstrated and companies take this into consideration when setting prices.

REFERENCES

Barral, P.E. (1985), *Ten Years of Results in Pharmaceutical Research Throughout the World (1975–1984)*, Paris: Prospective et Santé Publique.

Berlin, H. and B. Jonsson (1986), 'International dissemination of new drugs: a comparative study of six countries', *Managerial and Decision Economics*, 7(4), 235–42.

Branes, J.M. (2007), *Patent Technology: Transfer and Industrial Competition*, Hauppauge, NY: Nova Science Publishers.

Busfield, J. (2003), 'Globalization and the pharmaceutical industry revisited', *International Journal of Health Services*, 33(3), 581–605.

Business Insights (2009), 'The Japanese pharmaceutical market outlook to 2014: policy environment, market structure, competitive landscape, growth opportunities', London: Business Insights.

Coppinger, P.L., C.C. Peck et al. (1989), 'Understanding comparisons of drug introductions between the United States and the United Kingdom. Reply', *Clinical Pharmacology and Therapeutics*, 46(2), 139–45.

Danzon, P.M. and A. Epstein (2005), 'Launch and pricing strategies of pharmaceuticals in interdependent markets', University of Pennsylvania working paper, Philadelphia: University of Pennsylvania.

Danzon, P.M. and A.J. Epstein (2008), 'Launch and pricing strategies of pharmaceuticals in interdependent markets', NBER Working Paper No. W14041, Cambridge, MA: National Bureau of Economic Research.

Danzon, P.M. and J.D. Ketcham (2004), 'Reference pricing of pharmaceuticals for Medicare: evidence from Germany, the Netherlands, and New Zealand', in D.M. Cutler and A.M. Garber (eds), *Frontiers in Health Policy Research*, Vol. 7, Cambridge, MA: National Bureau of Economic Research, The MIT Press, pp. 1–54.

Danzon, P.M., Y. Wang et al. (2005), 'The impact of price regulation on the launch delay of new drugs – evidence from twenty-five major markets in the 1990s', *Health Economics*, 14, 269–92.

DG Competition (2009), 'Pharmaceutical sector inquiry final report', available at http://ec.europa.eu/competi-tion/sectors/pharmaceuticals/inquiry/staff_working_paper_part1.pdf, accessed 15 September 2009.

Garber, A.M. and J. Skinner (2008), 'Is American health care uniquely inefficient?', *The Journal of Economic Perspectives*, **22**(4), 27–50.

Grabowski, H.G. (1980), 'Regulation and the international diffusion of pharmaceuticals', in R.B. Helms (ed.), *The International Supply of Medicines*, Washington, DC: American Enterprise Institute for Public Policy Research, pp. 5–36.

Hassett, K.A. (2004), 'Price controls and the evolution of pharmaceutical markets', American Enterprise Institute, Washington, DC. Available at http://www.who.int/intellectualproperty/news/en/Submission-Hassett.pdf.

Kaitin, K.I., N. Mattison et al. (1989), 'The drug lag: an update of new drug introductions in the United States and in the United Kingdom, 1977 through 1987', *Clinical Pharmacology and Therapeutics*, **46**(2), 121–38.

Kessler, D.P. (2004), 'The effects of pharmaceutical price controls on the cost and quality of medical care: a review of the empirical literature', Stanford University, the Hoover Institution and the National Bureau of Economic Research, available at http://www.ita.doc.gov/td/chemicals/phRMA/PhRMA%20-%20 ANNEX%20C.pdf.

Kyle, M. (2007a), 'Pharmaceutical price controls and entry strategies', *The Review of Economics and Statistics*, **89**(1), 88–99.

Kyle, M.K. (2007b), 'Strategic responses to parallel trade', National Bureau of Economic Research, Working Paper No. 12968, available at http://www.nber.org/papers/w12968.pdf.

Lichtenberg, F.R. (1996), 'Do (more and better) drugs keep people out of hospitals?', *American Economic Review*, **86**, 384–8.

Lichtenberg, F. (2005), 'Impact of drug launches on longevity: evidence from longitudinal disease level data from 52 countries, 1982–2001', *International Journal of Healthcare Finance and Economics*, **5**, 47–73.

Parker, J.E.S. (1984), *The International Diffusion of Pharmaceuticals*, London: Macmillan.

Permanand, G. (2006), *EU Pharmaceutical Regulation: The Politics of Policy-making*, Manchester: Manchester University Press.

Pharmaceutical Manufacturers' Association (1993), *PMA Annual Survey Report: Trends in US Pharmaceutical Sales and R&D*, Washington, DC: PMA.

Schöffski, O. (2002), 'Diffusion of medicines in Europe', *Health Economic Research Zentrum*, University of Erlangen-Nuremberg, p. 9.

Tabata, Y. and C. Albani (2008), 'Globalising clinical development in Japan', *Journal of Commercial Biotechnology*, **14**(1), 13–8.

Thomas, L.G. (2001), *The Japanese Pharmaceutical Industry: The New Drug Lag and the Failure of Industrial Policy*, Cheltenham, UK and Northampton, MA, USA: Edward Elgar Publishing.

Uyama, Y., T. Shibata et al. (2005), 'Successful bridging strategy based on ICH E5 guideline for drugs approved in Japan', *Clinical Pharmacology & Therapeutics*, **78**(2), 102–13.

Vernon, J. (2005), 'Examining the link between price regulation and pharmaceutical R&D investment', *Health Economics*, **14**(1), 1–17.

Vogler, S. (2008), 'Pharmaceutical pricing and reimbursement information report', IPN Working Papers on Intellectual Property, Innovation and Health, Vienna, GÖG/ÖBIG, Austrian Health Institute. Available at http://ppri.oebig.at/Downloads/Publications/PPRI_Report_final.pdf.

Wardell, W.M. (1973), 'Introduction of new therapeutic drugs in the United States and Great Britain: an inter-national comparison', *Clinical Pharmacology & Therapeutics*, **14**(5), 773–90.

Wardell, W.M. (1974), 'Therapeutic implications of the drug lag', *Clinical Pharmacology & Therapeutics*, **15**(1), 73–96.

Wardell, W.M. (1978), 'The drug lag revisited: comparison by therapeutic area of patterns of drugs marketed in the United States and Great Britain from 1972 through 1976', *Clinical Pharmacology & Therapeutics*, **24**(5), 499–524.

Wertheimer, A.I. and T.M. Santella (2004), 'Pharmacoevolution: the advantages of incremental innovation', IPN Working Papers on Intellectual Property, Innovation and Health.

Wittner, P. (2004), *Growth Strategies in Generics: Innovative and Aggressive Strategies and their Impact on Branded Pharmaceuticals*, London. Business Insights.

WTO OMC (2003), 'TRIPS and pharmaceutical patents, Fact Sheet', available at http://www.wto.org/english/tratop_e/trips_e/tripsfactsheet_pharma_e.pdf, accessed 3 July 2009.

APPENDIX

Table 12A.1   Mean and median launch lags over time

	US & UK molecules (non-generic)					
	1995–2008		1984–1995		1960–1984	
	Mean	Median	Mean	Median	Mean	Median
Australia	3.598(*)	1.752	8.146(*)	4.838	18.143(*)	12.252
Austria	2.181(*)	0.999	6.514(*)	3.420	19.254(*)	9.415
Belgium	5.720(*)	2.667	9.137(*)	3.666	19.791(*)	8.501
Canada	3.431(*)	1.336	7.402(*)	4.000	13.257(*)	6.084
Finland	2.259(*)	0.999	7.397(*)	3.337	22.804(*)	13.999
France	2.903(*)	1.585	6.482(*)	3.329	16.558(*)	6.585
Germany	1.444	0.668	4.703(*)	2.001	11.576(*)	3.001
Greece	4.138(*)	2.166	7.798(*)	4.580	22.250(*)	14.412
Italy	2.927	1.749	6.227(*)	3.584	16.019(*)	6.253
Japan	7.885(*)	6.582	12.441(*)	9.673	21.218(*)	11.414
Netherlands	3.042(*)	0.750	5.726(*)	1.837	19.158(*)	7.247
Poland	4.402(*)	3.001	9.395(*)	7.335	27.980(*)	26.497
Portugal	8.521(*)	13.254	12.884(*)	8.830	25.436(*)	19.162
S. Africa	5.590(*)	3.168	7.877(*)	4.000	21.776(*)	20.246
Spain	6.318(*)	2.667	10.117(*)	5.840	19.309(*)	7.077
Sweden	2.809(*)	0.747	8.311(*)	4.167	27.842(*)	27.830
Switzerland	2.964(*)	1.413	5.842(*)	2.828	12.799(*)	4.085
Turkey	3.701(*)	4.000	9.381(*)	6.854	23.805(*)	21.852
UK	1.270	0.750	3.151	1.914	8.817	3.083
US	0.665	0.001	3.602	2.664	10.052	7.666
OVERALL	3.829(*)	1.667	7.636(*)	4.085	18.823(*)	10.587

Note: * Largest observed analysis time is censored; mean is underestimated.

Table 12A.2   Median delays and confidence intervals by period of first launch (generic molecules)

	Subjects	Median	Std err.	(95% conf. interval)	
1960–84	3924	26.83	0.54	25.75	27.83
1984–95	1688	14.58	0.23	14.00	14.92
1995–2008	869	7.83	0.31	7.33	8.58

Table 12A.3   *Mean and median launch delays for generic molecules that launched in USA and UK*

Country	1960–84			1984–95			1995–2008		
	Subjects	Median	Mean	Subjects	Median	Mean	Subjects	Median	Mean
Australia	199	24.586	27.460(*)	85	16.000	15.446(*)	42	8.085	7.425(*)
Austria	207	33.418	31.961(*)	86	14.001	16.248(*)	45	7.915	7.877(*)
Belgium	210	39.086	33.843(*)	89	17.084	18.075(*)	46	–	10.052(*)
Canada	200	17.333	22.390(*)	86	10.242	12.981(*)	40	6.916	6.560(*)
Finland	200	31.496	31.367(*)	89	16.000	16.553(*)	44	7.417	8.098(*)
France	205	29.752	31.178(*)	87	15.663	15.912(*)	44	8.914	8.610(*)
Germany	191	15.168	20.877(*)	83	12.167	12.768(*)	44	5.081	6.060(*)
Greece	200	32.838	30.055(*)	85	15.253	15.215(*)	46	8.413	9.261(*)
Italy	176	27.083	28.294(*)	85	16.999	16.817(*)	46	9.339	8.374(*)
Japan	181	18.412	24.920(*)	88	22.412	18.784(*)	45	11.496	9.782(*)
Netherlands	191	32.832	32.053(*)	71	13.413	15.386(*)	42	6.418	7.451(*)
Poland	193	29.495	30.611(*)	84	11.086	13.114(*)	41	7.168	7.858(*)
Portugal	209	–	35.085(*)	86	16.000	15.922(*)	45	11.496	9.259(*)
South Africa	154	31.247	32.282(*)	81	14.834	16.261(*)	42	8.832	8.911(*)
Spain	195	34.749	31.147(*)	83	13.919	16.110(*)	43	9.747	8.965(*)
Sweden	212	–	36.388(*)	90	15.001	16.578(*)	45	8.167	8.119(*)
Switzerland	201	29.248	30.654(*)	89	15.918	17.173(*)	45	–	10.530(*)
Turkey	209	28.413	29.481(*)	82	16.085	15.293(*)	39	9.832	8.767(*)
UK	194	18.168	18.619	80	11.250	10.596	42	4.252	4.486
USA	197	13.67	14.767	79	9.752	9.754	41	4.504	5.224
Total	3924	26.831	28.615(*)	1688	14.579	15.314(*)	869	7.833	8.117(*)

Note: * Largest observed analysis time is censored; mean is underestimated.

PART V

AGEING AND LONG-TERM CARE

13 Proximity to death and health care costs
Michael Murphy

1. DETERMINANTS OF HEALTH CARE COSTS

Health care costs depend on the characteristics of individuals such as sex, age and health/disability status as well as a range of other factors such as availability of facilities, health care technology and so on. Of these, the age and sex structure of the population is one of the less difficult components to predict (Lee and Miller, 2002). Per capita health care expenditure on both men and women rises sharply with age (Wanless, 2001, Figure 9.1) and therefore the future number of older people is often assumed to be an important determinant of overall costs, although the empirical macro-level evidence for this is not overwhelming (e.g. Getzen, 1992 and Barros, 1998). A simple widely used assumption is that demand for health care and health care costs remains constant within each sex and age group, so that changes in expenditure depend on changing numbers, especially in the age groups where use is the highest, which are expected to grow substantially in decades to come. For example, the number of people aged 80 and over in Western industrialised societies is projected to increase by a factor of over three between 2000 and 2050 (Table 13.1). This simple model may be modified to incorporate information about likely changes in health status or in the costs of treatment; in both cases there are arguments that changes could serve to increase or to reduce expenditure since it is unclear whether, for example, health status will improve or deteriorate. The most plausible scenario may be a combination of an increase of mild disability and a decrease in more serious disability in line with Manton's (1982) model of 'dynamic equilibrium', although there are divergent views. What is clear is that the older population will increase substantially in years to come.

However, studies for a number of decades have pointed out that costs of acute health care services, principally based on use of hospital services, are greater at any given age for those who die relatively shortly afterwards ('decedents') compared with those who survive ('survivors'). The implications of whether heath care costs are affected more by proximity to death rather than by age are potentially substantial in terms of likely additional costs associated with ageing populations. If age is the key driver, then increased longevity will lead to more years spent alive especially at the older, more expensive ages.

Table 13.1 Population aged 80 or over (thousands)

Year	Northern Europe	Southern Europe	Western Europe	Northern America
2000	3727	5044	6647	10408
2025	5687	10115	13212	17362
2050	9768	17606	22676	35813

Source: United Nations (2009).

On the other hand, if health care needs are mainly determined by experiences around the time of death, then the expected costs are likely to be less than anticipated for two main reasons. First, pushing back the age of death will reduce the number of deaths occurring in a given year and will also push the health care expenditure further into the future, which would be expected to make it cheaper since some of the costs can be discounted and developments in the intervening period might reduce costs. If this occurs, lifetime expenditure may not be substantially changed since an individual must die at some stage, but such changes will postpone current expenditure. Second, later age at death is beneficial in cost terms since in most, but not all, countries it has been found that acute health care costs in the last year of life are generally higher for people who die at younger than at older ages (Payne et al., 2007). This is probably due to a combination of factors, such as decisions that aggressive interventions are less worthwhile at older ages, and age discrimination (Brockmann, 2002). To the extent that expenditure is tied up with proximity to death rather than age, the implications are substantial; the increase in the size of the population aged 65+ in England and Wales between 2006 and 2051, 94 per cent, is expected to be twice that of the number of deaths at these ages, 43 per cent (Murphy and Martikainen, 2010, Table 2). Therefore the consequence of incorporating proximity to death in analyses is that the resource implications of ageing populations and increasing life-expectancy for the health care system are often interpreted as being less than might otherwise have been assumed. The evidence for this assertion will now be considered.

2.   EARLY STUDIES

An early study by Timmer and Kovar (1971) of expenses for hospital and institutional care during the last year of life of adults aged 25 and over who died in 1964 and 1965 found the median bill for such care was almost three times higher for decedents than for survivors ($691 compared to $259). A more detailed study by Lubitz and Prihoda (1984) confirmed the importance of proximity to death and led Fuchs (1984, p. 152) to conclude:

> Health care spending among the elderly is not so much a function of time since birth as it is a function of time to death. The principal reason why expenditures rise with age in cross-section (among persons aged 65 and over) is that the proportion of persons near death increases with age. Expenditures are particularly large in the last year of life, and, to a lesser extent, in the next-to-last-year of life. Among Medicare enrollees in 1976, the average reimbursement for those in their last year of life was 6.6 times (and in their next-to-last-year of life 2.3 times) as large as for those who survived at least two years.

Scitovsky (1984) provides a summary of these studies and in a later paper (Scitovsky, 1994) she reviewed further developments, mainly in the USA. In the intervening period, a number of issues became apparent: first that the earlier relative patterns of expenditure between decedents and survivors had remained almost constant even though expenditure on both groups had increased substantially. The second was that there were major differences in the relationship of expenditure to proximity to death by age in that while annual expenditure per survivor increased by 55 per cent between age groups 65–69 and 90 and over ($1455 to $2258), for decedents it fell by 42 per cent (from $15346 to $8888), so that the ratio of costs of decedents to survivors was 11 at ages 65–69 but only 4 at ages 90 and over. A second finding was that the costs in the last year of life differed substantially according to the cause of death, with costs for malignant neoplasms ($8021) being twice as high as for cardiovascular diseases ($4112) (kidney disease and chronic obstructive pulmonary disease (COPD) also had high costs). More detailed data on hospital expenditure became available for both longer and shorter periods before death and, even within the last year of life, costs were loaded close to the point of death, with over one-third of costs in the final year taking place in the final month of life.

A number of studies have confirmed these general findings such as that acute care in the last year of life accounted for about one-third of lifetime costs (some comparisons were with expenditure after age 65), which are summarised in Raitano (2006) and Payne et al. (2007). Many of these later studies were based on Medicare data, so include hospital and physician costs of those aged 65 and over, but give little information on items not covered such as expenditure on nursing home or other social care and drugs. One study from outside the USA by Roos et al. (1987) for Manitoba, Canada was based on a sample of 60 000 people drawn from the provincial health insurance scheme that was based on universal coverage without deductibles or co-payments (apart from a low board-and-lodging payment in nursing homes), so issues of cost and reimbursement were less relevant and the coverage of health care was more comprehensive. The authors used average number of days spent in hospital or nursing home as the indicator of service use, and also analysed physician visits. While the provider may be more concerned with the cost of provision, from the point of view of the user, number of days spent within the health care system may be a more meaningful indicator of their use of the health care system. Use of nursing homes rose much more rapidly with age than hospital use, with the annual average number of days spent in nursing homes by men rising from 4.0 (women 6.2) at ages 65–74 to 64.7 (women 107.5) at ages 85 and over (Roos et al., 1987, Table 3). The relative use of other health care services by decedents compared with survivors was considerably lower than for acute hospital use; among those aged 85 and over, decedents had three times as many days in nursing homes, and the ratio for physician visits was even lower, whereas for hospital care the ratio was seven to one. When the full costs of health care were calculated, the conclusion that costs around the time of death are lower for those who die later based on hospital data only was reversed: 'those dying at older ages have more rather than less expensive deaths, largely due to heavy nursing home use by the very elderly, at least in a health care system with no financial barriers to access nor usage limitations' (Roos et al., 1987, p. 245).

3.   STUDIES IN RECENT DECADES

As health care costs continued to increase substantially in developed countries, interest in the effect of proximity to death on costs increased. While most of the early studies were concentrated in the USA, the topic became of wider interest with studies around 2000 in Australia (Brameld et al., 1998), Britain (Wanless, 2001, 2002; Seshamani and Gray, 2004a, 2004b, 2004c), Canada (McGrail et al., 2000), the Netherlands (Polder et al., 2006), Denmark (Serup-Hansen et al., 2002), Germany (Schulz et al., 2004; Breyer and Felder, 2006), Sweden (Batljan and Lagergren, 2004) and Finland (Häkkinen et al., 2008). Interest in the topic in Europe was stimulated by a paper by Zweifel et al. (1999)

using a sample from two Swiss insurance funds (although they referred to only one of the earlier studies that had investigated the issue). They argued that ageing was a 'red herring' for future acute health costs since costs for survivors were independent of age. They used more sophisticated econometric techniques than earlier studies, which led to a series of methodological criticisms by specialists in this area, for example Salas and Raftery (2001), Dow and Norton (2002), Stearns and Norton (2004) and Seshamani and Gray (2004a, 2004b). However, the application of such models in a number of countries has served to confirm the robustness of earlier findings. For example, Polder et al. (2006) used Dutch health insurance data including 2.1 million persons (13 per cent of the Dutch population) linked at the individual level with data on the use of home care and nursing homes and causes of death. Health care costs in 1999 were €1100 per person on average, but costs per decedent were 13.5 times higher at €15000 in the last year of life. Most costs related to hospital care (54 per cent), followed by nursing home care (19 per cent). As in other studies, they also found that costs depend on the cause of death, which were twice as high for cancer (€19000) as for myocardial infarctions (€8000), and also that average costs for younger decedents were higher than for older ones (see also Wong et al., 2011).

Understanding of the underlying processes also improved; for example, most early studies were confined to investigating the relationship between closeness to death and costs to relatively short durations before death, but Seshamani and Gray (2004a, 2004b) used data from the Oxford Record Linkage Study (ORLS) from 1970 to 1999 to track hospital costs among a sample of 96000 individuals over a 20-year period, which showed that cost increases could be identified up to 15 years prior to death. This study confirmed the importance of proximity to death: hospital care costs in the final five years of life were ten times those for a person of the same age who survived, whereas the total increase in costs between age 65 and 85 was only 30 per cent.

4.   SOCIAL CARE COSTS AND PROXIMITY TO DEATH

Much less is known about the relationship of social care costs, including long-term care (nursing home) costs, with age and proximity to death (Roos et al., 1987). Social care costs, as with acute care costs, rise sharply with age, but it was less clear whether this is related primarily to age or to proximity to death. If the former is the case, the implications for demand for long-term care would be much more substantial than in the latter case. Spillman and Lubitz (2000) combined information on acute care from Medicare with estimated nursing home and other costs including prescription drugs and dental care, and they estimated total lifetime costs after age 65 based on age and proximity to death. The cost for a person dying at age 65 was $31000 but over $200000 for someone who dies at age 90; the latter figure was heavily influenced by high use of nursing homes at older ages. They also found that although Medicare (largely hospital) costs in the last two years of life fell from $37000 for those dying at age 75 to $21000 for those dying at age 95, this was more than offset by increases in nursing home costs from $6000 to $32000 (other expenses were relatively unimportant). McGrail et al. (2000) pointed out that most previous studies of the relationship of age and proximity to death to costs have been restricted to acute medical care, so they included both acute medical care and nursing and social care in a study of British Columbia. They also concluded that while the costs of acute care rise with age, proximity to death was the more important factor in determining costs, and that these costs fall with later age at death, but after combining health and nursing home costs, any savings on hospital costs of very old decedents are offset by increased long-term care costs. Yang et al. (2003) investigated the relative contributions of both age and time to death to health care expenditures for elderly Medicare beneficiaries and found that time to death is the main reason for higher inpatient care expenditures, whereas ageing is the main reason for higher long-term care expenditure (for which Medicaid was a major source of funding), but proximity to death retained an influence: for example, average nursing home expenditure around ages 85 to 90 was about twice as high for those who died within one year as those who survived, a similar ratio as was found for the Netherlands by Polder et al. (2006). These findings are confirmed in a number of studies from different countries and time periods: Scitovsky (1984, 1994), Schulz et al. (2004), Felder et al. (2006) and Murphy and Martikainen (2010), which also find that health care spending for women is consistently higher than that for men, even after adjustment for their higher longevity.

Inclusion of both acute and long-term care costs produces a much less optimistic scenario for expenditure than those studies confined only to acute hospital care since ageing has a relatively larger impact on social and nursing care costs than on acute medical care costs, even though a night spent in hospital is more expensive than one spent in a residential home.

Other areas of health care have been investigated, such as use of general practitioner services by long-term care residents by O'Neill et al. (2000), who found no age effect on the cost after controlling for time to death.

5.   PROXIMITY TO DEATH OR TIME TO DEATH?

While early studies compared decedents and survivors in the last year of life (or the last two in some cases), later data sets often permit longer-term effects to be assessed with costs being higher the closer to death (apart from very close to death, when treatment may be reduced). Higher death-related health costs and greater use of hospital services are not restricted to the last year of life and a negative relationship between health care costs and time to death up to 17 years before death had been identified (Batljan and Lagergren, 2004; Seshamani and Gray, 2004a; Lubitz et al., 1995). Recently, the effect of proximity to death has been shown to be important up to 30 years before death in the Danish centenarians study (Engberg et al., 2009, Table 2), where centenarians had spent only one day a year on average in hospital when they were aged 71–74.

Table 13.2   *Mean annual number of days in hospital at ages 71 to 74 per individual by age at death (years), Danish 1905 cohort*

Age at death	71–74	75–79	80–84	85–89	90–94	95–99	100+
Days	17.2	5.5	3.1	2	1.4	1.3	1

Source: Engberg et al. (2009), Table 2.

Table 13.3   Days spent in hospital and long-term care by proximity to death, Finland, 1998

| | Excess days of those dying compared with those surviving for at least 6 years: | | Days spent by those surviving for at least 6 years |
	in year of death	in years 2 and 3 prior to death	
Hospital			
Aged 65–69	51.1	32.2	0.5
Aged 90–99	100.4	107.4	3.1
Long-term care			
Aged 65–69	9.0	14.9	0.3
Aged 90–99	103.8	172.2	7.9

Source: Finnish 40 per cent sample described in Murphy and Martikainen (2010).

Concentration on the last year of life overstates the extent of differentials in acute care by age since patterns of use by proximity to death vary with age at death. While Medicare costs in the last year of life for people dying after age 90 are about half those of people in age group 65–75 (Bird et al., 2002), they are comparatively more for the second and third years before death (Shugarman et al., 2004). Older patients are typically disabled longer and their end-of-life expenditures are lower per year, but their illnesses often continue for more years (Spillman and Lubitz, 2000; Lubitz and Riley, 1993), so that people who die at 73 and 93, for example, cost Medicare nearly the same amount (Lubitz et al., 2003) and, of course, older people are much greater users of long term residential care.

Studies that include only costs by those who are or are not in their last year of life will also tend to overestimate the potential cost savings of postponing death for two reasons: first, non-acute costs are frequently not included and costs are higher in all years close to death, not just the last year itself. Second, these costs are relatively greater among older people: in Finland in 1998, people aged 90–99 who died within 12 months spent over 100 days more in hospital or long-term care than those who survived for at least six years, but these decedents spent even more additional days in hospital or long-term care in the two years before their last year of life than the survivors (Table 13.3).

6.   PROJECTIONS OF CARE USE AND COSTS INCLUDING PROXIMITY TO DEATH

A number of studies have pointed out that in the case of changing mortality, projection models of care costs based on proximity to death would be likely to show less substantial increases in expenditure than those based simply on age. Between 2006 and 2021, the annual number of deaths among people aged 65 and over in England and Wales is expected to fall by 4 per cent, whereas the population in this age group is expected to increase by one-third (Table 13.4). If expenditure were principally determined by the

Table 13.4   *Population (in thousands) and deaths (in hundreds), people aged 65 and over, England and Wales, 2006, 2021 and 2041*

	2006	2021	2041
Deaths	4422	4229	5846
Population	8611	11 449	15 643
of which 85 and over	1122	1739	3410

Source: Based on Office for National Statistics (2008).

number of people in proximity to death, then the number of deaths would be the key factor, whereas if it were age, then both the total number of people and the age distribution are important. With much more rapid growth of over 50 per cent expected by 2021 among the 'old old' population aged 85 and over, who have greater health care needs, this suggests *ceteris paribus* that costs would increase more than in line with population numbers.

While the main demographic factor influencing health care expenditure among older people is the larger numbers entering the old age group, the potential sensitivity of health care costs, especially acute health care costs, led Stearns and Norton (2004) to conclude that 'it is time for time to death' to be included in projections of future health care costs. This has already been done in a number of countries. These studies have usually attempted to identify the sensitivity to outcomes by comparing simple models with age-specific assumptions about rates of expenditure or service use and those that include rates disaggregated by both age and proximity to death while keeping other variables constant apart from changing mortality.

In the USA, Cutler and Sheiner (1998) estimated that Medicare spending per person between 1992 and 2030 would increase by 1 per cent per year with constant age-specific spending, but reduce by 3 per cent per year if costs were disaggregated by whether or not in the last year of life. Stearns and Norton (2004) produced a simulation of lifetime acute care costs for US population aged 65 and over with 1998 and a projected 2020 mortality regime under a simple model and an expanded model with proximity to death in the previous two years included. They found that projected acute health care expenditure would be 9 per cent less with 1998 mortality and 15 per cent lower with 2020 mortality levels in the expanded model as compared with the simple model.

For Britain, Wanless (2002, paragraph 5.34) estimated that including consideration of survivors and decedents would reduce the expected growth rate of NHS expenditure by about one-seventh compared with models that failed to do so over the period 2002 to 2022. On the other hand, Seshamani and Gray (2004c, p. 558) estimated that the rate of increase in hospital spending due to ageing in England would be halved over the period 2002–2026 by incorporating the end-of-life dimension:

> Using richer data and more refined methods than have hitherto been employed, this study strongly confirms that the pressure of population increases and ageing demographic structure on hospital expenditures will be partially countered by the postponement of death-related hospital costs to later in life – a finding consistent with emerging epidemiological evidence, and heartening for policy makers and physicians alike.

In part, the differences between these two studies arise from the restriction of Seshamani and Gray (2004c) to hospital costs where the 1 per cent of people dying in the year account for 29 per cent of hospital costs as well as the fact that they allowed for proximity-to-death effects at all durations rather than in the final year of life.

In Denmark, Serup-Hansen et al. (2002) included all ages, but only distinguished between decedents and survivors in the year. They applied these data and found that, in the period 1995–2020, acute health care costs would increase by 18.5 per cent with the simple method, but by 15.1 per cent when survivor status was included, a reduction of one-fifth. In Sweden, Batljan and Lagergren (2004) used a model that included both inpatient and outpatient care, but also incorporated proximity to death in eight groups (0 to 6 years and over 6 years before death), although they assumed that this pattern was constant for all ages. They estimated that the rise in combined inpatient and outpatient health care demand in Sweden in the period 2000–2030 based on a simple age-specific model would increase by 18 per cent, but this would be reduced by over one-third to an 11 per cent increase by including proximity to death (assuming a fixed pattern of costs). Polder et al. (2006) for the Netherlands found that including proximity to death led to a 10 per cent reduction in the growth rate of future health expenditure compared to conventional projection methods not including proximity to death.

Breyer and Felder (2006) applied a set of Swiss sex- and age-specific expenditure profiles of acute care expenditure (including medication) for persons in their last four years of life and for survivors to the official German population projections between 2002 and 2050. By 2030, the simple model would have implied increases of 14.05 per cent since 2002 and 11.45 per cent for the model including allowance for proximity to death. They point out that this difference is small compared to potential changes due to changing mortality or costs. Schulz et al. (2004) also make forecasts for Germany, not only for hospital care, where proximity to death of up to four years was included, but also for long-term care where proximity to death was judged to be less important and was therefore not included. They show that, with improving mortality, the number of hospital bed days needed would increase by 15.2 per cent if proximity to death were included but by 22.4 per cent if it were not, a reduction of about one-third. However, they also suggest that the number of people requiring long-term care over the same period will increase by 50 per cent.

Overall, the importance attributed to the relevance of proximity-of-death effects varies between authors. Zweifel et al. (2004, p. 652) argue that estimation methods that do not control for proximity to death will 'grossly' overestimate the effect of population ageing on aggregate health care expenditure, whereas other studies suggest that the impact is relatively small compared with factors such as overall population ageing, changes in health status, the cost inflation of health care and, in particular, whether social care in included in the calculations. A typical finding is that over the next two decades, the increase in acute care cost for older people might be about one-third lower after including proximity to death in calculations, but with a more comprehensive measure including residential care, this figure falls substantially. While proximity-to-death approaches have not been used routinely in official forecasts, there have recently been studies by the OECD (2006) and the Economic Policy Committee and European Commission (2009) that incorporate proximity to death in forecasts of health care, and proximity to death was used for forecasting British health care costs in a major government report on financing (Wanless, 2001, 2002). Inclusion of proximity to death is likely to become increasingly important in years to come in forecasting health care costs for older people, although the main conclusion is not that it will substantially affect overall costs, but it implies a shift from acute to social care.

7.   REASONS FOR THE DECLINE IN COSTS IN THE YEAR OF DEATH AT OLDER AGES

Acute health care costs in the last year of life are usually found to fall with higher ages at death, often substantially, so offsetting the additional health care experienced in the extra years of life by those who die at advanced ages. In some cases, it has thus been argued that the costs of population ageing have been overstressed and that lifetime health care costs may even decline. However, the 'surcharge' (i.e. the extra average cost associated with the final year of life as compared with a survivor of the same age) for social care will tend to compound the extra costs associated with later ages at death, and people who die at older ages use relatively more health care in years close to death apart from the last year of life. Oldest old patients receive less costly treatment for the same illness than younger patients, although they may stay in hospital longer. Health care is informally rationed according to the age of the patient, and age-related rationing appears to be more pronounced in Germany than in the USA (Brockmann, 2002). Initially, much of the interest in 'the high cost of dying' was concerned with the ethical rather than the financial implications in decisions about the appropriate treatment of those close to death, and this has continued in debates in areas such as the role of hospices for end-of-life care.

Proximity to death is not necessarily important in its own right but mainly reflects poor health status, which is a major determinant of both health care use and subsequent increased chance of death, but health status is frequently unavailable (Colombier and Weber, 2010). Proximity to death is a macro-level variable that can be easily calculated from standard population projections, but its use as an independent/explanatory variable for prior health care use is an example of a type of invalid reasoning 'conditioning on the future' and there are statistical issues such as endogeneity between survival and level of heath care spending. The cost of decedents and survivors with similar medical conditions are not very different (Hogan et al., 2001). Shang and Goldman (2008) show that when health status is included explicitly in models, proximity to death loses much of its explanatory power. The often-unstated assumption is that as average age at death increases, the age of need for health care will also increase if it is associated mainly with proximity to death rather than with age *per se*. Projection models that incorporate proximity to death in situations of improving mortality therefore implicitly assume improvement in health status at each age. This is the main reason why they show lower growth in health care costs than simple constant age-specific profile models in which population ageing results in higher proportions of the population in the oldest age groups and *ceteris paribus* a deterioration in the average health level and higher average health care use due to changing age composition.

It is likely that proximity to death will be increasingly used in forecasts of acute health care needs. However, many of the studies to date have been based on administrative records and contain little if any useful information on other important co-variates such as socioeconomic status, living arrangements and use of community services. More recently consumer-based sources such as Nordic population registers (Häkkinen et al., 2008; Murphy and Martikainen, 2010) rather than institutional records have started to be used, and these allow incorporation of a fuller range of drivers of both acute health and social care needs within a single framework.

8.   CONCLUSIONS

Acute health care costs of persons in the last year of their life can be six times higher than the costs of survivors. Medical spending during the last year of life tends to account for over a quarter of spending on older people. These conclusions are robust in that they hold in different time periods in various countries (Lubitz and Riley, 1993; Hogan et al., 2001; Hoover et al., 2002; Seshamani and Gray, 2004a, 2004b). Proximity to death is a useful analysis variable since it is easy to measure (albeit retrospectively) – at least in those countries where information on earlier circumstances can be linked to mortality data – and it reflects health status, a major determinant of health care use (Colombier and Weber, 2010). While some studies show the proportion of life spent in poor health increasing (an expansion of morbidity), others suggest the opposite (a compression of morbidity). Lack of clear trends makes it difficult to predict health status in the future, although, on balance, more experts expect a reduction in the proportion (although not in the absolute numbers) of people with poor health, especially the more severe types of poor health such as inability to undertake one or more activities of daily living or instrumental activities of daily living. In these conditions, it might be thought that later age at death would push back the onset of disability. However, even with optimistic assumptions about improvements, it is still likely that there will be no change in the proportion of people entering or time spent in nursing homes (Laditka, 1998), nor average lifetime health care costs (Lubitz et al., 2003). Thus, while the demand for health care might not increase wholly in line with numbers in the older population (Freedman et al., 2002; Lafortune and Balestat, 2007), health status improvement in the future may tend to reinforce the cost-lowering tendencies on acute care of proximity to death noted above, but studies that include long-term care suggest that this will be offset by increases in social care needs.

REFERENCES

Barros, P.P. (1998), 'The black box of health care expenditure growth determinants', *Health Economics*, **7**, 533–44.
Batljan, I. and M. Lagergren (2004), 'Inpatient/outpatient health care costs and remaining years of life – effect of decreasing mortality on future acute health care demand', *Social Science and Medicine*, **59**, 2459–66.
Bird, C.E., L.R. Shugarman and J. Lynn (2002), 'Age and gender differences in health care utilization and spending for Medicare beneficiaries in their last years of life', *Journal of Palliative Medicine*, **5**(5), 705–12.
Brameld, K.J., C.D.J. Holman, A.J. Bass, J.P. Codde and I.L. Rouse (1998), 'Hospitalisation of the elderly during the last year of life: an application of record linkage in Western Australia 1985–1994', *Journal of Epidemiology and Community Health*, **52**, 740–44.

Breyer, F. and S. Felder (2006), 'Life expectancy and health care expenditures: a new calculation for Germany using the costs of dying', *Health Policy*, **75**(2), 178–86.

Brockmann, H. (2002), 'Why is less money spent on health care for the elderly than for the rest of the population? Health care rationing in German hospitals', *Social Science and Medicine*, **55**, 593–608.

Colombier, C. and W. Weber (2010), 'Projecting health-care expenditure for Switzerland: further evidence against the "red-herring" hypothesis', *The International Journal of Health Planning and Management*, 10 October, DOI: 10.1002/hpm.1068.

Cutler, D.M. and L. Sheiner (1998), 'Demographics and medical care spending: standard and non-standard effects', NBER Working Paper No. 6866, Cambridge, MA: National Bureau of Economic Research.

Dow, W.H. and E.C. Norton (2002), 'The red herring that eats cake: Heckit versus two-part model redux', Triangle Health Economics Working Paper Series, 1, Chapel Hill, NC: University of North Carolina.

Economic Policy Committee and European Commission (EPC and EC) (2009), 'The 2009 Ageing Report: economic and budgetary projections for the EU-27 member states (2008–2060)', Working document, Forthcoming European Economy 2/2009 available at http://europa.eu/epc/pdf/2009_ageing_report.pdf.

Engberg, H., A. Oksuzyan, B. Jeune, J.W. Vaupel and K. Christensen (2009), 'Centenarians – a useful model for healthy aging? A 29-year follow-up of hospitalizations among 40 000 Danes born in 1905', *Aging Cell*, **8**, 270–76.

Felder, S., P. Zweifel and A. Werblow (2006), 'Population ageing and health care expenditure: is long-term care different?', *Schweizerische Zeitschrift für Volkswirtschaft und Statistik Sondernummer*, **142** S (special issue), 43–8.

Freedman, V.A., L.G. Martin and R.F. Schoeni (2002), 'Recent trends in disability and functioning among older adults in the United States: a systematic review', *Journal of the American Medical Association*, **288**(24), 3137–46.

Fuchs, V.R. (1984), '"Though much is taken": Reflections on aging, health, and medical care', *Milbank Memorial Fund Quarterly. Health and Society Special Issue: Financing Medicare: Explorations in Controlling Costs and Raising Revenues*, **62**(2), 142–66.

Getzen, T.E. (1992), 'Population aging and the growth of health expenditures', *Journals of Gerontology Series B Psychological Sciences and Social Sciences*, **47**, S98–S104.

Häkkinen, U., P. Martikainen, A. Noro, E. Nihtilä and M. Peltola (2008), 'Aging, health expenditure, proximity to death, and income in Finland', *Journal of Health Economics, Policy and Law*, **3**, 165–95.

Hogan, C., J. Lunney, J. Gabel and J. Lynn (2001), 'Medicare beneficiaries' costs of care in the last year of life', *Health Affairs*, **20**(4), 188–95.

Hoover, D.R., S. Crystal, R. Kumar, U. Sambamoorthi and J.C. Cantor (2002), 'Medical expenditures during the last year of life: findings from 1992–1996 Medicare current beneficiary survey', *Health Service Research*, **37**(6), 1625–42.

Laditka, S.B. (1998), 'Modeling lifetime nursing home use under assumptions of better health', *Journals of Gerontology Series B Psychological Sciences and Social Sciences*, **53**(4), S177–S187.

Lafortune, G. and G. Balestat (2007), 'Trends in severe disability among elderly people: assessing the evidence in 12 OECD countries and the future implications', OECD Health Working Papers 26, OECD Publishing. Available at http://ideas.repec.org/s/oec/elsaad.html.

Lee, R. and T. Miller (2002), 'An approach to forecasting health expenditures, with application to the U.S. Medicare system', *Health Services Research*, **37**(5), 1365–86.

Lubitz, J. and R. Prihoda (1984), 'The use and costs of Medicare services in the last two years of life', *Health Care Financing Review*, **5**, 117–31.

Lubitz, J. and G.F. Riley (1993), 'Trends in Medicare payments in the last year of life', *New England Journal of Medicine*, **328**, 1092–96.

Lubitz, J., J. Beebe and C. Baker (1995), 'Longevity and Medicare expenditures', *New England Journal of Medicine*, **332**(15), 999–1003.

Lubitz, J., L. Cai, E. Kramarow and H. Lentzner (2003), 'Health, life expectancy, and health care spending among the elderly', *New England Journal of Medicine*, **349**(11), 1048–55.

Manton, K.G. (1982), 'Changing concepts of morbidity and mortality in the elderly population', *Milbank Memorial Fund Quarterly. Health and Society*, **60**(2), 183–244.

McGrail, K., B. Green, M.L. Barer, R.G. Evans, C. Hertzman and C. Normand (2000), 'Age, costs of acute and long-term care and proximity to death: evidence for 1987/88 and 1994/95 in British Columbia', *Age and Ageing*, **29**, 249–53.

Murphy, M. and P. Martikainen (2010), 'Demand for long-term residential care and acute health care by older people in the context of the ageing population of Finland', in G. Doblhammer and R. Scholz (eds), *Aging, Care Need, and Quality of Life*, Wiesbaden: VS Verlag für Sozialwissenschaften, pp. 143–62.

Office for National Statistics (2008), *Population Projections by Age and Sex for the United Kingdom, Great Britain and Constituent Countries. National Population Projections 2006-based. Series PP2 No. 26*, Basingstoke: Palgrave Macmillan.

O'Neill, C., L. Groom, A.J. Avery, D. Boot and K. Thornhill (2000), 'Age and proximity to death as predictors of GP care costs: results from a study of nursing home patients', *Health Economics*, **9**, 733–8.

Organisation for Economic Co-operation and Development (2006), 'Projecting OECD health and long-term care expenditures: what are the main drivers?' Economics Department Working Papers No. 477. www.oecd.org/dataoecd/57/7/36085940.pdf.

Payne, G., A. Laporte, R. Deber and P.C. Coyte (2007), 'Counting backward to health care's future: using time-to-death modeling to identify changes in end-of-life morbidity and the impact of aging on health care expenditures', *The Milbank Quarterly*, **85**(2), 213–57.

Polder, J.J., J.J. Barendregt and H. van Oers (2006), 'Health care costs in the last year of life – the Dutch experience', *Social Science and Medicine*, **63**(7), 1720–31.

Raitano, M. (2006), 'The impact of death-related costs on health-care expenditure: a survey', Enepri Research Report No. 17. Ahead Wp7. February, www.enepri.org/files/Publications/RR17.pdf.

Roos, N.P., P. Montgomery and L.L. Roos (1987), 'Health care utilization in the years prior to death', *The Milbank Quarterly*, **65**(2), 231–54.

Salas, C. and J.P. Raftery (2001), 'Econometric issues in testing the age neutrality of health care expenditure', *Health Economics*, **10**, 669–71.

Schulz, E., R. Leidl and H.H. König (2004), 'The impact of ageing on hospital care and long-term care – the example of Germany', *Health Policy*, **67**(1), 57–74.

Scitovsky, A.A. (1984), '"The High Cost of Dying": What do the data show?', *The Milbank Memorial Fund Quarterly; Health and Society*, **62**(4), 591–608.

Scitovsky, A.A. (1994), '"The high cost of dying" revisited', *Milbank Quarterly*, **72**(4), 561–91.

Serup-Hansen, N., J. Wickstrøm and I.S. Kristiansen (2002), 'Future health care costs – do health care costs during the last year of life matter?', *Health Policy*, **62**, 161–72.

Seshamani, M. and A. Gray (2004a), 'Ageing and health-care expenditure: the red herring argument revisited', *Health Economics*, **13**, 303–14.

Seshamani, M. and A. Gray (2004b), 'A longitudinal study of the effects of age and time to death on hospital costs', *Journal of Health Economics*, **23**, 217–35.

Seshamani, M. and A. Gray (2004c), 'Time to death and health expenditure: improved model for the impact of demographic change on health care costs', *Age and Ageing*, **33**, 556–61.

Shang, B. and D. Goldman (2008), 'Does age or life expectancy better predict health care expenditures?', *Health Economics*, **17**(4), 487–501.

Shugarman, L.R., D.H. Campbell, C.E. Bird, J. Gabel, T.A. Louis and J. Lynn (2004), 'Differences in Medicare expenditures during the last 3 years of life', *Journal of General Internal Medicine*, **19**, 127–35.

Spillman, B.C. and J. Lubitz (2000), 'The effect of longevity on spending for acute and long-term care', *New England Journal of Medicine*, **342**(19), 1409–15.

Stearns, S.C. and E.C. Norton (2004), 'Time to include time to death? The future of health care expenditure predictions', *Health Economics*, **13**(4), 315–27.

Timmer, E.J. and M.G. Kovar (1971), 'Expenses for hospital and institutional care during the last year of life for adults who died in 1964 or 1965', Vital and Health Statistics, series 22, no. 11, March, Hyattsville, MD: US Department of Health, Education, and Welfare.

United Nations (2009), *World Population Prospects: The 2008 Revision Population Database*, http://esa.un.org/unpp/.

Wanless, D. (2001), *Securing our Future Health: Taking a Long-Term View: An Interim Report*, available at http://www.hmtreasury.gov.uk/Consultations_and_Legislation/wanless/consult_wanless_index.cfm.

Wanless, D. (2002), *Securing our Future Health: Taking a Long-Term View: Final Report*, available at http://www.hmtreasury.gov.uk/Consultations_and_Legislation/wanless/consult_wanless_index.cfm.

Wong, A., P.H. van Baal, H.C. Boshuizen and J.J. Polder (2011), 'Exploring the influence of proximity to death on disease-specific hospital expenditures: a carpaccio of red herrings', *Health Economics*, **20**(4), 379–400.

Yang, Z., E.C. Norton and S.C. Stearns (2003), 'Longevity and health care expenditures: the real reasons older people spend more', *Journals of Gerontology Series B Psychological Sciences and Social Sciences*, **58**(1), S2–S10.

Zweifel, P., S. Felder and M. Meiers (1999), 'Ageing of population and health care expenditure: a red herring?', *Health Economics*, **8**, 485–96.

Zweifel, P., S. Felder and A. Werblow (2004), 'Population ageing and health care expenditure: new evidence on the "red herring"', *The Geneva Papers on Risk and Insurance*, **29**(4), 652–66.

14 The health and social care divide in the United Kingdom

Catherine Henderson

1. INTRODUCTION

The health and social care 'divide' is a difficult issue. The problem has been depicted as a 'sterile argument about boundaries' that creates a poor experience of care, a poor quality of care and a poor use of public money, and the cause as a disproportionate focus on the needs of organisations (cf. 'Partnerships in action', Department of Health, 1998). Expressions of concern over such barriers and 'a culture of separatism' between the health and social care systems continue to pepper more recent ministerial discourse (Burnham, 2010; Hope, 2010). The 'divide' is a complex or even 'wicked' problem (Rittel and Webber, 1973) that can only be framed in terms of its proposed solutions, making it difficult to define and, therefore, to tackle. Other countries face similar challenges in addressing the question of how to bridge the health/social care boundary, a question that, however vexed, demands public and political attention in the face of growing demographic and budgetary pressures (Bergman et al., 1997; Leutz, 2005; Mur-Veeman et al., 2008).

The following section will consider the policy literature on health and social care relationships in the UK for an analysis of the causes of the divide before turning to a discussion of the consequences for the users of health and social care services and for the wider public. The rest of this chapter will consider the remedies proposed to 'bridge the divide' at the macro-, meso- and micro-levels, examining the international and UK-specific evidence.

2. CAUSES: HISTORICAL AND CURRENT

The divisions between health and social care services have a long history. It has been argued that the 'divide' between the services was carved out at the inception of the modern British welfare state by several mechanisms, financial, administrative and professional (Lewis, 2001). Clearly, access to the two services differs, as the NHS is free at the point of access, whereas most social services are subject to means-testing. Furthermore, the NHS is financed by general taxation and managed, ultimately, by central government in the person of the Secretary of State for Health, whereas social care is provided and/or purchased by social services departments and funded by a mixture of transfers from central government and local taxation (European Observatory on Health Care Systems, 1999; Comas-Herrera et al., 2004; Oliver, 2005).

Lewis (2001) identifies 'administrative' barriers between the services as springing from two key pieces of postwar legislation. The 1946 NHS Act gave the NHS responsibility

Table 14.1   Responsibilities of welfare and NHS authorities, according to Ministry of Health circulars, 1957

Welfare authorities	NHS
• The 'infirm (including the senile)' who required personal care • 'Otherwise active' residents in welfare homes with short or minor illness • Welfare home residents not expected to live long, who would not receive appropriate treatment if living in their own homes	• The 'chronic bedfast' needing 'prolonged nursing care' • 'Convalescent care' of those older patients who were not ready to be discharged home or to a welfare home • The 'senile, confused or disturbed patients who are, owing to their mental condition, unfit to live a normal community life in a welfare home'

Source: Adapted from Means et al. (2002).

for acute and continuing care. The 1948 National Assistance Act obliged councils to provide residential accommodation as well as home-based services, including home nursing and help. Crucially, it imposed a duty to provide 'residential accommodation for persons who by reason of age, infirmity or any other circumstances are in need of care and attention which is not otherwise available to them' (as given in Glasby and Littlechild, 2004). Lewis (2001) argues that subsequent government guidance in the 1950s reinforced this initial allocation of responsibilities, even though there were important areas of overlap: while councils were to look after those requiring 'care and attention', the NHS was to see to those requiring 'constant medical and nursing attention'. Means et al. (2002) point out that such clarifications drew a group that at one time would have been seen as having health needs into the realm of social care. That the populations to be covered by the two agencies could overlap substantially can be seen in Table 14.1.

These early decisions were followed by an accretion of legislation that progressively tightened the definitions of health and social services functions (thus reinforcing administrative boundaries) (Means et al., 2002; Glendinning and Means, 2004; Wanless et al., 2006). The medical profession has also played a part by exerting a powerful influence on the development of the NHS, swaying the Ministry's civil servants to allow the service to focus ever more narrowly on those with acute illness (Lewis, 2001). Differences in professional cultures are widely seen as having played (and continuing to play) a role in creating divisions between health and social care. Social workers and GPs, not just in the UK, have very different priorities: the former are more interested in their clients' current capabilities; the latter are more interested in the prospect of a future cure (Ikegami and Campbell, 2002). Such longstanding 'professional' barriers engender resistance among health and social care personnel to changes to their roles and may be difficult to tackle (Goodwin, 2002). Pessimism over professional barriers to interagency collaboration has often been expressed in the UK literature (see Hiscock and Pearson, 1999; Glendinning et al., 2002; Johnson et al., 2003).

The health service's increasing concentration on 'acute' care has been shaped by trends such as the tightening of public sector budgets in the 1970s and 1980s; and also by policy decisions in the 1980s to stimulate the private residential and nursing care market via social security payments (Player and Pollock, 2001; Means et al., 2002). Central government, for its part, has had an incentive to contain costs by shifting dependent populations by degrees from public sector providers (whether NHS or council-run) into (generally less expensive) independent sector care homes. Government policy has long favoured the independent sector (Player and Pollock, 2001): while in 1982, half of all care home places were in local authority-run homes, by 2002, that proportion had decreased to less than a tenth (Netten et al., 2005). The NHS, similarly, shed a large proportion of its 'geriatric' beds over the 1980s and 1990s, the numbers falling by 34 per cent between 1982 and 1995 (Hensher and Edwards, 1999). Some commentators have observed that the Health Service has consistently exerted more influence over government spending than local governments have been able to do. Means et al. (2002) describe health imperatives, such as addressing bed-blocking and the closure of long-stay hospitals, as playing a major part in the development of community social care over the 1970s and 1980s. Glendinning et al. (2005) see the NHS as having been dominant over social services during the past 25 years, bending local authority services to NHS demands for rapid 'throughput'.

To summarise, divisions between health and social care services can be seen to have arisen from the legislative foundations of the welfare state. These divisions have been exacerbated by the failure of central governments over many years to address the relationship between an increasingly 'acute' role for hospitals and budgetary pressures on social services departments, particularly in light of increasing levels of dependency within the population (related to demographics but also reduction of NHS continuing care provision – see Lewis, 2001; Glendinning and Means, 2004; Wanless et al., 2006). The introduction of competition or quasi-competition and other structural reforms has added a layer of complexity to already difficult relationships between health and social care (Hiscock and Pearson, 1999; Glendinning et al., 2005). Continual reforms and multiple competing directives and initiatives in recent years may also figure in impeding collaborative working (McMurray, 2007). Work by Lewis (2001) and Means et al. (2002) depicts an official narrative that has consistently justified the need to define the boundary between the services, ultimately driven by a desire to limit overall expenditure on older people with health or care needs; this is despite the substantial overlaps in the populations to be served by the separate agencies. Administrative, financial and professional arrangements in the post-1945 period have influenced the present organisation of health and social care, creating a profound impact on outcomes for the users of those services, as will be discussed.

3.   CONSEQUENCES FOR USERS OF SERVICES

Lewis (2001) contends that shortly after the 1945 settlement, an 'intermediate group' of older people evolved, occupying a 'no man's land', too sick for local authority care and too well for health care (Huws Jones, 1952, as cited by Lewis, 2001). This 'intermediate' population is not homogeneous. Some older people have high levels of need over the short term, some over the long term; some need a small amount of help and support. This group requires perhaps a third kind of care, neither purely 'social', nor purely 'health' care, and hence the need for something often known as 'long-term care', a potentially confusing term that requires some definition. The NHS, councils and the independent sector are all involved in the provision of long-term care. Long-term care typically involves assistance with tasks such as maintaining personal hygiene, dressing, feeding and toileting, and also with domestic tasks such as cleaning and shopping (Comas-Herrera et al., 2004). In the case of institutional care, continuing NHS care funding covers the total costs of the individual's care and care home accommodation. Local authority funding covers care and care home accommodation below a threshold of personal financial assets, above which, in England, the individual is liable for all the care home costs except those provided by a registered nurse, for which the NHS pays (Glendinning, 2007; Henwood, 2007). In Scotland, personal care provided by the home is also state-funded. Community-based care funded by local authorities is subject to eligibility criteria based on both needs and means (excluding capital assets), so that above a financial threshold, the individual must make co-payments in England, but, since 2003, not in Scotland[1] (Glendinning, 2007). The NHS can also provide community-based continuing care packages.

The consequences of 'boundary problems' for this intermediate group can be seen in terms of negative impacts upon equity and efficiency. The next section describes those consequences first for people in need of low levels of help and short-term help and then in more detail for those in need of high levels of care and support. The discussion will focus on the situation in England. In the other countries of the UK, policies on health and social care funding and provision have increasingly diverged from the English model (Hazell and UCL Constitution Unit, 2003; Greer, 2004).

3.1   Low-level Needs and Short-term Needs

Some older people live in their own homes, are not acutely ill and do not particularly need rehabilitation, but have 'low-level' needs such as perhaps one activities of daily living (ADL) limitation, typically difficulty with bathing; and/or difficulty with household tasks. At present, such people may not receive community nursing services or social services because they are not dependent enough to meet strict local authority risk and needs-based eligibility criteria; nor do they meet NHS criteria for nursing care. Also, local authorities are guided by legislation to arrange non-residential care services for disabled people,[2] but authorities can be narrow in their interpretation of the law (Mandelstam, 2009); thus they can decline to assist those with a short-term rather than 'permanent' need for assistance (for instance those being discharged from hospital).

There is evidence that some older people in these groups have significant unmet needs and that this is a growing problem, because eligibility criteria imposed by local authorities across England have tightened over recent years (Commission for Social Care Inspection, 2008). It has been estimated that about 15 per cent of those with low-level need, or 275 000 people, receive neither formal nor informal help (Forder, 2007), suggesting that there are problems of inequity.

Both those with low-level and short-term needs have been affected by the trend to scale back the availability of NHS beds and to restrict community nursing provision to meeting 'medical' needs. As responsibility for these groups progressively shifted to local government from the 1950s onwards (Means et al., 2002; Glendinning et al., 2005;

Health Select Committee, 2005), some care costs shifted to the end users. At the same time, eligibility for care from social services has also shrunken and, consequently, many older people have fallen victim to a lack of funding for rehabilitative services and non-residential community services (Audit Commission, 1997; Bridgen and Lewis, 1999; Lewis, 2001). Also, system-level failures to plan for services across the boundaries of care have resulted in older people being seen as 'bed blockers', remaining in an acute hospital bed when deemed no longer to require acute hospital care, because alternative services are difficult or slow to arrange (Audit Commission, 1997).

3.2   Long-term High Needs

There is a group of older people with relatively high levels of dependency and disability who are particularly likely to be in need of more intensive forms of long-term care. Disputes over long-term care funding have intensified over the past 20 years and have created a particular sense of injustice, as portrayed in the media, that there are people who have been deemed ineligible for continuing health care funding and forced to pay either some or all of their long-term care costs, sometimes by selling their own homes. As contentions over funding responsibilities have resulted in a series of highly public complaints and investigations (see The Health Service Ombudsman, 2003), occasionally coming in front of the courts, this group has experienced arguably the most acute and high-profile boundary-related problems in recent years and therefore recent developments in this area will be addressed in greater detail.

3.3   The Divide and Long-term Care

Before the Department of Health introduced new guidance on NHS continuing care funding in 1995, many years (38) had passed without any formal statements of the Health Service's role and responsibilities in providing long-term care (Lewis, 2001; Means et al., 2002). Yet, thereafter, the Department issued an increasing volume of guidance on the roles and responsibilities of health and social services agencies in the provision of long-term care, at an expanding level of detail, in the form of a series of clarifications, good-practice guides and checklists. In some cases the government was reacting to some form of legal challenge (the Coughlan and Pointon cases), in others to parliamentary scrutiny (reports by the Health Service Ombudsman for England), or to the recommendations of an inquiry (e.g. the Royal Commission on Long Term Care). As Henwood (2006) has remarked in her review of continuing care policy in England, the policy process in this arena has been strikingly driven by 'external developments'. The Royal Commission is a case in point. Tasked by the government in 1999 to report on funding options for the long-term care of older people, the Commission ultimately recommended making personal care free on the basis of the needs, but not the means, of individuals. The government's response (in the form of the NHS plan) was to reject this recommendation, opting instead to fund improvements to older people's services (Secretary of State for Health, 2000). However, it did adopt other recommendations. For example, it implemented a policy known as 'free nursing care' for those in non-NHS nursing homes who had previously had to pay for (non-NHS) nursing care as part of their fees, whereas those receiving NHS nursing care in NHS nursing homes had not had to pay for the service (Department of Health, 2001).

Thus the government had made considerable adjustments to continuing care policy by 2002; however, there remained unacceptable local variations in the implementation of the policy across the country, according to reports by the Health Service Ombudsman (2003, 2004). The effect of these marked local variations had been to 'cause injustice and hardship to some people' (Health Service Ombudsman, 2003, p. 8). Also, the government's guidance on 'free nursing care' introduced further complexities into the long-term care system, as the definition of the top band of the NHS contribution to the nursing element of care home fees was similar to that defining eligibility for continuing health care funding (Henwood, 2004).[3] In the former case, the user or council was liable for fees apart from the nursing element of care; in the latter, the NHS would pay all care and accommodation costs (Health Select Committee, 2005). New problems arose with each progressive clarification that the Department of Health sought to make of the respective responsibilities of the NHS and social services for long-term care provision in England (Henwood, 2006). And yet the government continued to defend the position that the NHS's responsibilities towards those with long-term care needs could be separated out from those of the social services. As Wanless et al. (2006) point out, the Department of Health 're-emphasised this separation' of responsibilities (ibid., p. 19) in the 'out of hospital' White Paper, *Our Health, Our Care, Our Say* (Department of Health, 2006). The government defended its course on the grounds of promoting local determination of care priorities 'by local people, through local government' (Department of Health, 2006, para. 4.8).

A contemporaneous strand of government policy of the time involved the 'personalisation' of social care, originally by promoting 'direct payments' to those eligible for care so that they could purchase their own support services, and later through the development of individual budgets (Department of Health, 2006). But here, too, the funding 'divide' posed further problems: if individuals with local authority funding to pay for care at home were subsequently granted an NHS continuing care package, they could lose valued 'personalised' services (Royal College of Nursing, 2008). They could also lose services purchased through direct payments, which could not legally be used to pay for health (BBC News, 2008).

In its eventual response to concerns that unacceptable regional variations existed in access to continuing care funding, the government introduced in 2007 a 'national' continuing care framework (Department of Health, 2007) for agreeing the responsibilities of NHS and councils' social services departments. The framework contained a continuing care decision support tool formed from a matrix of 11 need-related domains, rated by the complexity, lack of predictability and intensity of those needs. The tool has been criticised by those who use it as long and time-consuming, and the framework as inadequate to clarify eligibility for continuing care (Royal College of Nursing, 2008). Yet the most recent version of the tool has more domains (12) and could not be said to be 'simple'. Many commentators and regulators (South, 1999; Health Service Ombudsman, 2004; Glendinning, 2007; Commission for Social Care Inspection, 2008) have called for simple, transparent rules on eligibility for long-term care funding to replace the current system.

In spite of frequent revisions to the continuing care guidance, the issues have remained much the same. The geographical inequalities in continuing care funding have not been eradicated, given major variations between primary care trusts in the numbers of people considered eligible (Age Concern, 2008; Robins, 2008). It remains the case that very fine distinctions have to be made by those assessing for NHS continuing care eligibility, so that, as Wanless et al. observe, 'an apparently small change in diagnosis can have significant financial implications for a person' (Wanless et al., 2006, p. 247). The government itself has acknowledged that long-term care is fragmented into several funding streams (NHS, benefits, housing services and social services) (HM Government, 2009) and that people 'find it particularly difficult to understand where the boundary lies between NHS care and social care and what kind of conditions qualify for each' (ibid., p. 43).

A separate but related problem has been that adult social care legislation is presently a patchwork quilt of regulations that in places contradict each other, making it difficult to establish entitlements to social care (The Law Commission, 2010). There are presently plans to revise all such legislation: it is proposed to reorient eligibility decisions towards entitlements based on need, rather than on the definition of 'a disabled person or service user'. However, the proposals do not include plans to change the existing interface between health and social care in the assignment of responsibility for the provision of care home placements (The Law Commission, 2010). The new legislation could entrench the present divisions in law, at a point when there is a historic opportunity to change the system.

At the heart of the continuing care debate is a value judgement about the merits of a rights-based approach over the present resource-based or 'budget-constrained' approach (Brodsky et al., 2003). The present means-testing model of long-term care has little public support, according to one recent survey; there is a desire for 'a stronger "universal" element, determined by care need rather than by people's income or wealth' (Caring Choices, 2008). There is a lack of clarity over what rights citizens have in the UK to assistance, whether medical or social, with long-term care, and particularly personal care (see Dickinson et al., 2007).

In summary, governmental efforts to maintain the boundary between health and social services have resulted in a system for funding long-term care in England that is seen as overcomplicated and opaque. It poses problems for horizontal equity in allocating more resources to those people with high care needs when they also have 'health' needs, through NHS continuing care funding, than to those with only high care needs. It also risks creating vertical inefficiency in meeting the non-care needs of one group of people with long-term care needs, through NHS continuing care funding, rather than collecting revenue by charging them; those funds could be used to meet the long-term care needs of additional people (Collins, 2009).

4.   STRATEGIES FOR MITIGATING BOUNDARY PROBLEMS: BRIDGING THE 'DIVIDE'

Actions to bridge the gap between health and social care provision may be instituted at three levels. At the macro-level the government has the power to decide on the financing, direction (through guidance and legislation) and regulation of health and social care agencies (Glendinning, 2003). At the meso-, or 'local', level, health and social care agencies and teams cover areas defined by population size and geography (e.g. a council's adult services department, a primary care trust). These organisations have the ability to allocate resources from either local or central government, and have responsibility for strategic planning. At the micro-level, individual service users and carers have the potential to make decisions about the balance of health and social care services they wish to consume. Solutions introduced at one level are likely to have consequences at other levels. Moreover, solutions may cut across groups with low-level, short-term and long-term high needs, or help some groups more than others. There will be competing definitions of, perspectives on, and solutions to these 'wicked' boundary problems.

5.   MACRO-LEVEL

Lewis (2001) advances the thesis that the question of means-testing for social care must be addressed in order to solve other boundary issues (such as differences in professional cultures and priorities). If we agree with Lewis, addressing the financing of long-term care would solve other administrative and professional divisions that impede the seamless delivery of care to older people at all levels of need and dependency. Following this line of argument, addressing the issue of citizenship rights of access to both health and social care is fundamental to tackling the health and social care divide.

As Brodsky et al. (2003) make clear, there are pros and cons to the (relatively few) different options for funding long-term care. They emphasise the importance for governments of deciding whether to use either an entitlements (rights-based) or a 'budget-constrained' approach, as these approaches have different implications for equity, flexibility, coverage and support for informal carers. Rights-based approaches can protect access to services from the political process; however, the costs of such systems may be difficult to predict and to control. In contrast to the UK situation, embracing this approach would mean that eligibility criteria would no longer be set largely by official guidance, and implemented at the discretion of local health and social care bodies. It might be more difficult to rescind or to change the criteria once set down in law (Brodsky et al., 2003). Implementing legislation to clearly define benefits levels linked explicitly to levels of need would be a new step for the UK.

Wanless et al. (2006) explored the future costs of long-term care under different funding models, including models that involved establishing explicit entitlements to certain defined levels of care: the partnership model, social insurance, and private insurance; the free personal care model also confers universal, but not explicit, entitlements (see Box 14.1). In projections of both the free personal care model and partnership models,[4] more older people would access care than in the means-testing model (Wanless et al., 2006, p. xxxi). In contrast, the means-testing option was found to perform worse than these in terms of maintaining dignity and in relation to self-funders. The authors concluded that the partnership model performed best against certain criteria (including fairness, efficiency, choice, clarity and sustainability); free personal care performed better than other options but was the most expensive. Social insurance and limited liability models were also considered promising relative to other options, such as means-testing, private insurance, savings models and out-of-pocket payments.

BOX 14.1   FUTURE LONG-TERM CARE FUNDING OPTIONS CONSIDERED BY THE KING'S FUND REVIEW

Eight funding options:

- Abandoning aspects of means-testing (e.g. free personal care as in Scotland)
- Changing means-testing with fewer users paying charges
- A partnership model providing a universal minimum level of care, and incentives for private top-ups through matched funding
- A limited liability model capping individuals' potential private liability for social care costs, after a certain period or a specified financial limit
- Savings-based models, or care savings accounts with state contributions in the form of tax breaks
- A social entitlement model with a public sector version of insurance risk pooling
- Private long-term care insurance
- Out-of-pocket payments for long-term care

Source: Wanless et al. (2006).

It is also instructive to look at the evidence from other countries. Both Japan and Germany have implemented long-term care reforms in the recent past. In both countries, long-term care legislation addresses the link between levels of need and explicitly defined packages of benefits intended to meet those needs; in both, services are funded through social insurance schemes that provide 'universal' coverage. In Japan, long-term care is insurance-based: municipalities collect the premiums and act as insurers. Medical care is financed through social insurance (Ikegami and Campbell, 2002). Some services that would be classed as part of the NHS in the UK, such as community nursing and re-habilitation, are funded through long-term care insurance (Ikegami, 2007). Campbell and Ikegami (2003) argue that the Japanese model has permitted the integration of health and social services at an individual level, while offering users a greater choice of providers. They have also argued (Ikegami and Campbell, 2002) that, in general, insur-ance models have the advantage of an explicit entitlement that lends itself to cash and voucher payments and so may better satisfy individuals' preferences for health and social services, and encourage competition.

Glendinning (2007) argues that the UK should learn from the German model of long-term care. This model pays non-taxable benefits to those meeting functional dependency-based criteria, which do not differ by community or residential setting. The level of benefit is rated in three bands, increasing with dependency. The benefits for all those eligible do not vary by region or by individuals' means, because there is one set of eligibility criteria that can be administered in a consistent way across the country. Scheme membership is mandatory for adults and is income rated (Roth and Reichert, 2004; Rothgang and Igl, 2007). In Glendinning's view, the scheme provides 'high levels of horizontal equity between older people with similar levels of dependency, regardless of financial or social circumstances. Above all, eligibility confers access to a transparent level of public funding' (Glendinning, 2007, pp. 417–18).

Nonetheless, the design of a long-term care system needs careful thought. The establishment of a social insurance system does not *in itself* guarantee that social care will be provided seamlessly with health care. The design of the German long-term care system, with its separate health and long-term care funding systems and associated differences in entitlements, has contributed to problems in integrating the provision of German health and social care services (Kodner, 2003) and thus could be criticised for perpetuating boundary problems not dissimilar to those in England. Cost shunting between the German sickness funds (which cover health care) and long-term care insurers has occurred over rehabilitation in particular. The sickness funds, rather than the long-term care insurers, are responsible for assessing for and funding rehabilitation. Although rehabilitation might reduce the beneficiary's level of dependence and need for assistance, the savings would accrue to the long-term care insurers. There is thus little financial incentive for the sickness funds to recommend rehabilitation (Roth and Reichert, 2004; Rothgang and Igl, 2007). In contrast, the Japanese version of long-term care insurance appears to be more flexible in ensuring that preventive and rehabilitative services are provided because it covers some 'health' services. In Japan's recent reforms to try to contain costs, the coverage for those in the lowest dependency bands are limited to 'preventive' care, focused on preventing personal decline (Campbell et al., 2010).

Although it is not easy to imagine what would occur in practice in the English context, were means testing for some elements of social care to be abolished, we do have within the UK an example of a potential solution to the problems of the divide, in the Scottish policy of 'free personal care'.[5] Although it is important to be aware of the limits of comparability with the rest of the UK,[6] there are lessons to be learned from the way that the policy has played out.

The Scottish Executive initiated 'free personal care' (FPC) in 2002 (Dickinson et al., 2007), in response to a Scottish parliamentary committee report in 2000 that endorsed the Royal Commission for Long Term Care recommendation (Health and Community Care Committee of the Scottish Parliament, 2000). FPC in the Scottish context consists of fixed weekly payments (£145 per week in 2002/03) to care home residents over 65 years of age for the personal care component of costs; and open-ended payments to community care recipients (Bell et al., 2007).

Bell et al. (2007) suggest that FPC may have increased the efficiency of the health and social care system as a whole. If the costs of older people's services were to include health care costs, it is possible that the costs have been *falling* overall since the policy was introduced (ibid., p. 27). While demand for FPC has risen substantially, the authors do not find this trend to be explained by demographics, higher disability rates or informal care reductions. Rather, it might be due to cost shifting from the NHS to social care (for instance, with delayed discharges legislation and policies), as well as by the presence of previously unmet need.

There has been some encouraging evidence in terms of access and quality of care. Research from the early stages of implementation found that those who had most benefited from the policy were those with such conditions as dementia and also those who despite quite limited incomes would previously have been assessed as eligible to pay (Bell et al., 2007, p. 93). Also, service users benefited from more flexibility for their informal carers and a wider range of formal care providers (Bell et al., 2007). Costs also increased: homecare expenditure more than doubled between 1999 and 2005, from around £100million to £250million (Bell et al., 2007). More people have been able to access personal care services. Between 2002, when the policy was introduced, and 2005, there was a 10 per cent increase in the number of home care clients; of those receiving home care, the number receiving personal care rose by 62 per cent (Bell et al., 2006).

While the Scottish policy has reduced the financial burden on some older disabled people, there are limits to what is provided free of charge; similar to the situation with continuing care in England, the policy has not been well understood by the public and needs to be clarified (particularly in regard to those services not covered, such as care home accommodation) (Bell et al., 2007). Scottish experience suggests that the system may be more efficient, and more equitable. However, more is required than removing user charges for certain services to create a 'transparent' funding system for long-term care; also, the effect on collaboration between health and social care organisations and professionals, if any, has not yet been fully evaluated. There is little research evidence on whether the policy has lifted the administrative barriers, for instance by influencing the working practices of front-line staff in either health or social care (Dickinson et al., 2007). Some qualitative research at an early stage of the policy's implementation suggests that boundary disputes between health and social care continued to occur, in the context of budget pressures for both social and health agencies (Bell et al., 2006, 2007).

Long-term care in many countries suffers from a lack of integration across fragmented funding and service systems, and countries have typically attempted to address the problem through *ad hoc* and incremental reforms (Kodner, 2004; Mur-Veeman et al., 2008). The previous government's Green and White Papers on long-term care demonstrate its pursuit of such an incrementalist strategy (Lindblom, 1959; Smith and May, 1980) towards the integration of health and long-term care funding. In the Green Paper, *Shaping the Future of Care Together* (HM Government, 2009), it set out proposals considering five options satisfying the criteria that the system must be fair, easily understood, affordable, universal and flexible/personalised (see Box 14.2). In the White Paper, *Building the National Care Service* (HM Government, 2010), it proposed a comprehensive funding model for a new 'national care service'. It did not propose that long-term care funding should be consolidated into one stream, including that for some health services (not including acute health care funding), although it had commissioned research that did recommend this (Glendinning and Moran, 2009). Indeed, the White Paper contained no mention of NHS-funded or -provided continuing care, but it did set out plans for more 're-ablement' services via local authorities to be directed towards those with short-term needs and for the expenditure of £1.8 billion by the NHS to deliver social care in a more integrated system (HM Government, 2010, p. 129). In a previous move in this direction, the government had passed the Community Care (Delayed Discharge) Act 2003 (CCDDA), which eliminated user charges for the social services element of 'intermediate care' (Department of Health, 2001b). This legislation effectively introduced free personal care for six weeks for people with short-term needs, as long as they were eligible for the sort of restorative services usually offered as intermediate care, usually following

---

BOX 14.2   FUTURE LONG-TERM CARE FUNDING OPTIONS
            FOR A NATIONAL CARE AND SUPPORT SYSTEM

The government considered five funding options.

1. Pay for yourself – the government ruled this option out because it was widely seen as unfair.
2. Partnership – entitlement to state payment of a set proportion of basic care costs, on a sliding scale based on means. To cover the whole population.
3. Insurance – as with the partnership option in meeting a portion of costs, but voluntary insurance could cover additional care costs, either as a private or a social insurance scheme. Payment into the scheme could be before or after retirement or after death via a charge on the person's estate.
4. Comprehensive – all those over retirement age who had the means would have to pay into a compulsory social insurance scheme for over 65s. Based on need, for those qualifying, care would be free. The government would look at a separate scheme for working-age people.
5. Tax-funded, universal, for all ages – the government ruled out this option because of the burden on the working-age population.

Source: HM Government (2009).

---

discharge from hospital. The strategy was primarily directed at those with high short-term needs at the meso-level, as will be discussed. The previous government's proposals to implement the 'national care service' followed the same incrementalist path, now focusing on those with high long-term needs. The new service was to be taken forward in stages, starting in 2010 by providing free personal care to those with the 'greatest needs' and after 2015 providing 'high quality care for all adults in England with an eligible care need, free when they need it' (HM Government, 2010). A bill to implement this policy by amending the existing CCDA legislation was enacted in 2010[7] but did not set out the eligibility criteria to define what might constitute such needs. However, the provisions of the Act were not enforced by the new Coalition government, which rejected the previous government's strategy for social care reform as 'piecemeal' (Secretary of State for Health, 2010). Which funding option will offer choice and be affordable, sustainable and fair will now be a question for a new commission appointed to advise on long-term care funding in England (Department of Health, 2010).[8] Reflecting on the Scottish evidence, the previous government's strategy might have improved access to long-term care in England. However, it is just as important to establish transparent eligibility criteria, which it did not address.

Though not envisaged in the White Paper, some commentators have proposed that a further, politically difficult, change to long-term care funding would be to make those care home residents with NHS continuing care funding liable for the hotel costs of their stay on a means-tested basis (Henwood, 2006; Collins, 2009). It would level the playing field between those receiving long-term care funded by the NHS and those funded by councils, particularly for those in care homes. How much would be released is hard to estimate, as the government collects no statistics on NHS primary care trusts' expenditure on continuing care (Hansard, 2010), but Collins (2009) suggests that this would fund most of the cost of providing free personal care for all those in receipt of free nursing care payments, requiring modest additional funding of £212 million a year. It would also simplify administrative arrangements to set up integrated care services for those with long-term high needs (for instance when health and social care organisations set up jointly run care homes). It could make interdisciplinary working easier by enabling organisations to provide care without having to consider competing charging regulations.

In any major changes to the long-term care funding system, the implications for those with short-term needs would require careful consideration. It would be important to take into account the potential interactions between proposed long-term care funding reforms and existing legislation linking entitlements to the permanence of disability. For instance, a new system could focus on linking the individual's disability-related needs, as identified at the time of assessment, to her entitlements to appropriate services and funding, rather than to the permanence of her condition.[9] Agencies would be required to organise timely reassessments in order to adjust or remove services as the extent of the individual's disability changed.

6.   MESO- AND MICRO-LEVEL SOLUTIONS

In the UK, central government has in recent years sought to bridge the 'divide' at a local level by promoting 'joint working' arrangements between agencies and thereby to drive improvements in health and social care performance and more generally to promote more efficient, effective, seamless and equitable health and social care (see Department of Health, 1998, 2006b). Much of the English policy literature has advocated the adoption of such models as joint commissioning and integrated teams (see Department of Health, 2006b; Audit Commission, 1997).

The recent Labour governments implemented several important policies to promote joint working in the UK. One early move in this direction involved measures designed to dismantle some of the legal provisions that prevented NHS and social services departments from jointly commissioning and providing services. These measures, known as the Health Act Flexibilities (HAFs), were introduced in the Health Act 1999. HAFs gave health and social services bodies in England and Wales the powers to pool budgets, lead commission on behalf of other partners, and to integrate working arrangements (managing and employing health and social care staff within one organisation). The Act also enabled the creation of care trusts, integrated health and social care bodies responsible for commissioning and provision.[10] The government also introduced local partnership arrangements intended to promote collaborative strategic planning of services (including health and social care) at an area (local authority) level. These 'Local Strategic Partnerships' (LSPs) were implemented in England in 2001.[11] A new Care Quality Commission was established in 2009, consolidating previously separate social care and health inspectorates (Care Quality Commission, 2009). Thus the previous government, by stages, had gone some way towards dismantling some long-standing barriers between the services created by different performance management regimes and legal requirements, and sought to align the priorities of organisations responsible for health and social care (Department of Health, 2006a).

7.   PERSPECTIVES ON INTEGRATION OF HEALTH AND SOCIAL CARE SERVICES

The question arises whether it is sufficient to remove administrative barriers and to exhort health and social care organisations to develop partnerships in order to achieve joint working. The answer is likely to depend on one's outlook on joint working (whether 'optimistic', 'pessimistic' or 'realistic') (Sullivan and Skelcher, 2002). An optimist may see joint working as motivated by a desire to achieve a shared positive outcome and as driven by the altruism of those involved. Pessimists, on the other hand, may see joint working as motivated by organisational gain, since organisations or professional bureaucracies will seek to keep or increase the resources available through the collaboration (Sullivan and Skelcher, 2002). Hudson (2002) asserts that, in the pessimistic view taken in some of the sociological literature, the characteristics of professionalism pose formidable challenges to interprofessional collaboration. For instance, some professionals are accorded higher status than others (e.g. medicine versus nursing or social work), which can create tensions between members of multidisciplinary and multi-agency teams. Sullivan and Skelcher (2002) see a 'realistic' way between these approaches, one that considers the wider environment and the changes in a context in which collaboration can occur. From this perspective, altruism and self-serving motives may coexist. Local institutional factors or 'logics' may or may not facilitate collaborative working or satisfy these competing motivations. Thus all integration is to some extent local (Leutz, 2005), and lessons may not easily be generalised from one place to another.

Heenan and Birrell (2006) discern two lines of thinking about the future of integrated services between the NHS and social care services in the British literature on partnership working. Only structural integration at an organisational level can create the right conditions for joint working, runs one line of thought; a willingness to collaborate is more important than organisational structures, runs the other. Perhaps the two lines of thought are not so divergent. From an optimistic perspective, the drive to collaborate could end in structural integration, following a progression from informal, trusting relationships between members of organisations, to more formal arrangements and, ultimately, new structures, as organisations with shared goals merge (Sullivan and Skelcher, 2002).

8.   FORMS AND FEATURES OF INTEGRATED CARE

Models of integration between health and social care organisations as described in the literature fall somewhere on a continuum between the extremes of structural and collaborative (or network-type) relationships (Cameron and Lart, 2003; Kodner, 2003;

Leichsenring et al., 2004; Coxon, 2005; Ouwens et al., 2005; Kodner, 2006; Ramsay et al., 2009).

Integration takes different forms depending on the roles of the producers and the desired breadth of care production. 'Horizontal' integration can occur between professions or organisations producing complementary services (Leichsenring, 2004). 'Vertical' integration can take place when parts of the chain producing a care pathway are brought together (e.g. across primary, community health and social care, secondary care). Both horizontal and vertical integration can be achieved by more formal means (mergers) or more informal means (cooperation between groups of organisations or professionals with shared values). For instance, payers and providers, or groups of providers, can be formally vertically integrated, or integrated through networks such as 'chains of care' (Ramsay et al., 2009). One recent proposal for new integrated structures is to set up a health and social care commissioning body led by local government, which would be locally accountable, unlike the current, centrally accountable community health care organisations (primary care trusts) (Glasby et al., 2006).

The literature identifies a number of features of integrated care, such as case management and multidisciplinary professional teamwork and training. Financial mechanisms and incentives (such as capitated payments, or the 'pooling' of finances between organisations) can also support and promote effective and efficient integrated services (Cameron and Lart, 2003; Johri et al., 2003; Leichsenring et al., 2004; Coxon, 2005; Ouwens et al., 2005; Kodner, 2006). Kodner (2006), for instance, identifies four features accounting for the success of some North American programmes providing joined-up care to frail older people. These are: (1) an umbrella structure overseeing strategic and operational levels, monitoring costs and outcomes; (2) case management and multidisciplinary care with a single entry point; (3) organised networks of providers with standardised protocols for referrals, records and training; (4) financial incentives to promote rehabilitation and preventive approaches, to improve efficiency and integration. Johri et al. (2003) and Leichsenring et al. (2004) identify a single entry point to integrated services as an important mechanism to promote integrated services for older people. Leutz (1999) proposes three levels of integration processes, based on the US and UK evidence. In 'linkage', providers in both systems know who is responsible for paying for which services, eligibility and benefits, and follow coverage rules rather than engage in cost shunting. 'Coordination' involves a primary worker responsible for coordinating services and sharing information, and 'full integration', new services that pool resources from different systems to control benefits and services directly, and where team members can work from a shared record.

The majority of interventions proposed in the literature to allow users to enjoy seamless services are on the supply side. However, there are demand-side strategies that could be effective. Individuals may use their purchasing power, or be able to exercise choice through other means, for instance, choice of health and social care provider. As Ham et al. (2008) suggest, the use of individual budgets for long-term conditions could enable people to make links across agencies for themselves. Until recently, direct payments could not legally be made to purchase health services (Glendinning et al., 2008). There are now projects to test the implementation of personal health budgets in pilot areas of England (Department of Health, 2010a).[12]

9.   THE INTERNATIONAL AND UK EVIDENCE BASE

There is some evidence that 'structural' approaches may be effective. Ramsay et al. (2009) find that vertically integrating payer and provider has been perceived to improve partnerships, and possibly, to increase capacity, also to increase the focus on case management and on IT systems. Evidence of the impact of purchaser–provider integration on acute admissions and lengths of stay and costs is more mixed. Johri et al. (2003) and Leutz (1999, 2005) suggest that two models of vertically integrated care, the social health maintenance organisations (SHMOs) and PACE (Programme of All-inclusive Care for Elderly People), experienced patchy or slow-growing enrolment. SHMOs had disappointing outcomes in terms of utilisation, costs and patient well-being (Johri et al., 2003). Differences in financing mechanisms pose formidable barriers to integration. For example, Leutz (1999) observes that where health and social services have successfully integrated in the USA, they have been able to use their funding effectively by serving populations that can draw funding from only one source – for instance from private medical insurance plans, topped up with a private social care benefit, or by limiting eligibility to those on Medicaid. But Kodner (2006), reviewing three North American studies (of the US-based PACE programme, and two Canadian integrated care programmes, SIPA and PRISMA), finds the evidence for structural integration approaches 'promising'. He suggests that the PACE model, financed by risk-based capitation payments, has had good patient outcomes such as reduced hospital utilisation, improved health status, satisfaction with care and increased access to community-based services. An evaluation of the SIPA demonstration project (an example of vertical integration) suggests that a public, integrated programme with a single entry point can be effective (Johri et al., 2003) and improve outcomes increasing access to services and carers' satisfaction with services, and reducing the numbers of stays that result in 'bed-blocking' waits for nursing home placements.

Ramsay et al. (2009) surveyed the international literature on networks that create 'virtual' integration across acute health care and community health and social care, finding relatively little evidence of impact upon health outcomes and costs. While they did identify that networks can improve care provision, and communication across organisations, they also found that personnel involved in networks of care can be resistant to intended changes in practice and roles (Ramsay et al., 2009). In a similar vein, research from the PROCARE study found that some third of European models had never achieved 'real' collaboration in the eyes of the personnel involved in implementing them (Coxon, 2005, p. 20).

On the whole, reviews of the integration literature suggest that evidence is quite limited, with much more evidence on the effects of the processes of integration than on outcomes and on cost impacts in particular (Ouwens et al., 2005; Bowes, 2007; Ramsay et al., 2009). Cameron and Lart's (2003) systematic review of the literature on joint working between health and social services in the UK reveals little evidence of effectiveness in terms of impacts on the users of services, nor much new information on what hinders or promotes collaboration. Dowling et al. (2004), reviewing the literature on UK health and social care partnerships after 1997, find 'little hard evidence that they deliver improved outcomes for the users of those services'. Integrated care can be stuck in the 'boutique' projects stage, rather than becoming mainstream, and this makes it difficult to develop and to learn lessons from (Johri et al., 2003; Ramsay et al., 2009).

The lack of robust evidence on the impact of English joint working may be due to the small scale and limited scope of many partnership initiatives. Some recent studies (Brown et al., 2003; Davey et al., 2005; Lyon et al., 2006; Keating et al., 2008) have examined relatively modest co-location or 'placement schemes' (Cameron and Lart, 2003) to integrate provision in the English context, using some form of quasi-experimental pre-post design; interventions could be on as small a scale as co-locating a single social worker with a community nurse. The results of studies by Brown et al. (2003) and Davey et al. (2005) suggest that simply co-locating front-line staff of different agencies in the same offices may not be a sufficient condition for creating better outcomes. Both studies compared the status at follow-up (whether living at home, living in a care home or deceased) of those receiving collocated services and those receiving non-collocated services; neither detected significant differences in this outcome between the groups. However, co-location may improve service processes, for instance, in terms of increased contact between professionals from different agencies (Davey et al., 2005) and faster access for patients to assessments (Brown et al., 2003). The latter also suggest that a 'one-stop-shop approach' may also have had a positive impact on service delivery.

There is some evidence on the impact of the removal of barriers to joint commissioning and provision (using HAFs) on joint working within the broader context of mainstream services. Early research (Glendinning, 2003) focused on areas where partnerships were using the HAFs to integrate services for older people. Managers in these areas reported some benefits: HAFs increased the potential to access the resources of other partners and use pooled resources more effectively; enabled the construction of complex packages of care using local services; and reduced duplication of effort (e.g. in community equipment services). But more recent research on integrated intermediate care for frail older people (Phelps and Regen, 2008) suggests that HAFs could have had a greater impact in achieving effective partnership working and positive outcomes if local areas had been able to surmount a number of other barriers such as separate human resources policies; different IT systems; fears of unequal financial risks to partners involved in pooling funds; and different performance regimes. Apart from the last, these barriers remain largely unaddressed. Such barriers may be reasons why, as Leutz (2005) contends, programmes in the UK that have aimed to pool funds, share IT systems, and conduct common/single assessments, have undergone rather slow and patchy growth. The slow take-up of the care trusts model has been taken as sign of the problems in achieving full integration (Leutz, 2005; Ramsay et al., 2009). Even by 2010, only ten care trusts had been established (NHS Choices, 2010).[13] Small-scale developments and the removal of some administrative barriers may not have been sufficient to either facilitate, or at least to provide an evidence base on the effectiveness of, joint working in England.

On the other hand, it may be that administrative barriers do not hinder inter-agency collaboration too much if the will to collaborate is strong. Hudson (1999), reviewing joint commissioning research from the mid-1990s, finds that those who were determined to work together towards shared goals for joint commissioning were more likely to achieve their objectives than those whose energies were focused on setting up 'complex and cumbersome' structures around the task (Hudson, 1999, p. 365). This perspective is echoed in the conclusions of Phelps and Regen (2008): while intermediate care had a number of positive outcomes for older people, such as recovery of mobility and independence, these 'outcomes were the same whether the integrated team was using a HAF or not. It seems that it is the range of multidisciplinary staff working together to provide holistic care that makes the difference' (Phelps and Regen, 2008, p. 12).

For those in the other countries of the UK who might contemplate a structural solution to bridging the divide, the Northern Irish example does yield some evidence. In Northern Ireland (NI), there is one government department (Health and Social Services and Public Safety – DHSSPS) overseeing one health and social care board, five health and social care trusts and five local commissioning groups (Department of Health, Social Services and Public Safety, 2009). As in the rest of the UK, however, those receiving social care are subject to user charges (Department of Health Social Services and Public Safety, 2010). Heenan and Birrell (2006)[14] suggest that in the NI context a 'culture of integration' is as important as an integrated structure. Examining the extent to which integrated management has led to an integrated service, in the view of its senior managers, the authors found that while the integrated administrative structure could facilitate integrated working practices, a culture supportive of joint working was equally required. It was also found that education and training for health and social care workers continued to be delivered in professional silos, and was not conducive of integration. Studies comparing mental health services for adults and older people in Northern Ireland and England have reported, in a similar vein, that structural integration on its own does not ensure that integrated practice will result (Reilly et al., 2003, 2007). Research with older people who had experienced a hospital stay in Northern Ireland drew somewhat pessimistic conclusions about the success of the country's integrated management system (McCormack et al., 2008). Single assessment processes were not necessarily being achieved, despite the integration at a strategic level. Primary care workers, for instance, emphasised the divide between the hospital and the integrated community services. Linkages were still to be made to stop services from being 'organizationally focused rather than person centred' (McCormack et al., 2008, p. 112). Overall the Northern Irish picture appears somewhat positive at the meso-level but the benefits are less clear for patients and front-line workers in health and social care. That Northern Ireland cannot remove user charges for social care may be a barrier.

More research is needed on the impacts of joint working between health and social care in terms of the sub-populations most likely to benefit. The policy literature advocates integrated services for those with high needs in the short term, usually those being discharged from acute hospital (this is best exemplified in the policy on intermediate care – Department of Health, 2001b). Leutz (1999) suggests in general that there are only a few groups for whom 'full integration' is suitable: those with high needs, over the long term or where the condition is terminal; where the extent of self-direction may be weak, the scope of services broad, and the need for an urgent response may be frequent (e.g. at the transition between hospital and home). There is evidence for the effectiveness of some interventions that might fit under the rubric of intermediate care, as measured for instance by outcomes such as hospital readmissions (see Shepperd et al., 2009), but it is not possible to say what part integration plays in these (Phelps and Regen, 2008 excepted). It is unusual for the integration of services to be unpicked from the other aspects of the interventions in the trial literature. Indeed, measuring collaboration poses a number of challenges, not least the difficulty in adequately measuring effectiveness (El Ansari et al., 2001).

There has been particularly little research on the benefits of joint working between health and social care for those with low-level needs. For such service users, a group much larger than that requiring 'full' integration, there may be less costly, more quickly achieved routes to improving their experience of health and social care, via linkage and coordination (Leutz, 1999). Certainly the evidence on the impact of multisectoral partnership arrangements on public health outcomes for adult populations is sparse and the evidence that does exist is not robust (Smith et al., 2009). Evidence from the Partnerships for Older People (POPP) evaluation, examining partnerships between social care, health and voluntary agencies, showed some promising trends in terms of improvements in quality-of-life scores and decreases in unplanned hospital use by those using POPP services (Windle et al., 2009). The contribution of strategic partnerships *per se* to these outcomes, rather than, for instance, the injection of new funding to create the new services, is difficult to unpick. But in terms of process outcomes, the evaluation's qualitative results suggested that the partnerships most strengthened by the projects were between local government and voluntary organisations, rather than with health agencies.

In summary, moving some aspects of community health into a new long-term care system and implementing free personal care would be helpful in removing the financial barriers to integrating services. In combination with financial incentives such as capitated payment (Johri et al., 2003) for health and social care, this could create efficient and effective provision of care to people with high needs over the short and long term. Vertically integrated organisations would then have a common goal to use funds efficiently and to reduce institutional care. The Northern Irish example is incomplete, as Northern Ireland still charges for social care, but the system appears to have some advantages over the situation in the rest of the UK. The Northern Irish evidence points to potential problems when community health and social services are integrated, erecting a new boundary with acute care.

10.   CONCLUSION

This chapter has focused on the problems of the boundary between health and social care in England and some potential solutions to level or overcome the barriers.

10.1   Macro-level

There is evidence from Scotland that free personal care improves access to social care services; it is also possible that the policy is cost saving or cost neutral if the costs of both health and social care are taken into account. As has been discussed, there would be a need to support that policy with proper deliberation on the appropriate eligibility criteria. Research based on financial modelling has lent support to the adoption of a partnership model, guaranteeing a free basic level of care with matched state funding for private top-ups (Wanless et al., 2006); other research provides evidence in favour of social insurance as an entitlement option.

It is vital that the eligibility for long-term care is put on to a more transparent and equitable footing and that rules on payment for board and lodging in residential and nursing care settings should be the same, or very similar, between the two services. Long-term care benefits and their limits should be clearly defined. Thought needs to be given to how such changes would fit into new comprehensive adult social care legislation presently being considered. The solution will be complex and will require the public to understand what trade-offs will have to be made to make the system more equitable.

10.2   Meso- and Micro-levels

There is some evidence for structural integration and some that, if professional silos and culture are not addressed (for instance at an early stage in training), outcomes of integrated care will not improve as much for patients as they might.

Even though the evidence base could be stronger, there is a case for certain features of integrated care pilots that should be widely adopted because they are likely to make life easier for service users, despite potential professional resistance to integration efforts in some areas. For instance, collocation may improve access for users of services, as may single points of access/single service points and single points of contact, that is, case managers/coordinators, because this will also make it easier for service users to access appropriate services. There is some evidence that downward substitution to community health and social services can be effective (Johri et al., 2003) and also cost-effective (Windle et al., 2009).

New developments in personal budgets hold some promise for people with high needs to achieve the mix of health and social care services that they prefer.

NOTES

1. Older people needing personal care assistance can also apply for social security funding (known as attendance allowance), subject to eligibility criteria based on need not finances.
2. Under the National Assistance Act 1948, the disabled are those with sensory impairments, 'mental disorder' and 'permanent and substantial handicap' (Mandelstam, 2009).
3. At the time there were three bands. There is now only a single band for NHS-funded nursing care payments, as of 2007 (Department of Health, 2007).
4. This refers to projections under the 'current service' and 'core business' scenarios.
5. This does not include making such costs as accommodation in care homes, nor meal preparation in home settings, free of charge.
6. For instance, a benefit for those over 65 years of age, attendance allowance, cannot be claimed by care home residents in Scotland (Bell et al., 2006).
7. In the Personal Care at Home Act 2010.
8. Since this chapter was written, the report of the commission appointed to advise on long-term care funding in England has been published (Dilnot et al., 2011). This report can be accessed at: http://www. dilnotcommmission.dh.gov.uk/our-report/.
9. This is envisaged in the Law Commission's proposals to forgo 'a central definition of a disabled person' in new adult social care legislation (The Law Commission, 2010, p. 96).
10. Significantly, care trusts are modelled on NHS trusts, but with an obligation to represent councils within their governance arrangements (Glendinning and Means, 2004).
11. The local strategic partnership partners were placed initially under a duty to cooperate to produce community strategies (Department of the Environment, Transport and the Regions, 2001) and, later, to agree local priorities through 'local area agreements' (Office of the Deputy Prime Minister, 2005). Priorities were defined in terms of a set of jointly agreed central and local performance indicators, introduced in 2008. However, the LAAs and their associated targets were discontinued by the new Coalition government in 2010 (Department of Communities and Local Government, 2011).

12. Since this chapter was written, a number of interim reports on the personal health budgets evaluation have been published. These can be accessed at: https://phbe.org.uk/index.php.
13. There are 152 primary care trusts, of which five are care trusts (NHS Choices, 2010).
14. At the time of the research (2006), the Department of Health and Social Services and Public Safety oversaw four HSS boards, overseeing 11 CHSS trusts, seven hospital trusts, and one ambulance trust and several HSS agencies (Heenan and Birrell, 2006).

REFERENCES

Audit Commission (1997), *The Coming of Age. Improving Care Services for Older People*, London: HMSO.
BBC News (2008), 'GP fights for MS husband's care', available at http://news.bbc.co.uk/1/hi/wales/7199745. stm, accessed 14 July 2009.
Bell, D., A. Bowes et al. (2006), *Financial Care Models in Scotland and the UK*, York: Joseph Rowntree Foundation.
Bell, D., A. Bowes et al. (2007), *Free Personal Care in Scotland: Recent Developments*, York: Joseph Rowntree Foundation.
Bergman, H., F. Deland et al. (1997), 'Care for Canada's frail elderly population: fragmentation or integration?', *Canadian Medical Association Journal*, **157**(8), 1116–21.
Bowes, A. (2007), 'Research on the costs of long-term care for older people – current and emerging issues', *Social Policy and Society*, **6**(3), 447–59.
Bridgen, P. and J. Lewis (1999), *Elderly People and the Boundary between Health and Social Care 1946–91: Whose Responsibility?*, London: The Nuffield Trust.
Brodsky, J., J. Habib et al. (2003), 'Choosing overall LTC strategies: a conceptual framework for policy development', in J. Brodsky, J. Habib and M. Hirschfeld (eds), *Key Policy Issues in Long-term Care*, Geneva: World Health Organization, pp. 245–80.
Brown, L., C. Tucker et al. (2003), 'Evaluating the impact of integrated health and social care teams on older people living in the community', *Health & Social Care in the Community*, **11**(2), 85–94.
Burnham, A. (2010), Speech by the Rt Hon Andy Burnham, Secretary of State for Health, 18 January. Partnerships for Older People Projects event, Department of Health, London.
Cameron, A. and R. Lart (2003), 'Factors promoting and obstacles hindering joint working: a systematic review of the research evidence', *Journal of Integrated Care*, **11**(2), 9–17.
Campbell, J.C. and N. Ikegami (2003), 'Japan's radical reform of long-term care', *Social Policy and Administration*, **37**(1), 21–34.
Campbell, J.C., N. Ikegami et al. (2010), 'Lessons from public long-term care insurance in Germany and Japan', *Health Affairs (Millwood)*, **29**(1), 87–95.
Care Quality Commission (2009), *New Regulator for Health, Mental Health and Adult Social Care*, London: HMSO.
Caring Choices (2008), *Who Will Pay for Long-term Care?*, London: Caring Choices.
Collins, S. (2009), 'Options for care funding: what could be done now?', *Solutions: Lessons for Policy and Practice*, York: The Joseph Rowntree Foundation.
Comas-Herrera, A., R. Wittenberg and L. Pickard (2004), 'Long-term care for older people in the United Kingdom: structure and challenges', in M. Knapp, D. Challis, J.-L. Fernández and A. Netten (eds), *Long-term Care Resources: Matching Resources and Needs*, Aldershot, Hants: Ashgate Publishing, pp. 17–34.
Commission for Social Care Inspection (2008a), *Cutting the Cake Fairly. CSCI Review of Eligibility Criteria for Social Care*, London: Commission for Social Care Inspection.
Commission for Social Care Inspection (2008b), *The State of Social Care in England 2006–07*, London: Commission for Social Care Inspection.
Coxon, K. (2005), 'Common experiences of staff working in integrated health and social care organisations: a European perspective', *Journal of Integrated Care*, **13**(2), 13–21.
Davey, B., E. Levin et al. (2005), 'Integrating health and social care: implications for joint working and community care outcomes for older people', *Journal of Interprofessional Care*, **19**(1), 22–34.
Department of Communities and Local Government (2011), 'Local government: decentralisation', retrieved 13 March 2011, from http://www.communities.gov.uk/localgovernment/decentralisation/.
Department of Health (1998), 'Partnership in action (new opportunities for joint working between health and social services', A discussion document.
Department of Health (2001a), HSC 2001/017: *Guidance on Free Nursing Care in Nursing Homes*, London: Department of Health.

Department of Health (2001b), *National Service Framework for Older People*, London: Department of Health.

Department of Health (2006a), *The Future Regulation of Health and Adult Social Care in England*, London: Department of Health.

Department of Health (2006b), *Our Health, Our Care, Our Say: A New Direction for Community services*, retrieved from http://www.dh.gov.uk/en/Publicationsandstatistics/Publications/Publicationspolicyandguidance/Browsable DH_4127552.

Department of Health (2007), *The National Framework for NHS Continuing Healthcare and NHS-funded Nursing Care*, London: Department of Health.

Department of Health (2010a), *Direct Payments for Health Care: Information for Pilot Sites*, London: Department of Health.

Department of Health (2010b), Written Ministerial Statement: *Terms of Reference for the Commission on the Funding of Care and Support*, London: Department of Health.

Department of Health, Social Services and Public Safety (2009), 'Health and social care', retrieved 12 December 2009 from http://www.dhsspsni.gov.uk/index/hss.htm.

Department of Health, Social Services and Public Safety (2010), 'Care management, provision of services and charging guidance', Circular HSC (ECCU) 1/2010.

Department of the Environment, Transport and the Regions (2001), *Local Strategic Partnerships: Government Guidance*, London: DETR.

Dickinson, H., J. Glasby et al. (2007), 'Free personal care in Scotland: a narrative review', *British Journal of Social Work*, **37**(3), 459–74,

Dilnot, A., N. Warner and J. Williams (2011), *Fairer Care Funding: The Report of the Commission on Funding of Care and Support*, London: Commission on Funding of Care and Support. Available at: http://dilnot.dh.gov.uk/our-report/.

Dowling, B., M. Powell et al. (2004), 'Conceptualising successful partnerships', *Health and Social Care in the Community*, **12**(4), 309–17.

El Ansari, W., C.J. Phillips et al. (2001), 'Collaboration and partnerships: developing the evidence base', *Health and Social Care in the Community*, **9**(4), 215–27.

European Observatory on Health Care Systems (1999), *United Kingdom. Health Care Systems in Transition*, Copenhagen: European Observatory on Health Care Systems.

Forder, J. (2007), *Self-funded Social Care for Older People: An Analysis of Eligibility, Variations and Future Projections*, Canterbury: PSSRU.

Glasby, J. and R. Littlechild (2004), 'Creating "NHS local": a new relationship between PCTs and local government', Birmingham: Health Services Management Centre, University of Birmingham.

Glasby, J., J. Smith et al. (2006), 'Creating "NHS local": a new relationship between PCTs and local government', Birmingham: Health Services Management Centre, University of Birmingham.

Glendinning, C. (2003), 'Breaking down barriers: integrating health and care services for older people in England', *Health Policy*, **65**(2), 139–51.

Glendinning, C. (2007), 'Improving equity and sustainability in UK funding for long-term care: lessons from Germany', *Social Policy and Society*, **6**(03), 411–22.

Glendinning, C. and R. Means (2004), 'Rearranging the deckchairs on the Titanic of long-term care – is organisational integration the answer?', *Critical Social Policy*, **24**(4), 435–57.

Glendinning, C. and N. Moran (2009), *Reforming Long-term Care: Recent Lessons from Other Countries*, York: Social Policy Research Unit, University of York.

Glendinning, C., D. Challis et al. (2008), *Evaluation of the Individual Budgets Pilot Programme: Final Report*, York: Social Policy Research Unit, University of York.

Glendinning, C., A. Coleman et al. (2002), 'Partnerships, performance and primary care: developing integrated services for older people in England', *Ageing & Society*, **22**(2), 185–208.

Glendinning, C., B. Hudson et al. (2005), 'Under strain? Exploring the troubled relationship between health and social care', *Public Money & Management*, **25**(4), 245–51.

Goodwin, N. (2002), 'Creating an integrated public sector? Labour's plans for the modernisation of the English health care system', *International Journal of Integrated Care*, **2**.

Greer, S.L. (2004), 'Four way bet: how devolution has led to four different models for the NHS', London: The Constitution Unit.

Ham, C., J. Glasby et al. (2008), *Altogether Now? Policy Options for Integrating Care*, Birmingham: Health Services Management Centre, University of Birmingham: 12.

Hansard (2010), 'Continuing care: expenditure', Parliamentary Written Answers, *Daily Hansard*.

Hazell, R. and UCL Constitution Unit (2003), *The State of the Nations 2003: The Third Year of Devolution in the United Kingdom*, Exeter: Imprint Academic.

Health and Community Care Committee of the Scottish Parliament (2000), *16th Report: Inquiry into the Delivery of Community Care in Scotland*, Edinburgh: Scottish Parliament.

Health Select Committee (2005), *Sixth Report of Session 2004–05 on NHS continuing care*, 1.

Health Service Ombudsman (2003), *NHS Funding for Long Term Care. 2nd Report – Session 2002–2003*, London, The Stationery Office, 13 February.

Health Service Ombudsman (2004), *NHS Funding for Long Term Care: Follow up Report. 1st Report Session 2004–2005*, London: The Stationery Office.

Heenan, D. and D. Birrell (2006), 'The integration of health and social care: the lessons from Northern Ireland', *Social Policy & Administration*, **40**(1), 47–66.

Hensher, M. and N. Edwards (1999), 'The hospital of the future: hospital provision, activity, and productivity in England since the 1980s', *British Medical Journal*, **319**(7214), 911–14.

Henwood, M. (2004), *Continuing Health Care: Review, Revision and Restitution – Independent Research Review*, London: Department of Health.

Henwood, M. (2006), 'NHS Continuing care in England. Wanless social care review background paper', London: King's Fund.

Hiscock, J. and M. Pearson (1999), 'Looking inwards, looking outwards: dismantling the "Berlin wall" between health and social services?', *Social Policy and Administration*, **33**(2), 150–63.

HM Government (2009), *Shaping the Future of Care Together*, London: HMSO.

HM Government (2010), *Building the National Care Service*, London: HMSO.

Hope, P. (2010), Speech by Phil Hope, Minister of State for Care Services, 15 March, Dying to Talk Conference, Department of Health.

Hudson, B. (1999), 'Joint commissioning across the primary health care–social care boundary: can it work?', *Health and Social Care in the Community*, **7**(5), 358 66.

Hudson, B. (2002), 'Interprofessionality in health and social care: the Achilles' heel of partnership?', *Journal of Interprofessional Care*, **16**(1), 7–17.

Ikegami, N. (2007), 'Rationale, design and sustainability of long-term care insurance in Japan: in retrospect', *Social Policy and Society*, **6**(03), 423–34.

Ikegami, N. and J.C. Campbell (2002), 'Choices, policy logics and problems in the design of long-term care systems', *Social Policy and Administration*, **36**(7), 719–34.

Johnson, P., G. Wistow et al. (2003), 'Interagency and interprofessional collaboration in community care: the interdependence of structures and values', *Journal of Interprofessional Care*, **17**(1), 70–83.

Johri, M., F. Beland et al. (2003), 'International experiments in integrated care for the elderly: a synthesis of the evidence', *International Journal of Geriatric Psychiatry*, **18**(3), 222–35.

Keating, P., A. Sealy et al. (2008), 'Reducing unplanned hospital admissions and hospital bed days in the over 65 age group: results from a pilot study', *Journal of Integrated Care*, **16**(1), 3–8.

Kodner, D.L. (2003), 'Long-term care integration in four European countries: a review', in J. Brodsky, J. Habib and M. Hirschfeld (eds), *Key Policy Issues in Long-term Care*, Geneva: World Health Organization, pp. 91–138.

Kodner, D.L. (2004), 'Following the logic of long-term care: toward an independent, but integrated sector', *International Journal of Integrated Care*, **4** (Jan.–Mar.).

Kodner, D.L. (2006), 'Whole-system approaches to health and social care partnerships for the frail elderly: an exploration of North American models and lessons', *Health and Social Care in the Community*, **14**(5), 384–90.

Leichsenring, K. (2004), 'Developing integrated health and social care services for older persons in Europe', *International Journal of Integrated Care*, 1-15 DOI:

Leichsenring, K., A. Alaszewski et al. (2004), *Providing Integrated Health and Social Care for Older Persons: A European Overview of Issues at Stake*, Aldershot, Hants and Burlington, VT: Ashgate Publishing.

Leutz, W. (1999), 'Five laws for integrating medical and social services: lessons from the United States and the United Kingdom', *Milbank Quarterly*, **77**(1), 77–110, iv–v.

Leutz, W. (2005), 'Reflections on integrating medical and social care: five laws revisited', *Journal of Integrated Care*, **13**(5), 3–12.

Lewis, J. (2001), 'Older people and the health–social care boundary in the UK: half a century of hidden policy conflict', *Social Policy and Administration*, **35**(4), 343–59.

Lindblom, C.E. (1959), 'The science of "muddling through"', *Public Administration Review*, **19**(2), 79–88.

Lyon, D., J. Miller et al. (2006), 'The Castlefields Integrated Care Model: the evidence summarised', *Journal of Integrated Care*, **14**(1), 7–12.

Mandelstam, M. (2009), *Community Care Practice and the Law*, London: Jessica Kingsley.

McCormack, B., E.A. Mitchell et al. (2008), 'Older persons' experiences of whole systems: the impact of health and social care organizational structures', *Journal of Nursing Management*, **16**(2), 105–14.

McMurray, R. (2007), 'Our reforms, our partnerships, same problems: the chronic case of the English NHS', *Public Money & Management*, **27**(1), 77–82.

Means, R., H. Morbey et al. (2002), *From Community Care to Market Care? The Development of Welfare Services for Older People*, Bristol: Policy.

Ministry of Health (1957a), *Geriatric Services and the Care of the Chronic Sick*, HM (57)86.

Ministry of Health (1957b), *Local Authority Services for the Chronic Sick and Infirm*, Circular 14/57.

Mur-Veeman, I., A. van Raak et al. (2008), 'Comparing integrated care policy in Europe: does policy matter?', *Health Policy*, **85**(2), 172–83.

Netten, A., Robin Darton et al. (2005), *Understanding Public Services and Markets*, Report Commissioned by the King's Fund for the Care Services Inquiry. Kent: Personal Social Services Research Unit.

NHS Choices (2010a), 'All care trusts – what is a care trust?', retrieved 19 February 2010, from http://www.nhs.uk/servicedirectories/pages/caretrustlisting.aspx.

NHS Choices (2010b), 'What are primary care trusts (PCTs)?', retrieved 19 February 2010, from http://www.nhs.uk/chq/Pages/1078.aspx?CategoryID=68&SubCategoryID=153.

Office of the Deputy Prime Minister (2005), 'Local strategic partnerships: shaping their future', a consultation paper.

Oliver, A. (2005), 'The English National Health Service: 1979–2005', *Health Economics*, **14**(S1), S75–S99.

Ouwens, M., H. Wollersheim et al. (2005), 'Integrated care programmes for chronically ill patients: a review of systematic reviews', *International Journal of Quality Health Care*, **17**(2), 141–6.

Phelps, K. and E. Regen (2008), *To What Extent Does The Use Of Health Act Flexibilities Promote Effective Partnership Working and Positive Outcomes for Older People? Final Report*, Leicester: Leicester Nuffield Research Unit, University of Leicester.

Player, S. and A.M. Pollock (2001), 'Long-term care: from public responsibility to private good', *Critical Social Policy*, **21**(2), 231–55.

Ramsay, A., N. Fulop et al. (2009), 'The evidence base for vertical integration in health care', *Journal of Integrated Care*, **17**(2), 3–12.

Reilly, S., D. Challis et al. (2003), 'Does integration really make a difference? A comparison of old age psychiatry services in England and Northern Ireland', *International Journal of Geriatric Psychiatry*, **18**(10), 887–93.

Reilly, S., D. Challis et al. (2007), 'Care management in mental health services in England and Northern Ireland: do integrated organizations promote integrated practice?', *Journal of Health Services Research Policy*, **12**(4), 236–41.

Rittel, H.W.J. and M.M. Webber (1973), 'Dilemmas in a general theory of planning', *Policy Sciences*, **4**, 155–69.

Robins, J. (2008), 'Blind, immobilised, diabetic – but the NHS doesn't care', *The Observer*. London: Guardian News and Media.

Roth, G. and M. Reichert (2004), 'Providing integrated health and social care for older persons in Germany', in K. Leichsenring and A. Alaszewski (eds), *Providing Integrated Health and Social Care for Elder Persons: A European Overview of Issues at Stake*, in series 'Public Policy and Social Welfare', Vol. 28, Aldershot, Hants and Burlington, VT, Ashgate, pp. 269–327.

Rothgang, H. and G. Igl (2007), 'Long-term care in Germany', *Japanese Journal of Social Security Policy*, **6**(1), 54–84.

Royal College of Nursing (2008), *RCN response to DH on the Proposed Review of the National Framework for Continuing Care. To Department of Health*, London: RCN.

Secretary of State for Health (2000), *The NHS Plan: a plan for investment, a plan for reform*, London: Department of Health.

Secretary of State for Health (2010), *Government Response to the Health Select Committee Report on Social Care (Third Report of Session 2009–10)*, London: Department of Health.

Shepperd, S., H. Doll et al. (2009), 'Early discharge hospital at home', *Cochrane Database of Systematic Reviews*, DOI: 10.1002/14651858.CD000356.pub3.

Smith, G. and D. May (1980), 'The artificial debate between rationalist and incrementalist models of decision making', *Policy & Politics*, **8**, 147–61.

Smith, K.E., C. Bambra et al. (2009), 'Partners in health? A systematic review of the impact of organizational partnerships on public health outcomes in England between 1997 and 2008', *Journal of Public Health (Oxford)*, **31**(2), 210–21.

South, J. (1999), 'Eligibility criteria and entitlements: defining need for NHS continuing care', *Social Policy & Administration*, **33**(2), 132–49.

Sullivan, H. and C. Skelcher (2002), *Working Across Boundaries: Collaboration in Public Services*, Basingstoke: Palgrave, Macmillan.

The Law Commission (2010), 'Adult social care: a consultation paper', London: The Law Commission.

Wanless, D., J.L. Fernández et al. (2006), *Securing Good Care for Older People: Taking a Long-term View*, London: King's Fund.

Windle, K., R. Wagland et al. (2009), *National Evaluation of Partnerships for Older People Projects: Final Report*, Kent: PSSRU, University of Kent.

Websites

Age Concern, 'NHS failing older people needing continuing care local black spots exposed', 11 April 2008.
Health and Social Care in Northern Ireland, retrieved 12 December 2009 from http://www.hscni.net/index. php?link=trusts.

15 Barriers to and opportunities for private long-term care insurance in England: what can we learn from other countries?

Adelina Comas-Herrera, Rebecca Butterfield,
José-Luis Fernández, Raphael Wittenberg and
Joshua M. Wiener

1. INTRODUCTION

An ageing population, together with the rising cost of services, means that long-term care expenditures will increase greatly over the next several decades. Wittenberg et al. (2008) project that the numbers of disabled older people in England will more than double between 2005 and 2041, rising from around 2.40 million to around 4.95 million. They project that public expenditure on social care and disability benefits will need to rise from around 1.2 per cent of GDP in 2005 to around 2.0 per cent of GDP in 2041 to keep pace with demographic pressures and expected real rises in the unit costs of care. This raises serious questions about how this is to be funded.

In light of increasing fiscal constraints, policy makers are particularly keen on mechanisms for incentivising private contributions to the care system, for instance by increasing use of the private long-term care insurance market. In spite of their advantages in terms of the pooling of risks of needing long-term care, there have been substantial difficulties in the development of private long-term care insurance products in England.

In many countries, especially where the public long-term care system plays only a residual or 'safety-net' role, individual and family resources pay for a substantial proportion of long-term care costs, often out of pocket at the point of need. The Personal Social Services Research Unit (PSSRU) estimates that in England in 2006 nearly 40 per cent of social care expenditure was funded privately by individuals and their families (Comas-Herrera et al., 2010). About a quarter of that expenditure was as a result of user fees for publicly subsidised care and the rest was expenditure by people who faced the full cost of their long-term care (self-funders).

Recent estimates suggest that the expected average lifetime costs of care for people aged 65 or more in England, including hotel costs for those in care homes, were £50 300 in 2009/10, £34 300 for men and £64 800 for women (Fernández and Forder, 2010, p. 11). However, averages do not give a full picture of the financial risk that long-term care can present for some families. Around a third of people aged 65 and over will spend little on care. For a small proportion of people, however, long-term care costs will represent so-called 'catastrophic' levels of expenditure: 7 per cent of people aged 65 will face lifetime care costs of at least £100 000, and 5 per cent of at least £200 000. In England, dependent people in residential care homes are often required to deplete their assets, including having to sell their homes to contribute to their care costs.[1] Buckinghamshire County

Council, for instance, estimated that 15 per cent of the self-funders in their area deplete their capital every year (Birchley, 2010). Partnership Insurance, a firm specialised in immediate needs annuity products, has estimated that meeting the costs of care of people who deplete their assets in England costs nearly £1 billion a year (Partnership, 2010). In some of the cases where individuals are unable to continue to pay privately for their care, the transition into the public support system leads to a move to a cheaper care home.

Because not everyone will need care, and many people will need care for only a short period, in principle, some form of risk pooling through insurance seems a more attractive way of financing long-term care than individual savings. Risk pooling would mean that people who would be self-funders, or would be required to pay co-payments under the current scheme, could limit the amount that they would have to pay for their care to a lower, known amount. This would mean that those people who require care for long periods (and whose care costs exceed the average in the insurance pool) would be prevented from having to spend down their assets or go without the care they need.

Despite the very substantial levels of private expenditure involved in funding long-term care in England, the market for private long-term care insurance is very small. Only 22 000 people had private long-term care insurance in 2008 (Association of British Insurers, 2009). Instead, care is usually publicly funded for those with few resources and funded from the income, savings and housing assets for those with resources. At present, no pre-funded long-term care insurance is being sold in England. There are two companies selling immediate needs care annuities.[2]

There are a number of countries where the markets for long-term care are substantially bigger than that in England. The two countries with the biggest markets for long-term care insurance are the USA and France. In the USA, about 10 per cent of the population aged 60 and over have private long-term care insurance (Brown and Finkelstein, 2009); it has been estimated that in total there are around 7 to 8 million policy holders. There are currently around 3 million policy holders in France (FFSA, 2010), which represents about 24 per cent of the population aged 60 and over.

There are substantial private long-term care insurance markets in other countries too. Swiss Re reported that, in 2007, Germany had the third-largest private insurance market (Swiss Re, 2008), comprising mandatory private long-term care insurance and private supplementary long-term care insurance, which represented about 15 per cent of the in-force premiums volume in 2007. Nearly 1 million German people were covered by supplementary long-term care insurance in Germany in 2006 (PKV, 2007), which is sold as a supplement (or top-up) to the benefits of the social long-term care insurance system.

The size of the private long-term care insurance market in Israel is relatively large compared to other countries because half the adult population have private long-term care insurance (Brammli-Greenberg and Gross, 2010) and policy holders are often unaware that they are covered. This is predominantly bought with other forms of health insurance. The market for long-term care insurance grew quite rapidly in Italy in 2007 and 2008; after a new collective wage agreement for insurance and bank employees that provided automatic compulsory long-term care coverage (funded, totally or partially, by employers), the number of people covered by long-term care insurance grew very rapidly, to approximately 355 000 in 2009 (Rebba, 2010).

This chapter is part of a research project titled 'How can private long-term care insurance supplement state systems? The UK as a case study', funded by the AXA Research

Fund and involving researchers from the London School of Economics, the University of East Anglia, the Nuffield Foundation and the Universitat de Barcelona.[3] The chapter is an early summary of an ongoing literature review, combined with interviews with international experts in private long-term care insurance (including academics, policy makers and insurance representatives).

The chapter begins by considering the rationale for insuring against the costs of long-term care, arguing that there appears to be a strong rationale for the purchase of long-term care insurance by individuals (Section 2). It then considers the barriers to the development of an efficient long-term care insurance market (Section 3), followed by Section 4, which considers the types of insurance products available. The final two sections consider the effects that the underlying public system can have on the structure and success of private long-term care insurance schemes, and what the state can do to encourage the development of private long-term care insurance (Sections 5 and 6).

2.   RATIONALE FOR INSURING AGAINST THE COSTS OF LONG-TERM CARE

The potential cost to the individual of long-term care, when not insured against its cost, is highly uncertain. Insurance works as a mechanism for pooling the risks of catastrophic costs, so that the risks of all the people insured by the scheme are collectively borne by the insurance scheme. This works only when the loss of the group as a whole can be predicted (i.e. when the costs, on average, are broadly certain). When group costs are known, statisticians and actuaries can calculate the contribution that should be made by each insured individual, in exchange for the security of knowing that the group will cover the costs of their care should they need it. The insurance scheme therefore receives premium contributions from all its enrollees and makes payments to those who suffer the risk specified in the policy. This allows individuals to pool risks, despite some future uncertainties.

There are a number of rationales for using long-term care insurance to finance long-term care. Insurance, unlike reliance on individual or family savings, redistributes costs from those with lesser to those with greater care needs. By pooling risks and reducing the uncertainty faced by an individual, risk-averse individuals would be better off purchasing an actuarially fair insurance policy. In principle, insurance is also a more efficient approach than private savings because it removes the need for every single individual to save up to the maximum possible lifetime cost of their care (see, e.g., Barr, 2010 and Rivlin and Wiener, 1988). Finally, in theory, long-term care insurance could also potentially promote choice, independence and dignity.[4]

The potential role for private long-term care insurance is highly dependent on the characteristics of public sector coverage for long-term care in that particular country (see, e.g., Foubister et al., 2006). Where the public sector role is to act as a safety net for people who cannot afford to pay for their own care (as, e.g., in England and the USA), only people without enough resources to pay for their own care needs are covered by the public system. In those countries, private insurance can potentially substitute for the lack of public coverage by protecting against the probability of having to pay for care in the event of needing it, or, for people who are at the point of needing care, against the catastrophic costs involved in requiring a very long duration of care (preventing asset depletion).

Where the public sector offers full (or near full) coverage of the risks and costs of long-term care, the role for private insurance is nearly non-existent. In some countries, however, the public sector offers partial universal coverage so that everyone is entitled to a certain level of publicly funded care (given a certain level of need). Usually these systems also offer means-tested benefits for people who cannot cover the rest of the costs of their care. In countries with this type of 'quasi-universal' public coverage (for example Germany, France and Spain), private long-term care insurance is often marketed as a 'top-up', or complement, to the public system.

3. BARRIERS TO THE DEVELOPMENT OF PRIVATE LONG-TERM CARE INSURANCE

Despite there being a clear rationale for the role of private long-term care insurance, there is a substantial body of theoretical work on the economics of long-term care insurance (see, e.g., Barr, 2010 for a recent review) that lists several conditions under which private insurance will be inefficient or non-existent. These market failures lead to doubts about how far voluntary private insurance is feasible as the principal means to finance long-term care. This section briefly discusses the theoretical barriers to private insurance and reviews the evidence about the effect of these barriers. We distinguish broadly between supply barriers that affect the risk to insurers and as a result the costs of premiums and types of products on offer, and demand barriers.

3.1 Supply Barriers

Insurers face major risks when providing long-term care insurance, which can be summarised under three headings: uncertainty about future costs; adverse selection; and insurance-induced demand.

Uncertainty about the future numbers of people needing care and the unit costs of care
Economic theory has long identified as one of the fundamental conditions for an insurance market to work well that the risk insured should be independent and have a known distribution (Barr, 2010). This is not the case for long-term care, which is complicated by the fact that insurance is often purchased decades in advance of its use.[5] The Association of British Insurers (ABI) identify five major sources of uncertainty: the probability of living to an advanced age;[6] probability of needing care; length of time care is needed; future indexation of benefits; and investment returns (ABI, 2010, p. 5). Other important sources of uncertainty include the future extent of public coverage, the type of services that will be available and preferred by future cohorts of older people, and future rates of lapse.

Unlike the risk at the individual level, these group risks are subject to uncertainty, with the distribution of probability unknown. This means that insurers cannot forecast expenditures with any certainty, and therefore cannot set actuarially fair premiums based on expected lifetime costs with certainty. This has a major effect on the insurance products available and their affordability.

Adverse selection

Economic theory suggests that people who know they are more likely to need care are more likely to wish to buy premiums; this is particularly a problem when people buy policies later in life and therefore may have more information on their individual probability of needing long-term care. If insurance were predominantly bought by those with higher risk, to compensate for the high levels of benefit payouts insurance companies would need to increase the prices of premiums. Higher premiums could make insurance even less attractive to people with better risk, exacerbating the problem. To combat adverse selection, insurers seek to protect themselves by using medical screening and rejecting applicants who represent a bad risk. In the USA, 15 to 20 per cent of those who apply for coverage are denied (Tumlinson et al., 2009, p. 12).

The evidence suggests that people who buy long-term care insurance do tend to perceive themselves at higher risk of needing care than those who do not purchase (see, e.g., Courbage and Roudaut, 2008; Schaber and Stum, 2007; Sloan and Norton, 1997). Some authors interpret this as a confirmation of the presence of adverse selection. However, it could just be a result of having better information about the risks. Also, Mellor (2000) warns that this increased awareness about the risk of needing care may be a result of having purchased insurance. Finkelstein and McGarry (2003) examined the relationship between insurance coverage and the likelihood of entering a nursing home and found no relationship. They argue that people are more likely to opt into an insurance scheme for long-term care if they (a) have private information that suggests that they are more likely than average to require long-term care in the future, or (b) have a higher preference for insurance than the average individual (i.e. are more risk-averse). They suggest that these two tendencies work in opposite directions and may cancel each other out. Interpreting the empirical evidence from the USA is complicated by the fact that there is medical underwriting that screens out people with known risks by not allowing them to purchase policies.

In the USA, men and women pay the same premiums,[7] irrespective of the fact that women have a much higher risk of needing long-term care. Adverse selection would suggest that women, when facing the same price, would be much more likely to buy long-term care coverage than men. However, Brown and Finkelstein (2009, p. 13) show that there is almost no difference in the rates of purchase of long-term care insurance by men and women (10.1 and 10.7 per cent, respectively), even though they estimate that men are implicitly being charged between 25 and 50 cents per dollar more than women for the same benefits. It is important to consider, though, that women on average earn less than men over their lifetime, potentially making the insurance premiums less affordable for them (Holdenrieder, 2006).

Another way in which adverse selection could have an impact, in principle, would be if individuals chose to cancel the insurance held with an insurer if they obtained new information suggesting that they were at lower risk (Brown and Finkelstein, 2007; Hendel and Lizzeri, 2003). This has been described as the 'dynamic contracting' problem: under a voluntary insurance scheme, individuals may opt out when they receive more information on the likelihood of requiring long-term care, so that good risk types may be inclined to leave the insurance pool over time. This could affect the pool of risk types held by the insurer. Critics of this proposition argue that, in practice, individuals rarely receive information that they are at lower risk. Recent US evidence suggests that the primary reason for terminating the policies is financial, and that individuals who cancel their insurance (or 'lapse') are likely to be in poorer health (Konetzka and Luo, 2011). However, evidence from a sample of Spanish long-term care policy holders, who faced much lower premiums than those in US policies, suggests that people who lapsed had better health histories than those who remained (Pinquet et al., 2010).

Insurance-induced demand

When people are covered by long-term care insurance they experience care services either free or at a low cost, which may encourage them to use more care than they would in the absence of insurance. Insurance-induced demand for care could also lead to market failure for long-term care insurance. Scanlon (1992) argues that the issue of moral hazard is more pronounced in the market for long-term care insurance (compared to health insurance) because it is difficult for the insurer to detect an individual's preference for receiving care from family members, as opposed to formal services. It is therefore difficult to predict how individuals' preferences might change when insured. Insurers are likely to introduce co-payments to limit the effects of insurance-induced demand. Controlling for disability level and other variables, analyses by Cohen et al. (2000) show that people with insurance were using significantly higher amounts of care.

Although insurance companies use high prices in excess of an actuarially fair premium and medical underwriting to protect themselves from the risks they face, they also use other mechanisms. For example, a study by Brown and Finkelstein (2007) found that most policies in the USA have an 'elimination period' or deductible (typically 30 to 100 days), which is the number of days a person has to receive care before insurance payments commence. This measure aims to minimise the effect of insurance-induced demand. A number of measures have also been taken to reduce the intertemporal risk faced by insurers by shifting the risk to the individuals. For example, policies in the USA typically provide payments equal to the cost of care, but only up to a specified maximum daily benefit (most frequently $100 per day in 2002, substantially below the average daily cost of $143 per day in a shared room in a nursing home). In addition, about 60 per cent of policies have a daily benefit maximum that is fixed in nominal terms and does not increase over time with inflation. Most policies also specify a maximum 'benefit period', often one to five years, which caps the total number of days that an individual can receive benefits.

Another important supply issue that was mentioned by interviewees in all the countries covered so far in this study (England, Austria, Spain, Italy, France and the USA) was that a regulatory framework for long-term care insurance is a major barrier to the development of the private long-term care insurance market.

3.2   Demand Barriers

From a consumer's point of view, private long-term care insurance is not an attractive product to buy because of high costs and poor affordability, unrealistic risk perceptions, misconceptions about the generosity of the public care system and low preference for insurance. The saying in the USA is that long-term care insurance 'is sold, not bought'.

High costs and poor affordability

It has been shown that, even if long-term care insurance premiums that covered the full costs of care were actuarially fair, they would still be unaffordable for large sections of the population (Wiener et al., 1994). In practice, policies at an actuarially fair price are unlikely to be offered in the market for long-term care insurance. Private insurers protect their companies from uncertainty about the future, insurance-induced demand and the potential for adverse selection by increasing the cost of the premiums (or curtailing benefits in some way). Evidence suggests that the prices of typical long-term care insurance policies are substantially more than those of other private insurance products (Brown and Finkelstein, 2007). This limits even more the affordability and attractiveness of insurance products to potential purchasers.

As discussed earlier, different types of insurance and different ways of selling have a major impact on their cost. In the USA in particular, the administrative costs of private long-term care insurance are very high, in great part because in the USA the vast majority of long-term care insurance policies are sold at an individual level. The proportion of the premium that is accounted for by benefits is known as the loss ratio. In general, individually sold private long-term care insurance in the USA is believed to have a loss ratio of about 60 per cent.[8] This means that, for each £1 spent on the insurance premium, the individual receives back, on average, 60p in benefit. Employer-sponsored long-term care insurance is believed to have a loss ratio of around 70 per cent. The loss ratio for employer-sponsored long-term insurance is assumed to be higher because, for example, group markets may be able to take advantage of economies of scale. Employers are also likely to bear some of the costs of administering the policy themselves, for example collecting premiums through payroll deductions and helping to market the policies (Wiener, 1998).

Le Bihan and Martin (2010) argue that monitoring and predicting the outgoings of insurance schemes is more difficult when assistance is in the form of in-kind benefits, which may result in policies where the benefits in kind (as is more common in the USA[9]) have higher administrative costs than those that offer cash benefits (as is predominant in France and other European countries). Taleyson (2003) and Kessler (2008) also argue that because of the type of insurance product design in France (cash benefits, as opposed to reimbursement of provider fees, and the fact that benefits are triggered by fixed thresholds of disability often based on the same disability scales and thresholds as the public system), the administrative costs of long-term care insurance in that country are considerably lower than those in the USA.

It has been estimated that only 10 to 20 per cent of older people in the USA can afford good-quality private long-term care insurance (Wiener et al., 1994). Crown et al. (1992) add that although there is potential for the market for long-term care insurance to be significant, this might involve individuals in the 65–69 age group spending up to 50 per cent of their discretionary income on such insurance.[10]

Risk perception and misconceptions and uncertainty about public system coverage

A common explanation for the lack of long-term care insurance purchasing is that individuals ignore low-frequency, high-severity events that have not occurred recently (Kunreuther et al., 1978). A recent experiment in Germany suggests that increased awareness of risk is likely to result in higher rates of purchase of long-term care insurance (Zhou-Richter et al., 2010), with about 30 per cent of interviewees who were previously not willing to purchase (supplementary) long-term care insurance in the past indicating a willingness to purchase after being informed about the risk associated with long-term care. Courbage and Roudaut (2008) also found that having provided informal care positively affected the probability of contracting long-term care insurance in France.

Experts from the USA, England and Italy interviewed for this project emphasised that a very important barrier to the purchase of private insurance is that people wrongly believe that they are covered by the public long-term care or health care systems. Thus they see no need to purchase additional coverage. A study of non-buyers of long-term care insurance in the USA shows that 20 per cent of non-buyers considered the statement 'If I need long-term care services, I believe that Medicare (and Medicaid) will pay' an important or very important reason they did not buy long-term care insurance (LifePlans, 2007). However, it appears that US initiatives to educate people about their risks of long-term care and extent of public coverage have had some effect, because in 1990 the percentage answering that they believed Medicare and Medicaid would cover them was 58 per cent.

Also, when there are expectations that the public system will be reformed to provide additional public coverage, people may be reluctant to buy insurance to avoid over-insuring. Insurance companies may also be more reluctant to market their policies if they expect substantial changes. The latest figures from France show that growth in the numbers of people who buy private long-term care insurance has slowed significantly: whereas in 2005 the market grew by 12 per cent, in 2009 it only increased by 1 per cent (FFSA, 2010). Experts suggest that the French market is stagnating because of uncertainties related to the public framework for long-term care (Le Corre, 2010) because, since at least 2007, a major reform has been expected (Le Bihan and Martin, 2010).

Low preference for insurance
In addition to underestimating the probability that they will need care (and as a result resisting buying a product that they do not expect to need), long-term care (particularly in care homes) is not a 'product' that people have a desire to consume. This is exacerbated by frequent reports of cases of very poor quality of care in the media (see, e.g., recent articles in the *Guardian*, 2010 and in *The Times*, 2009). It can be expected that people will resist buying a product that they do not wish to use.

Brown and Finkelstein (2009) add to this point, arguing that insurance against long-term care essentially transfers wealth from a period where the individual is active and healthy to a period where the individual has problems with carrying out activities of daily living and so requires care. They argue that if an individual places more value on consumption in the healthy state, then equating marginal utilities across the states may not lead to equal consumption over the two periods. In such a case, the purchase of insurance would not be welfare optimising. Whether this hypothesis holds perhaps depends on how debilitating the individual expects the 'unhealthy' state to be, and his or her expectation of the contribution that care might make to improving his or her quality of life. Offering a care package that is tailored to the individual's needs (e.g. offers a choice between informal, domiciliary, assisted living and residential care) may increase the utility that the individual places on receiving care.

Particularly at younger ages (when pre-funded insurance products can be bought at a lower price) there are major competing demands on people's incomes, such as mortgages, child care, saving for general retirement income and saving for children's university fees.

Various other explanations have been put forward as to why people may not have very strong preferences for private long-term care insurance. In a widely quoted article, Pauly (1990) argued that the main reason people purchase long-term care insurance is to protect bequests. However, he argued that even if an individual receives positive utility from leaving a bequest, if he prefers informal care over formal care, he still may prefer not to purchase long-term care insurance, because private insurance may remove family members' incentives to provide informal care to protect the bequest. Pauly (1990) therefore argues that even in a market with actuarially fair prices and perfect information, opt-in rates are likely to remain low. Empirical evidence for this differs in its conclusions. Sloan and Norton (1997) find that marital state and number of children are not related to the purchase of long-term care insurance, suggesting that demand is not motivated by bequest or exchange motives (i.e. older people exchanging informal care for the bequest). However, other studies have shown that being married is positively associated with purchasing insurance (Brown and Finkelstein, 2009; Cramer and Jensen, 2006), but only when assets fall within the middle range (Courbage and Roudaut, 2008). Having children and higher numbers of children were also found to be associated with purchasing insurance when using the French sample of the SHARE survey by Courbage and Roudaut (2008). However, Schaber and Stum (2007), in the USA, found that people who bought long-term care insurance tended to have smaller family sizes. The LifePlans study on 'who buys long-term care insurance' shows that, in practice, there are many factors at play behind the decision to buy long-term care insurance. It found that although asset protection was the most important reason people bought long-term care insurance, guaranteeing that they could afford services, ensuring choice of services and protecting a family's standard of living were very important factors as well (LifePlans, 2007).

Mistrust of private insurers

Mistrust of private insurers has been mentioned by interviewees as a major factor in the low demand for long-term care insurance, particularly in the USA and Italy. The main reason for concern in the USA seems to be the lack of consumer protection against premium increases[11] and the fact that if policy holders drop their policies (or 'lapse', often as a result of economic difficulties), they are not entitled to any benefits (this issue is often referred to as the lack of 'nonforfeiture benefits').

In contrast, at the time of needing care, a recent US study has shown that people covered by comprehensive long-term care insurance are rarely denied benefits and have a good choice of care settings. Interestingly, the authors of the study conclude that their findings do not support 'widespread suspicion or fears that private long-term care insurance companies routinely deny legitimate claims' and also do not support 'concerns that private long-term care insurance benefits are typically inadequate to cover a substantial share of long-term care costs in the settings where claimants have chosen to reside' (Doty et al., 2010, p. 620).

4.   LONG-TERM CARE INSURANCE PRODUCTS

Existing public long-term care coverage is a major determinant of the types of private long-term care insurance offered. Foubister et al. (2006), Taleyson (2003), Mayhew et al. (2010) and Le Bihan and Martin (2010) discuss various aspects of this topic. Building on their work, it seems useful to distinguish between the following types of insurance products:

- Full long-term care insurance
- Top-up long-term care insurance
- Immediate needs annuities
- Disability-linked annuities
- Combined long-term care and life insurance.

4.1   Full Long-term Care Insurance

This type of insurance is predominantly found in countries with a safety-net type of public coverage of long-term care. It is normally designed as a substitute for the public system, for those who are not covered by it (Foubister et al., 2006). It is typically a reimbursement product, with some limits to the daily or monthly benefits. These products are normally medically underwritten, excluding people with chronic illnesses or disability. This is the predominant type of private insurance in the USA. Until recently this type of insurance was available in the UK, but only a very small number of people bought it. There are currently no such products on offer in the UK. The administrative costs for this type of policy, particularly if sold at individual level, are typically very high because of the costs of detailed medical underwriting, expenses incurred managing the reimbursements, agent fees and marketing costs.

4.2   Top-up or Supplementary Long-term Care Insurance

This type of insurance usually coexists with a partial universal public coverage of the costs of long-term care. The insurance is normally for cash benefits that are fixed given a certain level of disability (which in some cases, such as in Spain, is sold specifically as a complement to the public long-term care system, even using the same assessment criteria as the public long-term care system; see, e.g., INESE, 2010), making the underwriting process relatively cheap. This type of insurance is available in France, Germany, Spain, Israel and Italy, among other countries. It is relatively cheap to administer, especially in comparison with full long-term care insurance.

Immediate needs annuities
Immediate needs annuities cover people at the point of needing care and insure against the duration of care needs (to avoid catastrophic costs of care). People may buy this coverage to limit how much their estate will be depleted, or to ensure that their assets are not depleted to the point of needing to rely on publicly funded care (which may involve a move to a cheaper care home). The premium is calculated considering the individual's health and choice of care home. The fees are reimbursed directly to the care providers, who are normally happy to accept a predetermined rate of growth for the insured person's care fees. This product fits well with home equity release. It is currently the only form of private long-term care insurance available in England.

The rate of coverage is low relative to the numbers of self-funders who could potentially afford it. The main provider of these annuities in England, Partnership, is currently investing in increasing awareness of this product by campaigning to improve the financial advice available to older people and their families, particularly at the point of entering a care home. They estimate that out of 53 000 people who had to pay care fees in 2009 in England, only 7000 received appropriate financial advice. Research on the net benefit and affordability of immediate needs annuities suggests that, while there will always be a limit on the suitability of these annuities for less wealthy people, around 40 per cent of all self-funders in England (assuming they had at least a modest degree of risk aversion) would both benefit from and be able to afford them (Forder, 2011).

Disability-linked annuities

This is a type of annuity in which the payments could increase if the beneficiary became disabled. The additional funds could be used to pay for long-term care services. Different benefit levels could be defined, according to the level of disability. Murtaugh et al. (2001) show that combining an income annuity with disability coverage has the potential to reduce the cost of both products, compared to purchasing them separately, and calculate that this could be useful to more potential purchasers. They showed that minimal underwriting, excluding only those who would be eligible for benefits at purchase, would increase the potential market to about 98 per cent of 65-year-olds, compared with only 77 per cent under usual underwriting practice. Such a product would be targeted to people with substantial savings at retirement. A major obstacle to this product in the USA is the current regulatory framework because combining an annuity with disability insurance would require complying with two different sets of regulations (Warshawsky, 2007).

Combined long-term care and life insurance

This type of insurance is a combination of a life insurance policy and disability annuity, where the benefit is paid at death if there has been no need for long-term care, or as monthly payments from the onset of the need for care until death (Mayhew et al., 2010). These contracts are available in France (Le Bihan and Martin, 2010) and Italy (Rebba, 2010).

5.   THE RELATIONSHIP BETWEEN PUBLIC FINANCING AND PRIVATE LONG-TERM CARE INSURANCE

The underlying state-funded system has a major impact on the design and success of any private insurance scheme for long-term care. The types of insurance products offered by private sector insurers are determined, to a large extent, by the public scheme in operation within a country. For example, in France, all individuals have access to some support from the state under the Allocation personnalisée à l'autonomie. For those with an income below some fixed amount, the state funds their entire care package. Above that income level, the proportion of the costs of care that the state funds declines as the individual's income increases, with individuals with a monthly income greater than €2720 paying 90 per cent of their care package. Le Bihan and Martin (2010) estimate that dependency costs are, on average, €2500 per month, with the public allowance contributing around €500. Private insurance may therefore be purchased to complement the contributions from the public system. Le Bihan and Martin (2010) estimate that private insurance may pay for an additional €300 towards the cost of dependency, on average.

In contrast in the USA, where Medicaid only covers people's costs of long-term care if they have an income below some threshold or if they incur large long-term care costs relative to their income, private insurance products on offer are substitutive.

An important aspect of the relationship between private insurance and the public system is whether the public system is a primary payer or a secondary (safety-net) payer. If it is a primary payer, the public system does not take into account private insurance benefits when applying the means test. In such systems, which normally involve a universal needs-based entitlement, private insurance benefits tend to be used to top up the public entitlement; this is the case, for example, in France.

If the public system is a secondary payer, then insurance benefits have to be paid first. In systems where access to public care is means-tested and the public system is a secondary payer, people who buy insurance may be 'pushed' over the means test, even if they would have been eligible otherwise. In the USA, Medicaid is the secondary public payer of long-term care costs, which means that the insurance policy has to pay benefits first, even if the individual is otherwise eligible for Medicaid. Brown and Finkelstein (2009) argue that the Medicaid programme crowds out private insurance demand. They have calculated that, even if comprehensive private insurance were available at actuarially fair prices, nearly two-thirds (60th percentile) of the wealth distribution would still not wish to purchase insurance because of Medicaid. Medicaid's crowd-out effect is a result of the 'implicit tax' that Medicaid imposes on the purchase of private policies: part of the premium that individuals pay for the purchase of private policies goes to pay for benefits that may end up duplicating benefits that Medicaid would have paid for in the absence of insurance.[12] Because Medicaid is means-tested, private insurance also reduces the probability of becoming eligible for Medicaid in the first place. Brown and Finkelstein (2009) argue that a possible solution would be that Medicaid becomes the primary payer and allows the asset test threshold to vary with wealth. However, they acknowledge that although this could stimulate demand, it may not necessarily make a big difference to the overall purchase of long-term care insurance policies because other factors would still limit demand.

6.   HOW CAN THE PUBLIC LONG-TERM CARE SYSTEM ENCOURAGE WIDER LONG-TERM CARE INSURANCE?

There are a number of ways in which the public sector can promote demand for long-term care insurance. On the demand side, the state might make premiums cheaper through making policies tax-deductible (or providing tax credits), offering opt-outs from public or social contributions to people who purchase private insurance, increasing awareness of the risks of long-term care through educational programmes, clarifying entitlements to public support, ensuring that independent specialist financial advice for long-term care is more widely available, making sure that benefits are tax-exempt, and encouraging access to group-based policies (which tend to be cheaper). Alternatively, the state might target the supply side, by improving the regulatory framework and taking on part of the risk faced by insurers, for example by defining the level of public coverage in a way that limits the risk to long-term care insurance providers. The state might also choose to intervene more directly by making private long-term care insurance compulsory, or creating a public insurance system.

6.1   Encouraging Demand for Insurance

Government has a number of tools at its disposal to encourage the demand for private long-term care insurance, ranging from helping make insurance more affordable, to educating the population about the risk of long-term care, to improving regulation to improve the degree to which people trust private insurance companies.

6.2   Tax Incentives

In many countries there are tax incentives for the purchase of long-term care, and benefits received through long-term care insurance are generally tax-free. In the USA, since 1996, long-term care insurance premiums have been treated as health insurance when calculating an individual's federal income tax liability. Individuals may deduct a portion of their medical and long-term care expenses (including insurance premiums) from their adjusted gross income under highly limited circumstances[13] (Courtemanche and He, 2008). At the state level, there is wide variation in the tax treatment of long-term care premiums. Some states provide individual tax deductions; others provide tax credits to employers who offer group policies (Stevenson et al., 2009; Wiener et al., 2000). In Spain, long-term care insurance premiums are tax-deductible, but the maximum amount that can be deducted is calculated in conjunction with deductions for pensions, so the amount of the deduction is limited. In Italy there are both income tax credits of 19 per cent (maximum amount of €1291.14 per year) and tax exemptions for group policies, for both employees and employers. Premiums paid by employers are totally exempted from regional business taxes (Rebba, 2010). In France, there has been some discussion about introducing tax incentives for middle-income households to encourage the purchase of long-term care insurance policies (Le Bihan and Martin, 2010).

The evidence strongly suggests that tax relief, at least at the level that has been implemented in the USA, will only have a small impact on uptake because of price inelasticity (Brown and Finkelstein, 2009; Courtemanche and He, 2008; Cramer and Jensen, 2006). Courtemanche and He (2008) also found that the loss in tax revenue from granting the federal tax incentive in the USA exceeds the reduction in Medicaid expenditures, suggesting that from a fiscal point of view it is not cost-effective to use tax subsidies to expand the private long-term care insurance market. Stevenson et al. (2009) and Goda (2010) also found that the effects were very small. Goda's analysis suggests that the effects of state tax incentives in the USA are concentrated among the high-income and wealthy population. It is possible that bigger tax incentives could have a bigger impact on the market. Wiener (2011) argues that, because tax subsidies are unlikely to increase substantially the proportion of people with private insurance, most of the tax subsidies go to people who would have bought insurance without the incentive.

6.3   The Public System Takes on Part of the Risk of Long-term Care

Another way in which the public sector could reduce the cost of private long-term care insurance is by effectively taking part of the risk. The partnership schemes, which were originally introduced in four US states more than 15 years ago, have this effect (Wiener, 2001). These partnerships generally allow policy holders to keep an extra dollar in financial assets for each dollar that their insurance policies pay in benefits. Wiener (2011, p. 14) gives the example that, in Connecticut, persons with state-approved private long-term care insurance policies that pay \$150 000 in benefits can keep \$152 000 in financial assets and still qualify for Medicaid once the insurance policy has paid all of its benefits. Essentially, the US partnership model offers asset protection to induce people to buy insurance. In 2005 the partnership schemes were extended to other US states. Nevertheless, the uptake of partnership policies in the USA has been slow (GAO, 2005). Wiener (2011, p. 15) suggests that this is because asset protection may not be as decisive a factor for the purchase of long-term care as this policy assumed it to be. Factors such as retaining autonomy and independence and having a choice of providers may be playing an important role, which suggests that purchasers of private long-term care insurance are not particularly interested in having easier access to the Medicaid system. Indeed, most private long-term care insurance is marketed as a way of avoiding Medicaid.

In countries where the public sector currently only plays a safety-net role with regard to long-term care, the state could also take on some of the risk by introducing a universal entitlement to needs-tested long-term care, which may have the effect of encouraging people to buy top-up long-term care insurance products that supplement the public coverage. Because top-up insurance only needs to cover part of the risk of long-term care, the premiums for long-term care insurance tend to be more affordable than the premiums for comprehensive insurance and therefore could be purchased by higher numbers of people (see, e.g., Bolancé et al., 2010 for an empirical exploration for Spain). The current proposals for long-term care reform in Italy seem to be converging on a long-term care system formed by a national scheme providing basic levels of long-term care services, defined explicitly and guaranteed across the country, and complementary private insurance schemes covering the costs of long-term care not funded by the public scheme (Rebba, 2010).

6.4   Promoting Awareness of the Risk of Needing Care and of the Extent of Public Coverage

Another approach to promote private long-term care insurance is to promote awareness of the financial risks of long-term care. A number of US states participate in a federal programme to educate people about the need to plan for long-term care. The empirical evidence suggests that higher awareness about long-term care insurance and the risks of needing care increase the probability of buying insurance (see, e.g., Long Term Care Group Inc. and LifePlans Inc., 2006). For example, even controlling for income and wealth, people with higher levels of education are more likely to buy private long-term care insurance (Courbage and Roudaut, 2008; Cramer and Jensen, 2006; Mellor, 2000).

Reforms of the public long-term care system that simplify and clarify the entitlements to publicly funded care, particularly in countries with fragmented care systems, could also encourage people who become aware that they are not covered, fully or partially, by the public system to plan how they will meet their costs of care.

The most recent report produced by the French senate discussing the forthcoming reforms to the long-term care system suggest that the new reform will actively seek to improve the complementarity between public support and private insurance. The new system would also involve maintaining the current public system, but with the introduction of a recovery on inheritance, which may reduce the number of people seeking public care (Le Bihan, 2011).

Finally, experts from France suggested in interviews that in countries where adult children are liable for the costs of their parents' long-term care (as is the case in France, Germany and Austria), there is a stronger incentive for people with moderate wealth to purchase insurance, to protect their children from having to pay for their care if they run out of assets. However, it is unlikely that such a policy would be acceptable in countries where there is no tradition of adult children being financially responsible for their parents.

6.5   Encouraging the Supply of Insurance at Lower Prices

Encouraging employment-related insurance
Without requiring major reforms, the encouragement of employment or group-based long-term care insurance products, which, as discussed in the previous sections, are substantially cheaper to administer, has the potential to increase the number of people covered by private insurance.

In Italy, as part of the new collective wage agreements for insurance and bank employees that include automatic employment-related coverage for long-term care, the number of people holding long-term care policies has increased very rapidly. Coverage for employees of the banking and insurance sectors is provided by employer-based, professional, mutual aid and integrative health care funds, either directly or through insurance companies. Premiums are funded by payroll deductions and are low and uniform, based on group profiles (which, in this case, are white-collar workers) and there is no individual underwriting (Rebba, 2010).

However, governments need to ensure that employment-based and other group insurance policies are portable and people are not dropped from their policies when their employment ends, as the Israeli experience has highlighted (Chernichovsky et al., 2010). This issue has also been flagged in Italy, particularly with regard to the portability of group long-term care plans with wealth accumulation mechanisms.

The US CLASS Act has created a new voluntary public long-term care insurance programme, administered by the federal government (Miller, 2011; Wiener, 2010). The CLASS Act involves no medical underwriting (although there is a five-year waiting period before individuals can be eligible for benefits), premiums will vary by age and people with low incomes or students will be subsidised by other enrollees. The benefits will be in the form of cash. Although enrolment is voluntary, all people who work for participating employers will be automatically enrolled unless they choose to opt out. This is a public insurance scheme, although insurance premiums are the only source of finance. No more than 3 per cent of premiums may be used to pay for administrative costs. The design of the CLASS Act poses some interesting challenges for those who run it, particularly with regard to the choice of the initial premiums because they will have to be at a level that is high enough to guarantee the sustainability of the scheme even if few people enrol, yet low enough to attract a sufficient number of people to join (see, e.g., Wiener, 2010 and Tumlinson et al., 2010).

Finally, improving the regulatory framework for long-term care insurance has been mentioned in interviews as a major area in which the public sector could make an impact on the development of long-term care insurance products that perform better. For example, making it easier for people to draw on housing equity to purchase care protection has been cited in England. In the USA and Italy, improving portability of insurance and protection against the growth of premiums are major issues.

6.6 Compulsory Private Insurance

The public sector could intervene to make long-term care insurance compulsory. Barr (2010) suggests that compulsory private long-term care insurance would recognise the evidence from behavioural economics that people do not always make decisions that are in their own best interest. It would also avoid the problems associated with adverse selection, the differential expected lifetime costs of care by gender,[14] and people being denied insurance coverage because of poor health. It may also result in cheaper premiums because there would be no need for medical underwriting or marketing costs. Depending on how premiums are set under a compulsory private insurance scheme, it may also allow for some income redistribution. For example, if premiums were unrelated to risk factors, insurance would redistribute wealth from those with low needs to those with high needs. If premiums were related to income, then insurance would redistribute wealth from people with high incomes to people with low incomes.

A compulsory insurance system raises a number of practical challenges that would need addressing. First, there is the issue of how to fund the premiums of those who cannot afford them. Should they be covered by public funds, or should they be covered by other people's premiums? Second is the issue of whether the premiums should be determined at an individual level, with medical underwriting and all the costs involved, or whether they should be determined at the population level.

Whilst compulsion is not itself inconsistent with an important role for private sector provision, a compulsory private system does raise the issue of how premiums are met for those unable to pay the premiums themselves. Mandatory premiums would require a form of subsidy for those unable to afford the private insurance premium.

The state would clearly need to play an important role in addressing these fundamental issues, which raises the question of whether such a system would be, effectively, a public system delivered by private insurance companies, and whether this would be the most efficient way to fund long-term care.

The Eldershield plan in Singapore offers an interesting example of a partnership between public bodies and private players (de Castries, 2009). The scheme, which began in 2002, is based on private insurance with automatic enrolment for persons aged between 40 and 69. It is possible to opt out during the first three months. If one opts out, neither subsidies from public bodies nor preferred underwriting conditions are provided in the future. Product design and claims management are the responsibility of private insurance. Products are standardised with a lifetime guarantee of an annuity in case of needing long-term care. Communication and prevention responsibilities are shared between government and insurers.

Premiums, which differ by gender, are set at the age of entry into the scheme and do not increase as people age, to give people an incentive not to opt out. The current annual premiums for Eldershield 400 at age 40 are $174.96 for men and $217.76 for women (Ministry of Health, 2011). When the system was first introduced, as older people would have faced higher premiums, the Singapore government financed a share of the premium for those aged 55 to 69. A large awareness campaign of risks was carried out to promote the plan and the products. The opt-out rate has decreased from 38 per cent in 2002 (the year the scheme was launched) to 14 per cent in 2006 (de Castries, 2009, p. 31).

The Singaporean government also has a programme called 'Interim Disability Assistance for the Elderly' (IDAPE), which provides financial assistance to people who are not eligible for Eldershield because of their age or pre-existing disabilities. It is also administered by a private insurance provider.

Based on the Eldershield example, de Castries (2009) proposes a cooperative public/private partnership, with automatic enrolment and the freedom to opt out. Some public subsidies could help with the transition generation and help the low-income population to fund their premiums, making the cover affordable for everyone. A simplified underwriting would be set up to reduce discrimination related to health status. Near universal coverage would spread the risk efficiently. De Castries argues that such a system would be positive in terms of social justice and would provide robust funding of the risk, consistent with its long-term nature. It would provide an incremental financing source for the economy and ensure that individual solvency is confronting this risk.

7.   CONCLUSIONS

The evidence from other countries suggests that private long-term care insurance on its own is unlikely to contribute significantly to the financing of long-term care, in terms of coverage or in terms of proportion of total expenditure on long-term care. Buying private long-term care insurance is complex and involves purchasing protection against events far in the future and involves many uncertainties. In addition, changes in the public funding of long-term care may result in people being overinsured if the public system becomes more generous, or underinsured if it becomes less so (Barr, 2010). Only a minority of the population could reasonably afford long-term care insurance that covered them for the full costs of long-term care, unless they purchased it early in life (or possibly through the use of housing equity). Yet early in life people have other priorities and may not be well informed about the risk of long-term care and about the arrangements for public funding of long-term care. The use of housing equity is hampered by a lack of efficient and flexible financial products.

There are also major equity issues to consider concerning relying on private insurance to finance long-term care to any great degree. Private long-term care insurance policies are regressive in that only wealthier people are able to afford the premiums. Numerous studies conducted in the USA find evidence of a strong association between income and assets and the probability of owning insurance (see, e.g., Brown and

Finkelstein, 2009; Schaber and Stum, 2007). Some of the research suggests that the relationship between wealth and purchase of insurance is not linear (Courbage and Roudaut, 2008; Cramer and Jensen, 2006; Mellor, 2000). This research suggests that people in the middle of the wealth distribution are more likely to buy insurance than those at the bottom (who may not be able to afford it and are covered by the public schemes anyway), or the very wealthy (who have enough assets to self-insure and may be less risk-averse).

Additionally, groups of people with a higher probability of needing care, who are also likely to have lower incomes, would also be expected to pay higher private premiums (Holdenrieder, 2006) or are unable to purchase it at all, making private long-term care insurance yet more regressive when compared to alternative financing mechanisms, unless there are premium subsidies.

Despite these difficulties, the experience of other countries suggests that private insurance for long-term care could play a bigger role in the financing of long-term care. Across many countries, the system of financing and providing long-term care is mixed, combining family, market and state 'poles of protection' (Le Bihan and Martin, 2010, p. 393; Rebba, 2010), with a role for private insurance as a supplement to the public long-term care system.

In countries where most of the private financing of long-term care (to meet the costs of self-funding, co-payments, or payments for services not covered by the public system) is drawn from savings and sometimes housing equity, with no pooling of risk or redistribution, there may be scope for private insurance, perhaps in partnership with the public sector, to improve the efficiency and equity of the private financing of long-term care.

Relying on private long-term care insurance as the main source of long-term care financing would require very substantial subsidies or compulsion. Although the private long-term care insurance markets appear to have encountered important difficulties (mostly a result of lack of affordability) in countries with safety-net types of systems where private long-term care policies are expected to cover the full costs of care, in countries with universal public benefits that cover part of the costs of long-term care, private long-term care insurance, particularly when sold at a group (or employer) level, appears to be finding a niche as a top-up or supplementary product.

ACKNOWLEDGEMENTS

This chapter draws on research funded by the Department of Health and research funded by the AXA Research Fund. It does not, however, represent the views of the Department of Health or of the AXA Research Fund. Adelina Comas-Herrera, Raphael Wittenberg and José-Luis Fernández are beneficiaries of a financial contribution from the AXA Research Fund as part of 'The AXA Research Project on How can private long-term care insurance supplement state systems? The UK as a case study'. The researchers are very grateful to long-term care insurance experts who completed a questionnaire, commented on previous drafts of this chapter and spoke to them at length.

NOTES

1. Usually this applies to people who were living alone before moving to a care home. Some councils offer the possibility of deferring the costs of an individual's care under a 'deferred payment agreement'. These are loans, provided by the local authority, that cover those costs of care and accommodation that individuals are unable to fund themselves from their income. The loan is set against the home of someone who has gone into residential care. Under a deferred payment agreement, the local authority pays the costs of residential care, and places a lien on the person's home. When the person dies, the debt is repaid from the person's estate. Deferred payment agreements are not universally available, and are subject to the discretion of local authorities.
2. Immediate needs annuities are insurance products purchased at the point of need and provide a stream of funds for the duration of the period of disability.
3. More information about this project is available from http://www.pssru.ac.uk/axa/index.php.
4. Interviews with insurers highlighted that prepaid private long-term care insurance policies in England, when they were available, were often purchased by single or widowed people without close relatives who wanted to ensure that arrangements would be made on their behalf to guarantee them good-quality care should they need it.
5. For example, in the USA, the average age of buyers was 61 in 2005 (LifePlans, 2007).
6. A representative from an insurance company we interviewed gave the example of the impact that a cure for all cancers would have on the future numbers of people needing long-term care.
7. Although in the USA and France there is no gender differentiation, in other countries, such as Austria, Italy, Spain and the UK, men and women can be charged different premiums. In Spain, for example, the cost of buying a particular policy that pays out €1000 per month in case of severe dependency, if spread over ten years, would be €265 per month for men and €492 per month for women (INESE, 2010).
8. Note that the loss ratio for long-term care insurance is less than for acute health care insurance in the USA. This is likely to be, at least in part, because the take-up rate for employer-sponsored long-term care insurance is only about 5 to 8 per cent of people eligible in the USA, compared to 80 to 90 per cent for acute care insurance, so there are fewer economies of scale. In contrast, Medicare, the government health insurance programme for older people in the USA, spends about 3 per cent of its total expenditures on administration, substantially lower than that seen in the private sector.
9. In the USA insurers assume that not everyone wants a stranger coming into their house to provide paid services, but everyone wants cash. As a result, private long-term care insurance benefits have higher premiums than in-kind benefit policies (Stevenson et al., 2010).
10. For example, the 2008 annual premiums for a policy with $150 per day, three years' comprehensive coverage, 5 per cent automatic compound inflation protection, 90-day elimination period, from the three major insurers in the USA range from $1485 to $1701 for people aged 40, to $4359 to $4680 for people aged 70 (Tumlinson et al., 2009, p. 6).
11. There have been several recent large premium increases in the USA. Genworth Financial is seeking an 18 per cent increase on older policies held by about 25 per cent of its customers. John Hancock has filed for permission to raise premiums for about 80 per cent of its customers by an average of 40 per cent. It has also temporarily stopped offering new long-term care insurance plans through employers while it recalculates premiums (Lieber, 2010). John Hancock Financial said it would ask state regulators for an average 40 per cent increase for about 850 000 of its 1.1 million policy holders (Tergsen and Scism, 2010).
12. In practice it is likely that people do not make such accurate judgements about the impact of purchasing insurance on their Medicaid eligibility status, but that they simply do not buy private insurance because they believe they are already covered by Medicaid.
13. In the USA, premiums are only deductible if total out-of-pocket health care expenditures exceed 7.5 per cent of adjusted gross income. The recent health reform bill raises that percentage to 10 per cent. If total out-of-pocket health care expenditures are less than the threshold, then none of the cost of the premium can be deducted. However, on the employer side, all contributions towards the cost of private long-term care insurance premiums are tax-deductible, but few employers contribute towards the cost of the policies, even when they offer them to their employees.
14. If insurance is mandatory, there is little or no distortionary effect from charging men and women a premium based on joint probabilities. Second, there are obvious political difficulties from imposing on women a significantly higher contribution rate than on men, all the more because the differential is, and is likely to remain, very large. The use of unisex tables can therefore be defended as a simple value judgement (Barr, 2010, p. 15).

REFERENCES

Association of British Insurers (2009), Personal communication, 16 September.

Association of British Insurers (2010), *Long-Term Care Market Overview*, December.

Barr, N. (2010), 'Long-term care: a suitable case for social insurance', *Social Policy and Administration*, **44**(4), 359–74.

Birchley, P. (2010), 'Support for self-funders', Local Government Association, http://www.lga.gov.uk/lga/core/page.do?pageId=15205050, accessed 17 February 2010.

Bolancé, C., R. Alemany and M. Guillén (2010), 'Prediction of the economic cost of individual long-term care in the Spanish population', Documents de treball XREAP2010-8 i Documents de l'Institut de Recerca d'Economi Aplicada, http://www.pcb.ub.es/xreap/aplicacio/fitxers/XREAP2010-8.pdf, accessed 18 February 2011.

Brammli-Greenberg, S. and R. Gross (2010), *Private Long Term Care Insurance in Israel*, JDC-Brookdale Institute and Bar Ilan University.

Brown, J.R. and A. Finkelstein (2007), 'Why is the market for long-term care insurance so small?', *Journal of Public Economics*, **91**, 1967–91.

Brown, J.R. and A. Finkelstein (2009), 'The private market for long-term care insurance in the United States: a review', *The Journal of Risk and Insurance*, **76**(1), 5–29.

Chernichovsky, D., M. Koreh, S. Soffer and S. Avrami (2010), 'Long-term care in Israel: challenges and reform options', *Health Policy*, **96**(3), 217–25.

Cohen, M., M. Weinrobe and J. Miller (2000), *Multivariate Patterns of Informal and Formal Caregiving Among Privately-Insured and Non-Privately Insured Disabled Elders Living in the Community*, Washington, DC: Office of the Assistant Secretary for Planning and Evaluation, US Department of Health and Human Services, http://aspe.hhs.gov/daltcp/reports/2000/multanal.pdf, accessed 28 January 2011.

Comas-Herrera, A., R. Wittenberg and L. Pickard (2010), 'The long road to universalism? Recent developments in the financing of long-term care in England', *Social Policy and Administration*, **44**(2), 375–91.

Courbage, C. and N. Roudaut (2008), 'Empirical evidence on long-term care insurance purchase in France', *The Geneva Papers on Risk and Insurance*, **33**, 645–58.

Courtemanche, C. and D. He (2008), 'Tax incentives and the decision to purchase long-term care insurance', *Journal of Public Economics*, **93**, 296–310.

Cramer, A.T. and G.A. Jensen (2006), 'Why don't people buy long-term care insurance?', *Journal of Gerontology: Social Sciences*, **61B**(4), S185–S193.

Crown, W.H., J. Capitman and W.N. Leutz (1992), 'Economic rationality, the affordability of private long-term care insurance, and the role of public policy', *The Gerontologist*, **32**(4), 478–85.

de Castries, H. (2009), 'Ageing and long-term care: key challenges in long-term care coverage for public and private systems', *The Geneva Papers on Risk and Insurance*, **34**, 24–34.

Doty, P., M.A. Cohen, J. Miller and X. Shi (2010), 'Private long-term care insurance: value to claimants and implications for long-term care financing', *The Gerontologist*, **50**(5), 613–22.

Fernández, J.-L. and J. Forder (2010), 'Impact of changes in length of stay on the demand for residential care services in England', Report commissioned by Bupa Care Services, PSSRU Discussion Paper 2771, Canterbury: PSSRU.

FFSA (2010), *Les contrats d'assurance dépendance en 2009*, http://www.ffsa.fr/ffsa/jcms/p1_80891/les-contrats-dassurance-dependance-en-2009?cc=fn_7350, accessed 21 January 2011.

Finkelstein, A. and K. McGarry (2003), 'Private information and its effect on market equilibrium: new evidence from long-term care insurance', NBER Working Paper No. 9957.

Forder, J. (2011), 'Immediate needs annuities in England', PSSRU Discussion Paper 2776, PSSRU: Canterbury.

Foubister, T., S. Thomson, E. Mossialos and A. McGuire (2006), *Private Medical Insurance in the United Kingdom*, Copenhagen: European Observatory on Health Systems and Policies.

Goda, G.S. (2010), 'The impact of state subsidies for private long-term care insurance on coverage and medicaid expenses', NBER Working Paper 16406, http://www.nber.org/papers/w16406.pdf, accessed 26 January 2011.

Government Accountability Office (GAO) (2005), *Overview of the Long-Term Care Partnership Program*, GAO-05-1021R, http://www.gao.gov/new.items/d051021r.pdf, accessed 4 February 2010.

Guardian News (2010), 'Care homes forcing elderly to have feeding tubes fitted', available from http://www.guardian.co.uk/society/2010/jan/06/care-homes-elderly-feeding-tubes, accessed 18 February 2011.

Hendel, I. and A. Lizzeri (2003), 'The role of commitment in dynamic contracts: evidence from life insurance', *Quarterly Journal of Economics*, **118**(1), 299–327.

Holdenrieder, J. (2006), 'Equity and efficiency in funding long-term care from an EU perspective', *Journal of Public Health*, **14**, 139–47.

INESE (2010), http://www.inese.es/formacion/detalle_formacion/-/asset_publisher/gwB2/content/seguro-de-dependencia-prima-uniforme, accessed 11 March 2010.

Kessler, D. (2008), 'The long-term care insurance market', *The Geneva Papers on Risk and Insurance*, **33**, 33–40.

Konetzka, R. and Y. Luo (2011), 'Explaining lapse in long-term care insurance markets', *Health Economics*, **20**(10), 1169–83.

Kunreuther, H., R. Ginsberg, L. Miller, P. Sagi, P. Slovic, B. Borkan and N. Katz (1978), *Disaster Insurance Protection: Public Policy Lessons*, New York: John Wiley.

Le Bihan, B. (2011), Personal communication.

Le Bihan, B. and C. Martin (2010), 'Reforming long-term care policy in France: private-public complementarities', *Social Policy and Administration*, **44**(4), 392–410.

Le Corre, P.-Y. (2010), 'Revamping French LTC insurance – heading for a mature sustainable market', Presentation at the Geneva Association's 7th Health and Ageing Conference, US and French Long-Term Care Insurance Markets Development, Paris, 18–19 November.

Lieber, R. (2010), 'When a safety net is yanked away', *New York Times*, 12 November, http://www.nytimes.com/2010/11/13/your-money/13money.html?pagewanted=1&_r=1&emc=eta1, accessed 2 January 2011.

LifePlans (2007), 'Who buys long-term care insurance? A 15-year study of buyers and non-buyers, 1990–2005', prepared for America's Health Insurance Plans by LifePlans, Inc., http://www.ahipresearch.org/PDFs/LTC_Buyers_Guide.pdf, accessed 18 February 2011.

Long Term Care Group Inc. and LifePlans Inc. (2006), *Final Report on the 'Own your future' Consumer Survey*, US Department of Health and Human Services, Assistant Secretary for Planning and Evaluation, Office of Disability, Aging and Long-Term Care Policy, http://aspe.hhs.gov/daltcp/reports/2006/OYFsurvey.pdf, accessed 26 January 2011.

Mayhew, L., M. Karlsson and B. Rickayzen (2010), 'The role of private finance in paying for long-term care', *The Economic Journal*, **120**, F478–F504.

Mellor, J. (2000), 'Private long-term care insurance and the asset protection motive', *The Gerontologist*, **40**(5), 596–604.

Miller, E.A. (2011), 'Flying beneath the radar of health reform: the Community Living Assistance Services and Supports (CLASS) Act', *The Gerontologist*, **51**(2), 145–55.

Ministry of Health (2011), http://www.moh.gov.sg/mohcorp/hcfinancing.aspx?id=356, accessed 20 February 2011.

Murtaugh, C., B. Spillman and M. Warshawsky (2001), 'In sickness and in health: an annuity approach to financing long-term care and retirement of income', *Journal of Risk and Insurance*, **68**(2), 225–54.

Partnership (2010), http://www.partnership.co.uk/press/2010/June/Press Release 7 June 20101/, accessed 17 February 2011.

Pauly, M.V. (1990), 'The rational nonpurchase of long-term care insurance', *The Journal of Political Economy*, **98**(1), 153–68.

Pinquet, J., M. Guillen and M. Ayuso (2010), 'Commitment and lapse behavior in long-term care insurance: a case study', Ecole Polytechnique, cahier de recherche no. 2010-30, http://hal.archivesouvertes.fr/docs/00/54/18/21/PDF/cahier_de_recherche_2010-30.pdf, accessed 28 February 2011.

PKV (2007), Zahlenbericht der privaten Krankenversicherung 2006/2007. Verband der privaten Krankeversicherung e.V. Köln (as quoted in Zhou-Richter et al., 2010).

Rebba, V. (2010), 'Long-term care in Italy: a role for private insurance?', Long-Term Care 2010: International Conference on Evidence-based Policy in Long-term Care, London School of Economics and Political Science, Personal Social Services Research Unit (PSSRU), London, 9 September.

Rivlin, A.R. and J.M. Wiener, with R.J. Hanley and D.A. Spence (1988), *Caring for the Disabled Elderly: Who will Pay?* Washington, DC: The Brookings Institution.

Scanlon, W.J. (1992), 'Possible reforms for financing long-term care', *Journal of Economic Perspectives*, **6**, 43–58.

Schaber, P.L. and M.S. Stum (2007), 'Factors impacting group long-term care insurance enrollment decisions', *Journal of Family and Economic Issues*, **28**, 189–205.

Sloan, F.A. and E.C. Norton (1997), 'Adverse selection, bequests, crowding out and private demand for insurance: evidence from the long-term care market', *Journal of Risk and Uncertainty*, **15**, 201–19.

Stevenson, D.G., R.G. Frank and J. Tau (2009), 'Private long-term care insurance and state tax incentives', *Inquiry*, **46**(3), 305–21.

Stevenson, D.G., M.A. Cohen, E.J. Tell and B. Burwell (2010), 'The complementarity of public and private long-term care coverage', *Health Affairs*, **29**(1), 96–101.

Swiss Re (2008), 'Innovative ways of financing retirement', *Sigma* 4/2008, http://media.swissre.com/documents/sigma4_2008_en.pdf, accessed 17 February 2011.

Taleyson, L. (2003), 'Private long-term care insurance – international comparisons', *Health and Ageing* No. 08. The Geneva Association.

Tergsen, A. and L. Scism (2010), 'Long-term care premiums soar', *Wall Street Journal*, 16 October, http://

online.wsj.com/article/SB10001424052748703298504575534513798604500.html, accessed 2 January 2011.

Times online (2009), 'Care homes: a system in crisis', available from http://women.timesonline.co.uk/tol/life_and_style/women/the_way_we_live/article5511395.ece, accessed 18 February 2011.

Tumlinson, A., C. Aguiar and M.O. Watts (2009), 'Closing the long-term care funding gap: the challenge of private long-term care insurance', The Kaiser Commission on Medicaid and the Uninsured, http://www.kff.org/insurance/upload/Closing-the-Long-Term-Care-Funding-Gap-The-Challenge-of-Private-Long-Term-Care-Insurance-Report.pdf, accessed 18 February 2011.

Tumlinson, A., W. Ng and E. Hammelman (2010), 'The circular relationship between enrollment and premiums: effects of the CLASS Act', in Bringing CLASS to Long-Term Care Through the Affordable Care Act. *Public Policy & Aging Report*, **20**(2), 28–30.

Warshawsky, M.J. (2007), 'The life care annuity: a proposal for an insurance product innovation to simultaneously improve financing and benefit provision for long-term care and to insure the risk of outliving assets in retirement', Working Paper No. 2 Georgetown University Long-Term Care Financing Project.

Wiener, J.M. (1998), 'Can private insurance solve the long-term care problems of the baby boom generation?', Testimony before the Senate Special Committee on Aging, http://www.urban.org/url.cfm?ID=900278, accessed 17 November 2010.

Wiener, J.M. (2001), 'The limits of the partnership for long-term care', in N. McCall (ed.), *Who Will Pay for Long-Term Care? Insights from the Partnership Programs*, Chicago, IL: Health Administration Press, pp. 243–59.

Wiener, J.M. (2010), *Implementing the CLASS Act: Six Decisions for the Secretary of Health and Human Services*, Research Triangle Park, NC: RTI Press, available at http://www.rti.org/pubs/pb-0002-1009.pdf.

Wiener, J.M. (2011), *Long-Term Care Reform Options in Hawaii*, Final Report prepared for the Hawaii Long-Term Care Commission.

Wiener, J.M., L.H. Illston and R.J. Hanley (1994), *Sharing the Burden: Strategies for Public and Private Long-Term Care Insurance*, Washington: The Brookings Institution.

Wiener, J.M., J. Tilly and S.M. Goldenson (2000), 'Federal and state initiatives to jump start the market for private long-term care insurance', *Elder Law Journal*, **8**(1), 57–99.

Wittenberg, R., L. Pickard, J. Malley, D. King, A. Comas and R. Darton (2008), *Future Demand for Social Care, 2005 to 2041: Projections of Demand for Social Care for Older People in England*, Report to the Strategy Unit (Cabinet Office) and the Department of Health, PSSRU 2514.

Zhou-Richter, T., M.J. Browne and H. Gründl (2010), 'Don't they care? Or, are they just unaware? Risk perception and the demand for long-term care insurance', *The Journal of Risk and Insurance*, **77**(4), 715–47.

PART VI

BEHAVIOUR AND HEALTH PRODUCTION

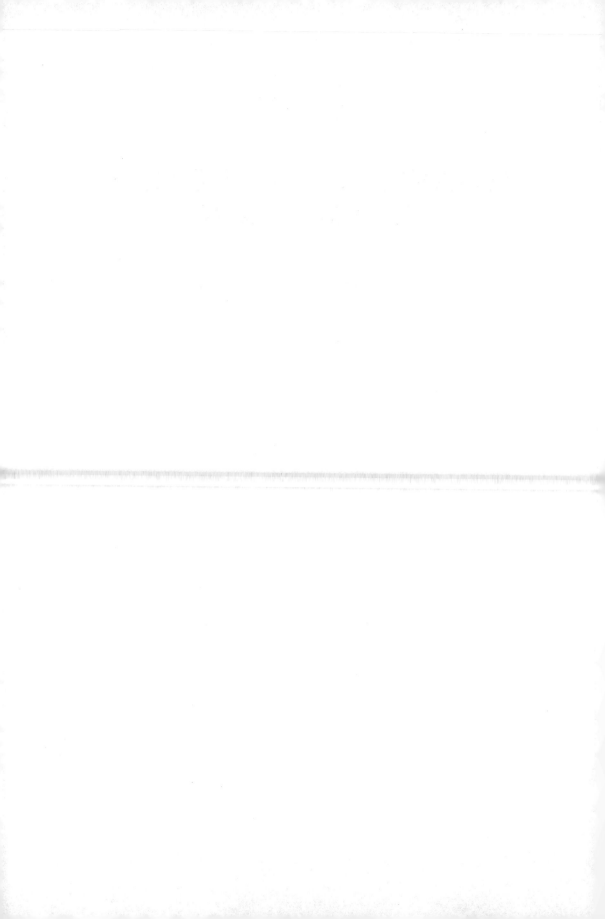

16 Historical trends of mortality and its implications for health policies in England and Wales: the cause-of-death approach

Mariachiara Di Cesare and Michael Murphy

1. INTRODUCTION

Developed countries have experienced a substantial increase in life expectancy in the last century due to lower levels of mortality including a shift from dying at younger ages to older ages (Janssen and Kunst, 2004). This shift has been both a cause and a consequence of a changing pattern in causes of death from communicable diseases to chronic and degenerative diseases (Omran, 1971, 1998; Charlton and Murphy, 1997).

The increasing importance of overall and cause-specific mortality patterns, especially among older people, has gained interest especially for the impact – in terms of costs, policies and actions – on the health and social care system (WHO, 2008). Acute care costs for the last year(s) of life (which account for a major part of lifetime health expenditures; see Chapter 13) differ according to the cause of death, reflecting earlier patterns of morbidity (Polder et al., 2006; Pierce and Denison, 2010; Scitovsky 1984, 1994). For example, causes such as unexpected, fatal heart attacks have low costs compared to cancers. Analysis of cause-of-death trends can indicate the interaction of health, economic and social factors with technology and medical knowledge to monitor the present and suggest appropriate policies for the future.

Health policies based on use of cause-specific mortality data have to rely on data mainly from death certification for continuous monitoring of mortality over time. Nowadays, most developed countries have essentially complete civil registration systems, with at least 90 per cent of death events registered (Mahapatra et al., 2007). Nevertheless, the analysis of long-time mortality series may be affected by various factors that can lead to inconsistency over time and hamper or bias the identification of the real levels and the time patterns of cause-specific mortality.

Factors such as the preferred specific causes that are recorded on death certificates in particular periods of time, or definitions of the leading cause of death linked to doctor's experience, tend to undermine the integrity of cause-of-death time series, making it harder to decide whether a reported increase in a specific cause of death is the consequence of a real increase in the number of deaths from that cause or simply reflects a higher propensity to certificate it (Logan, 1950). These external knowledge and 'fashion' factors may have a different impact at national and sub-national levels; therefore establishing the validity of trends in broad causes of death may be problematic even if there are no differences in the classifications used – for example, variations between countries observed in ischemic heart disease could be partly explained by differential coding of such diseases (Murray and Lopez, 1996).

The International Classification of Diseases (ICD), adopted at the beginning of the twentieth century with the purpose of providing a consistent classification and comparability of causes of death within and across countries (WHO, 2009; Charlton and Murphy, 1997), has been revised frequently (ICD-1 to ICD-10). These subsequent revisions have been necessary to keep pace with medical knowledge and discoveries in both disease nomenclature and aetiology (Griffiths and Brock, 2003; Anderson et al., 2001), which have consistently improved the allocation of death to specific causes over time, as indicated by the reduced use of the ill-defined cause-of-death category, and recently the increasing tendency to code Alzheimer's disease rather than simple dementia. New codes have been introduced through the ICD versions due to the identification of new diseases such as HIV/AIDS. Revisions include changes in coding rules as well as in the number of codes (Janssen and Kunst, 2004): for example, ICD-2, used during the decade 1911–20, had 300 categories, while in the last two revisions, ICD-9 and ICD-10 had 5000 and 10 000 respectively (WHO, 2009). These modifications have led to inconsistency over time, making it harder to establish the real trend of cause-specific mortality, as noted almost 70 years ago by Janssen (1938). Moreover, changes in coding rules have been introduced from time to time within a particular ICD with instantaneous effects on the cause mortality levels (Griffiths and Brock, 2003) and without any consistency within countries. For example, during the ICD-5 period in England and Wales, a change was introduced in the selection of the principal cause of death in accordance with the general practitioner's preference (Logan, 1950) rather than by the simple order of occurrence on the death certificate. A temporary change in the rules for selecting the underlying cause of death affected cause-specific mortality trends in the ICD-9 period in the UK, leading to a discontinuity in some causes in years 1984–92. Similarly, a change in the coding rule 3 – which allowed a condition reported in both Parts I and II of the death certificate to be the leading cause of death rather than the underlying condition selected – led to changes in the distribution of deaths by cause (Brock et al., 2006).

Although the quality of registration data is high in developed countries, increasing proportions of deaths occur at older ages from non-communicable diseases, often characterised by high levels of co-morbidity, which makes it more difficult to assign a single underlying cause of death (WHO, 2006).

All these factors have to be taken in consideration when assessing recorded trends in cause-specific mortality. A substantial literature exists on generating consistent series by use of bridge (or concordance) tables between ICD revisions (Dunn and Shackley, 1944; Faust and Dolman, 1964; Klebba and Dolman, 1975; Klebba and Scott, 1980; Anderson et al., 2001; Janssen and Kunst, 2004; NCHS, 2009; Meslé and Vallin, 1996; Wolleswinkel-van de Bosch et al., 1996). However, it is not possible to obtain completely consistent long-run historical time series, given the range of potentially confounding exogenous factors.

With these caveats in mind, the next section shows how consistent cause-of-death series may be used to assess trends in mortality over extended periods in England and Wales.

2.   ANALYSIS OF PAST TRENDS OF MORTALITY IN ENGLAND AND WALES

Analysis of changes over time in cause-of-death patterns led Omran (1971, 1998) to define the epidemiological transition theory. According to Omran, all societies experience three stages: the 'age of pestilence and famine'; the 'age of receding pandemics'; and the 'age of degenerative and man-made diseases'. In the first phase the levels of mortality are high and life expectancy is between 20 and 40 years; in the second phase it rises to 50 years; while in the third it tends to stabilise at a maximum of about 75 years.

Omran's generalisations have been criticised (Mackenbach, 1994): although based on the evolution of causes of death, they analyse the general levels of mortality. According to Gaylin and Kates (1997), subgroups of the population may sometimes show diverging rather than converging epidemiological profiles as suggested by Omran. Moreover, the achievements in the treatment and prevention of cardiovascular diseases (which were not foreseen by Omran) have led to higher life expectancy, leading authors (e.g. Rogers and Hackenberg, 1987) to define a fourth stage of the epidemiological transition, which Olshansky and Ault (1986) named the 'age of delayed degenerative diseases'. In recent decades, the problem of infectious diseases has gained attention among the scientific community and the general public (Caselli, 1991; Barrett et al., 1998; Sanders et al., 2008), suggesting another new phase in the epidemiological transition. One example of the interaction between emerging and re-emerging diseases is the synergistic relation between AIDS and tuberculosis (Rieder, 1994; Smallman-Raynor and Phillips, 1999). Although overstating the inevitability of progression through predetermined stages, the epidemiological transition framework remains widely used as a model from which exceptions and anomalies can be more easily identified and assessed as in the case of England and Wales.

In contrast to the nineteenth century, deaths in England and Wales are now mainly due to chronic and degenerative rather than to communicable diseases, following the much more rapid decline in communicable than non-communicable disease deaths (Charlton and Murphy, 1997). This transition took place during the nineteenth and twentieth centuries but different factors were responsible for it in the two periods. The reduction of mortality observed during the second half of the nineteenth century can be largely explained by a decrease in five groups of causes of death: tuberculosis; typhus, typhoid and continuing fever; scarlet fever; cholera, dysentery and diarrhoea; and smallpox (McKeown and Record, 1962), although Preston (1976) argued that decline in rheumatic heart disease was also important. Half of the gain in life expectancy at birth by the end of the nineteenth century was due to the reduction of infectious diseases, of which almost two years of life expectancy was gained due to the fall of respiratory tuberculosis (Caselli, 1991). Factors such as increases in living standards (affecting tuberculosis), positive balance between infectious virulence and human resistance to it (affecting scarlet fever), and improved sanitation (affecting typhus–typhoid and cholera group) have been identified as possible factors driving the changing nineteenth-century mortality pattern (McKeown and Record, 1962; Logan, 1950).

During the first half of the twentieth century infectious diseases continued to decrease, with medical measures (such as immunisation), reduced exposure to infection and improved nutrition identified as key factors in this reduction (Logan, 1950; McKeown et al., 1975; Charlton and Murphy, 1997). However, during the second half of the century there were occasional periods when mortality even among non-infectious diseases increased among groups such as working-age men (Aylin et al., 1999).

Figure 16.1 shows age-specific overall mortality rates for selected years between 1911 and 2007 in England and Wales. Improvements during the first half of the twentieth century were mainly concentrated among children and young adults. In recent decades, mortality among these age groups has generally continued to improve, but substantial reductions in mortality at older working ages and above have also occurred. The declines in both fertility and mortality during the past century have led to increases in the proportion of deaths occurring at older ages (Griffiths and Brock, 2003). In 2007, only 0.8 per cent of male deaths and 0.6 per cent of female deaths occurred before the first birthday, compared with 28 per cent and 23 per cent respectively in 1901, whereas the proportion of deaths at ages 75 and over increased from 10 per cent for males and 13 per cent for females in 1901 to 58 per cent and 74 per cent respectively by 2007. A consequence of the lower mortality of females than males is that a higher proportion of deaths occurs at older ages.

Figure 16.2 shows changes in the cause-of-death patterns using eight broad groups of cause of deaths based on Preston et al.'s (1972) cause-of-death classification. The corresponding ICD-10 codes are shown in Table 16.1 (consistent bridging coding has been used throughout the ten ICD versions). Infectious and parasitic diseases (at the bottom of the figure) decrease in importance over time: at the beginning of the twentieth century they accounted for half of all deaths, but only 6 per cent among males and 9 per cent among females by 2007. The proportion of deaths due to influenza, pneumonia and bronchitis decreased rapidly during the first half of the twentieth century, then slackened and stabilised (except for discontinuities during the ICD-9 due to a temporary change in coding rules) at around 5 per cent of deaths for males and 7 per cent for females.

In contrast, the group of degenerative diseases gained relative importance over time, the proportion increasing from around 230 out of every 1000 deaths in 1901 to 686 (for males) and 625 (for females) per 1000 by 2007. Among these causes, cardiovascular diseases started to decline in importance from the 1970s, when they accounted for about half of all deaths to just over one-third by 2007 (both sexes combined). Neoplasms have become more prominent over the past 100 years: in 1901 they accounted for only 39 of every 1000 deaths among males and 65 per 1000 among females, compared with 300 and 250 per 1000 in 2007 respectively.

The relative importance of the third main group, external causes (accidents and violence), has tended to decrease over time, accounting for about 4 per cent of deaths in the last decade, although since they often occur early in life, they will be more important when indicators such as years of potential life lost are considered.

Analysis of cause-of-death trends in the last century in England and Wales clearly shows that changes occurred both in the overall burden of diseases and in particular causes. However, simple changes in coding rules can lead to unexpected changes in mortality trends, which may be particularly problematic for more detailed causes of death coding. This may be illustrated by the case of Alzheimer's disease and other dementias as an example of the way mortality trends are affected by ICD coding changes and improvements in medical knowledge.

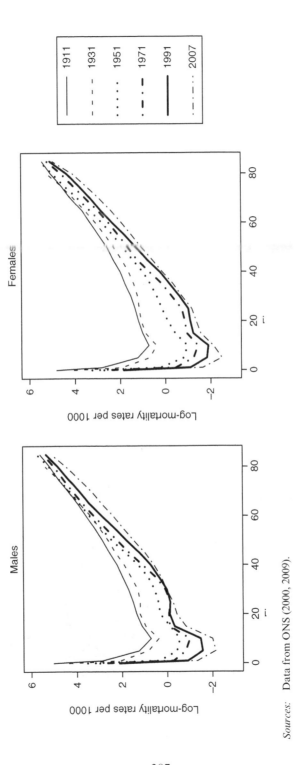

Sources: Data from ONS (2000, 2009).

Figure 16.1   Log-mortality rates (per 1000), males and females, England and Wales, 1911, 1931, 1951, 1971, 1991 and 2007

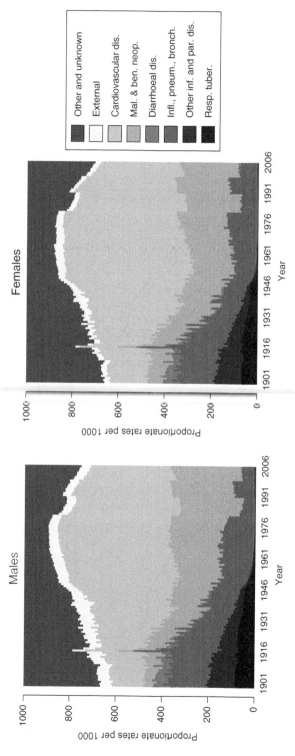

Figure 16.2 Proportionate rates per 1000 deaths from all causes, males and females, England and Wales, 1901–2007

Table 16.1   ICD-10 codes for 12 selected causes of death

Respiratory tuberculosis	A15-A16
Other infectious and parasitic diseases	A00-B99 (minus A15-A16, A044-A049, A071-A09)
Malignant and benign neoplasma	C00-D48
Cardiovascular diseases	I00-I99
Influenza, pneumonia, bronchitis	J10-J22, J40-J42
Diarrhoea, gastritis, enteritis	A044-A049, A071-A09
External causes	V01-Y89
Other	Residual

3.   ALZHEIMER'S AND DEMENTIA: A PROBLEMATIC CAUSE OF DEATH

Dementia is defined as the 'loss of intellectual abilities (cognitive function) of sufficient severity to interfere with social or occupational functioning' (American Psychiatric Association, 1994), which has a disproportionate impact on capacity of independent living (Knapp and Prince, 2007). It is characterised by a strong age-dependence, which means that the social and economic costs arising from this group of diseases/deaths will certainly increase in the future, due to population ageing (Lowin et al., 2001). In contrast to the next most common form, vascular dementia due to small strokes that affect blood flow to areas of the brain related to memory and thinking, the precise causes of Alzheimer's disease, the most common type of dementia (Torpy et al., 2004), are not known. Risk factors such as family history and age have been identified (Mathers and Leonardi, 2000; Torpy et al., 2004); although findings on the effects of lifestyle factors such as alcohol consumption or smoking are mixed, recent studies suggest that smoking increases the risk of dementia (Anstey et al., 2007).

Table 16.2 shows the ICD codes selected for the construction of the time series for the main group of dementia cause of death. Trends for Alzheimer's disease are available only from 1979 (ICD-9), when specific codes were introduced. Different studies use slightly different groups of codes; these are consistent with the codes used by ONS in ICD-9 and ICD-10 for identifying senile and pre-senile organic psychotic conditions (including Alzheimer's), and in ICD-6 to ICD-10 for a WHO study (Janssen and Kunst, 2004).

In 1911 the total number of deaths coded as 'senile dementia' was 847; by 2007 this number increased to 20 645 (vascular dementia, unspecified dementia, Alzheimer's disease, senility, degeneration of brain). In 1911 the proportion of female deaths was slightly greater than for men: around 56 per cent of deaths were of women, a figure that had increased to 71 per cent by 2007.

Men and women showed similar levels of recorded Alzheimer's disease mortality until 1992 (left panel in Figure 16.3), but the gap increased subsequently, leading to a higher standardised death rate (SDR) of around 25 per cent for women in the last six years. The secular trend shows clearly how changes in the ICD coding have a strong impact, especially between ICD-8 and ICD-9, and ICD-9 and ICD-10. Within ICD-9 the

Table 16.2   Concordance table used for bridging nine revisions of the international
Classification of Diseases – main groups of dementia

Code	Description
ICD10 (2001–present)	
G30	Alzheimer's
G31.1	Senile degeneration of brain
F01	Vascular dementia
F03	Unspecific dementia
ICD9 (1979–2000)	
331.0	Alzheimer's
331.2	Senile degeneration of brain
290	Dementia
ICD8 (1968–78)	
290	Senile and pre-senile dementia
293	Psychosis associated with other cerebrovascular condition (with cerebral arteriosclerosis/with other cerebrovascular disturbance)
ICD7/ICD6 (1950–67)	
304	Senile psychosis
305	Pre-senile psychosis
306	Psychosis with cerebral arteriosclerosis
ICD5 (1940–49)	
162b	Senility with mention of senile dementia
ICD4 (1931–39)	
162a	Senile dementia
ICD3 (1921–30)	
164(1)	Senile dementia
ICD2 (1911–20)	
154a	Senile dementia

temporary change in the rules to select the underlying cause of death in Britain (Griffiths and Rooney, 2006; Kirby et al., 1998) led to an apparent sharp increase in death rates from dementias during the period 1984–92, resulting in a substantial transfer of deaths from the influenza–pneumonia–bronchitis group to the Alzheimer's disease and dementia group (Figure 16.3). Another noteworthy fact is the increasing tendency to record Alzheimer's as the disease process underlying dementia (Griffiths and Rooney, 2006), and a consequent increase in the recorded level of Alzheimer's disease is apparent over the last 30 years.

The analysis of this specific case clearly shows how the whole group of dementia-related causes of death is strongly affected by exogenous factors unrelated to the underlying level of the disease itself. There is a propensity to make the diagnosis of dementia more frequently now than in the past and to code Alzheimer's disease explicitly as the specific type of dementia. Recorded levels of mortality are affected, as previously

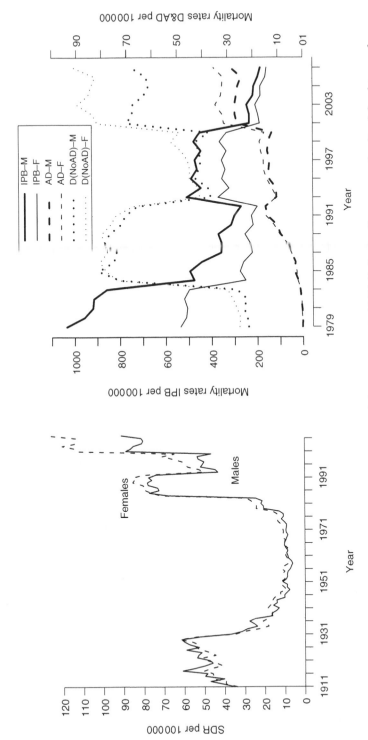

Figure 16.3 Age-standardised death rates from all types of dementia, 1911–2007 (left panel); age-standardised death rates from dementia without Alzheimer's disease (D(NoAD)), Alzheimer's disease (AD) and influenza–pneumonia–bronchitis (F) aged 60+ (right panel), England and Wales

underlined, both by changes in coding rules and practices and by the level of accuracy in death coding due to improvements in medical knowledge and diagnosis.

Mortality improvement in general and changes in the burden of diseases represent a real challenge for public policies, especially for the health, social care and pensions systems. A range of factors, such as those illustrated in the case of dementia and related diseases, affects recorded mortality trends, which have to be analysed with caution especially if used for forecasting purposes, a topic that will now be considered.

4.   FORECASTING MORTALITY

Cause-of-death forecasts are increasingly important due to the implications of changing cause-of-death patterns for health and social care costs predictions since, for example, formal and informal care costs in the period before death vary substantially according to the cause of death (Crimmins, 1984; Tabeau et al., 1999; Scitovsky, 1994; Polder et al., 2006).

In recent decades a range of methods for mortality forecasting has been developed (e.g. Lee and Carter, 1992; Booth et al., 2002; Renshaw and Haberman, 2006; Heathcote and Higgins, 2001; Girosi and King, 2008; for a review see Booth and Tickle, 2008).

The Lee–Carter model is the most widely used method for forecasting future mortality, so it will be briefly described. For each sex and for a particular cause of death (Booth et al., 2002), the model is:

$$\ln m_{xt} = \alpha_x + \beta_x k_t + \varepsilon_{xt}$$

where m_{xt} is the death rate at age x in year t, k_t is an index of the overall level of mortality at time t, α_x is the average pattern of mortality by age across years, β_x is the relative speed of change at each age, and ε_{xt} is the residual at age x and time t. The α_x values are calculated as the average of $\ln m_{xt}$ values over the time period over which the model is fitted, and β_x and k_t values are estimated by singular value decomposition. To obtain a unique solution, constraints are imposed: conventionally the estimated β_x values are set to sum to 1, and the estimated k_t values to sum to zero. The Lee–Carter model therefore consists of a base model of age-specific death rates with a dominant time component and a fixed relative age component, and a time-series model for the time component. The model incorporates an adjustment to the k_t estimates so that fitted number of deaths matches the observed total deaths in each year; this gives greater weight to ages at which numbers of deaths are high, thereby partly counterbalancing modelling on the logarithmic scale.

The k_t time series are forecast using a standard **ARIMA** time-series model, usually a simple random walk with drift model (Booth et al., 2006):

$$k_t = k_{t-1} + d + e_t$$

where d is the average annual change (drift) in k_t and e_t are uncorrelated error terms.

The Lee–Carter model is widely used because of advantages such as: no subjective judgement involved; forecasting based on long-term trends; and availability of confidence intervals (Lee and Carter, 1992) that provide estimates of forecast uncertainty. The model has been proved to be reliable and accurate in situations in which historical trends are characterised by linear trends in age-specific death rates. This is mainly because the drift model is appropriate for forecasting linear trends but it also appears to be reasonably robust in situations of unpredictable change (Booth et al., 2006). A series of variants to the original Lee–Carter model has been developed (Lee and Miller, 2001; Hyndman and Ullah, 2007; De Jong and Tickle, 2006; Booth et al., 2002) with superior results in some but not all empirical applications (Di Cesare and Murphy, 2009).

The Lee–Carter model analyses data by age and time period, but increasingly forecasting models tend to include the effects of possible cohort as well as period forces (Pollard, 1998; Renshaw and Haberman, 2006; Currie, 2006; Carstensen, 2006). Such approaches may be particularly appropriate for cases where there is a clear-cut underlying cohort mechanism, such as in the case of lung cancer where a cohort's earlier smoking patterns will be a key determinant. The cohort approach for forecasting mortality allows incorporation of contextual (period) and historical (cohort) factors (Tabeau, 2001). In the case of official UK overall mortality forecasts, a cohort effect – based on the evidence of a rapid improvement in mortality for the cohorts born around 1930s – has been assumed to be the main driver of future mortality (Murphy, 2009).

5. SUMMARY

In practice, the main source of comparable data on morbidity across time and space is cause-specific mortality, although its limitations for this purpose must be recognised, and a range of other indicators of population health is also required. Some major diseases such as arthritis are not life-threatening, and therefore not reflected in cause-of-death statistics, which therefore do not reflect the burden of disease from such causes. While it has been impossible to eliminate all inconsistencies, considerable effort has gone into providing comparable cause-of-death data across time and space, and such data remain a key component of the health information system.

REFERENCES

American Psychiatric Association (1994), *Diagnostic and Statistical Manual of Mental Disorders, DSM-IV, Fourth edition*, Washington, DC: American Psychiatric Association.

Anderson, R.N., A.M. Miniño, D.L. Hoyert and H.M. Rosenberg (2001), 'Comparability of cause of death between ICD–9 and ICD–10: preliminary estimates' (National Center for Health Statistics), *National Vital Statistics Reports*, **49**(2), 1–32.

Anstey, K.J., C. von Sanden, A. Salim and R. O'Kearney (2007), 'Smoking as a risk factor for dementia and cognitive decline: a meta-analysis of prospective studies', *American Journal of Epidemiology*, **166**(4), 367–78.

Aylin, P., K. Dunnell and F. Drever (1999), 'Trends in mortality of young adults aged 15 to 44 in England and Wales', *Health Statistics Quarterly*, **1**, 34–9.

Barrett, R., C.W. Kuzawa, T. McDade and G.J. Armelagos (1998), 'Emerging and re-emerging infectious diseases: the third epidemiological transition', *Annual Review of Anthropology*, **27**, 247–71.

Booth, H. and L. Tickle (2008), 'Mortality modelling and forecasting: a review of methods', ADSRI Working Paper, No. 3, http://adsri.anu.edu.au/pubs/ADSRIpapers/ADSRIwp-03.pdf.

Booth, H., J. Maindonald and L. Smith (2002), 'Applying Lee–Carter under conditions of variable mortality decline', *Population Studies*, **56**(3), 325–36.

Booth, H., R.J. Hyndman, L. Tickle and P. de Jong (2006), 'Lee–Carter mortality forecasting: a multi-country comparison of variants and extensions', *Demographic Research*, **15**(9), 289–310.

Brock, A., C. Griffiths and C. Rooney (2006), 'The impact of introducing ICD-10 on analysis of respiratory mortality trends in England and Wales', *Health Statistics Quarterly*, **29**, 9–17.

Carstensen, B. (2006), 'Age-period-cohort models for the Lexis diagram', *Statistics in Medicine*, **26**, 3018–45.

Caselli, G. (1991), 'The key phases of the European health transition', *Polish Population Review*, **7**, 107–25.

Charlton, J. and M. Murphy (1997), *The Health of Adult Britain, 1841–1994*, London: HMSO.

Crimmins, E.M. (1984), 'Life expectancy and the older population. Demographic implications of recent and prospective trends in old age mortality', *Research on Aging*, **6**(4), 490–514.

Currie, I.D. (2006), 'Smoothing and forecasting mortality rates with P-splines', paper given at the Institute of Actuaries, June, http://www.ma.hw.ac.uk/~iain/research/talks/Mortality.pdf.

De Jong, P. and L. Tickle (2006), 'Extending Lee–Carter mortality forecasting', *Mathematical Population Studies*, **13**(1), 1–18.

Di Cesare, M. and M. Murphy (2009), 'Forecasting mortality, different approaches for different cause of deaths? The cases of lung cancer; influenza, pneumonia, and bronchitis; and motor vehicle accidents', *British Actuarial Journal*, **15**, Supplement, 185–211.

Dunn, H.L. and W. Shackley (1944) 'Comparison of the cause-of-death assignments by the 1929 and 1938 revisions of the International List: deaths in the United States, 1940', Vital Statistics Special Reports, **19**, 153 277, www.odo.gov/noho/data/iod1_5.pdf.

Faust, M.M. and A.B. Dolman (1964), 'Comparability ratios based on mortality statistics for the sixth and seventh revision: United States, 1958', *Vital Statistics Special Reports Selected Studies*, **51**(4), Hyattsville, MD: National Center for Health Statistics.

Gaylin, D.S. and J. Kates (1997), 'Refocusing the lens: epidemiological transition theory, mortality differentials, and the AIDS pandemic', *Social Science and Medicine*, **44**(5), 609–21.

Girosi, F. and G. King (2008), *Demographic Forecasting*, Princeton, NJ: Princeton University Press.

Griffiths, C. and A. Brock (2003), 'Twentieth century mortality trends in England and Wales', *Health Statistics Quarterly*, **18**, 5–17.

Griffiths, C. and C. Rooney (2006), 'Trends in mortality from Alzheimer's disease, Parkinson's disease and dementia, England and Wales, 1979–2004', *Health Statistics Quarterly*, **30**, 6–14.

Heathcote, C. and Higgins, T. (2001), 'A regression model of mortality, with applications to the Netherlands', in R. Tabeau, A. Van Den Berg Jeths and C. Heathcote (eds), *Forecasting Mortality in Developed Countries Insights from a Statistical, Demographic and Epidemiological Prospective*, Dordrecht: Kluwer Academic Publishers, pp. 59–82.

Hyndman, R.J. and M.S. Ullah (2007), 'Robust forecasting of mortality and fertility rates: a functional data approach', *Computational Statistics and Data Analysis*, **51**(10), 4942–56.

Janssen, F. and A.E. Kunst (2004), 'ICD coding changes and discontinuities in trends in cause-specific mortality in six European countries, 1950–99', *Bulletin of World Health Organization*, **82**(12), 904–13.

Janssen, T.A. (1938), 'Comparability of mortality statistics', *Journal of the American Statistical Association*, **33**(202), 399–403.

Kirby, L., P. Lehman and A. Majeed (1998), 'Dementia in people aged 65 years and older: a growing problem?', *Population Trends*, **92**, 23–8.

Klebba, A.J. and A.B. Dolman (1975), 'Comparability of mortality statistics for the seventh and eighth revisions of the international classification of diseases, United States', National Center for Health Statistics, Data Evaluation and Methods Research Series, 66. http://www.cdc.gov/nchs/data/series/sr_02/sr02_066.pdf.

Klebba, A.J. and J.H. Scott (1980), 'Estimates of selected comparability ratio based on dual coding of 1976 death certificates by the eighth and ninth revisions of the International Classification of Diseases', *Monthly Vital Statistics Report*, **28**(11), www.cdc.gov/nchs/data/mvsr/supp/mv28_11s.pdf.

Knapp, M. and M. Prince (2007), *Dementia UK. The Full Report*, London Alzheimer's Society. http://alzheimers.org.uk/site/scripts/download_info.php?fileID=2.

Lee, R.D. and L.R. Carter (1992), 'Modeling and forecasting U.S. mortality', *Journal of the American Statistical Association*, **87**(419), 659–71.

Lee, R.D. and T. Miller (2001), 'Evaluating the performance of the Lee–Carter method for forecasting mortality', *Demography*, **38**(4), 537–49.

Logan, W.P.D. (1950), 'Mortality in England and Wales from 1848 to 1947', *Population Studies*, **4**, 132–78.

Lowin, A., P. McCrone and M. Knapp (2001), 'Alzheimer's disease in the UK: comparative evidence on cost-of-illness and of health services research funding', *International Journal of Geriatric Psychiatry*, **16**, 1143–48.

Mackenbach, J.R. (1994), 'The epidemiologic transition theory', *Journal of Epidemiology and Community Health*, **48**, 329–31.

Mahapatra, P., K. Shibuya, F. Coullare, F.C. Notzon, C. Rao and S. Szreter (2007), 'Civil registration systems and vital statistics: successes and missed opportunities', *The Lancet*, **370** (9599), 1653–63.

Mathers, C. and M. Leonardi (2000), 'Global burden of dementia in the year 2000: summary of methods and data sources', *Global Burden of Disease* 2000, Geneva: World Health Organisation, http://www.who.int/healthinfo/statistics/bod_dementia.pdf.

McKeown, T. and R.G. Record (1962), 'Reasons for the decline of mortality in England and Wales during the nineteenth century', *Population Studies*, **16**(2), 94–122.

McKeown, T., R.G. Record and R.D. Turner (1975), 'An interpretation of the decline of mortality in England and Wales during the twentieth century', *Population Studies*, **29**(3), 391–422.

Meslé, F. and J. Vallin (1996), 'Reconstructing long-term series of cause of death – the case of France', *Historical Methods*, **29**, 72–87.

Murphy, M. (2009), 'The "golden generations" in historical context', *British Actuarial Journal*, **15**(Supplement), 151–84.

Murray, C.J.L. and A.D. Lopez (1996), *The Global Burden of Disease: A Comprehensive Assessment of Mortality and Disability from Diseases, Injuries, and Risk Factors in 1990 and Projected to 2020*, Cambridge, MA: Harvard School of Public Health (Global Burden of Disease and Injury Series).

NCHS (2009), 'Comparability across revisions for selected causes', http://www.cdc.gov/nchs/nvss/mortality/comparability_icd.htm.

Olshansky, S.J. and B. Ault (1986), 'The fourth stage of the epidemiologic transition: the age of delayed degenerative diseases', *The Milbank Quarterly*, **64**(3), 355–91.

Omran, A.R. (1971), 'The epidemiologic transition: a theory of the epidemiology of population change', *The Milbank Memorial Fund Quarterly*, **49**(4), 509–38.

Omran, A.R. (1998), 'The epidemiologic transition theory revisited thirty years later', *World Health Statistics Quarterly*, **51**, 99–119.

ONS (2000), '20th century mortality (England and Wales 1901–2000)', CD-ROM.

ONS (2009), '21st century mortality', http://www.statistics.gov.uk/statbase/ssdataset.asp?vlnk=6922.

Pierce, J.R. and A.V. Denison (2010), 'Accuracy of death certifications and the implications for studying disease burdens', in Victor R. Preedy and Ronald R. Watson (eds), *Handbook of Disease Burdens and Quality of Life Measures*, New York: Springer, Part 1 (1.2), pp. 329–44.

Polder, J.J., J.J. Barendregt and J.A.M. van Oers (2006), 'Health care costs in the last year of life – the Dutch experience', *Social Science & Medicine*, **63**, 1720–31.

Pollard, J.H. (1998), 'Keeping abreast of mortality change', Actuarial and Demography Research Paper Series, No. 002/98, http://www.afas.mq.edu.au/research/research_papers/1995-1998_research_papers.

Preston, S.H. (1976), *Mortality Patterns in National Populations: With Special Reference to Recorded Causes of Death*, New York: Academic Press.

Preston, S.H., N. Keyfitz and R. Schoen (1972), *Causes of Death: Life Tables for National Populations*, New York: Seminar Press.

Renshaw, A.E. and S. Haberman (2006), 'A cohort-based extension to the Lee–Carter model for mortality reduction factors', *Insurance: Mathematics and Economics*, **38**, 556–70.

Rieder, H.L. (1994), 'Tuberculosis and human immunodeficiency virus infection in industrialised countries', in P.D.O. Davies (ed.), *Clinical Tuberculosis*, London: Chapman and Hall, pp. 227–40.

Rogers, R.G. and R. Hackenberg (1987), 'Extending epidemiologic transition theory: a new stage', *Social Biology*, **34**, 234–43.

Sanders, J.W., G.S. Fuhrer, M.D. Johnson and M.S. Riddle (2008), 'The epidemiological transition: the current status of infectious diseases in the developed world versus the developing world', *Science Progress*, **91**(1), 1–37.

Scitovsky, A.A. (1984), '"The high cost of dying": What do the data show?', *Milbank Memorial Fund Quarterly*, **62**(4), 591–608.

Scitovsky, A.A. (1994), '"The high cost of dying" revisited', *Milbank Quarterly*, **72**(4), 561–91.

Smallman-Raynor, M. and D. Phillips (1999), 'Late stages of epidemiological transition: health status in the developed world', *Health and Place*, **5**(3), 209–22.

Tabeau, E. (2001), 'A review of demographic forecasting models for mortality', in E. Tabeau, A. Van Den Berg Jeths and C. Heathcote (eds), *Forecasting Mortality in Developed Countries: Insights from a Statistical, Demographic and Epidemiological Prospective*, Dordrecht: Kluwer Academic Publishers, pp. 59–82.

Tabeau, E., P. Ekamper, C. Huisman and A. Bosch (1999), 'Improving overall mortality forecasts by analysing cause of death, period and cohort effects in trends', *European Journal of Population*, **15**(2), 153–83.

Torpy, J.M., C. Lynm and R.M. Glass (2004), 'Dementia', *Journal of the American Medical Association*, **292**(12), 1514.

WHO (2006), 'Counting the dead is essential for health', *Bulletin of the WHO*, **84**(3), 170–71.

WHO (2008), 'The global burden of disease. 2004 update', WHO, http://www.who.int/healthinfo/global_burden_disease/2004_report_update/en/index.html.

WHO (2009), 'History of the development of the ICD', http://www.who.int/classifications/icd/en/HistoryOfICD.pdf.

Wolleswinkel-van de Bosch, J.H., F.W. van Poppel and J.P. Mackenbach (1996), 'Reclassifying causes of death to study the epidemiological transition in Netherlands, 1875–1992', *European Journal of Population*, **12**, 327–61.

17 Risk research and health-related behaviours
Caroline Rudisill

1. INTRODUCTION

The way in which individuals perceive risks matters when making choices about health-related behaviours such as smoking, food consumption, alcohol intake, pharmaceutical use and vaccination uptake. Understanding how individuals perceive risks informs health prevention programmes such as public health awareness campaigns as well as ways to successfully convey the risks and benefits associated with medicines and vaccines.

The causal links between many health-related risks and associated behaviours have been well established. For example, the relationship between tobacco use and lung cancer was established over 50 years ago (Doll and Hill, 1950; Levin et al., 1950; Mills and Porter, 1950; Schrek et al., 1950; Wynder and Graham, 1950). Knowledge about the association between liver disease and drinking has also been well recognised (Pequignot et al., 1978; Saunders et al., 1981), as has the relationship between sun exposure and various types of skin cancer (Armstrong and Kricker, 2001; Elwood and Jopson, 1997). The same is true for the relationship between unprotected sex and sexually transmitted diseases, drunk driving and car accidents, as well as illicit drug use and addiction.

Given the overwhelming evidence regarding many health-related behaviours, individuals' decisions to continue pursuing such activities present concern over humans' risk assessment abilities. Humans sometimes make choices that result in unambiguously poorer outcomes, such as over-eating that leads to a myriad of health concerns, over unambiguously better outcomes, such as healthy eating that reduces the chances of multiple conditions such as coronary heart disease and diabetes. Individuals also might decide not to take a medicine because they have heard about related side effects, when in fact the safety and efficacy profile of the drug make any potential costs of taking it worth the likely health benefits gained.

Risk perceptions are of increasing interest within the health policy field because, compared to studies looking only at 'actual risks', it is often the perception of risks that is most 'determinant' in influencing behaviour, as individuals appear to make decisions based upon their unique mental models for assessing the risks of an action. Risk perceptions rather than actual risks determine health-related behaviour, and consequently the dissemination of risk information is closely dependent on risk information sources.

Public health policy aims to reduce the preventable exposure to health risks and improve population health. One of the ways that policy achieves this goal is by helping the public develop and adapt their perceptions of health risks. Understanding the cognitive processes individuals use when making decisions about their behaviour augments efforts to correctly inform the public about risks. The study of risk perceptions and health-related behaviours focuses on the determinants of what makes individuals behave as they do and thus allows for practical application in policy setting. Understanding the drivers behind individual behavioural decision making allows for the tailoring of communication policies to provide information in a way that portrays risk messages in a complete and helpful manner.

While individuals have the responsibility of making health-related decisions, governments often play a crucial role in ensuring that these decisions are well informed. Yet public action might fail without investigating information sources' effectiveness in influencing individual risk perceptions. Given the constraints placed on national budgets for health promotion among populations, understanding what types of messages and which delivery vehicles effectively inform individuals' behavioural decisions helps to shift funding towards modes that will achieve health policy objectives (Viscusi, 1992a).

This chapter will set out a framework for examining perceptions of risks about health-related behaviours. It begins by setting risk perceptions research within the context of expected utility theory, prospect theory and subsequent developments in the field of behavioural economics. The next sections discuss the influences of cognitive biases, rational addiction models and theories behind information uptake on risk research. The chapter also extensively examines the application of Bayesian learning frameworks to risk perceptions research and builds a theoretical framework for thinking about the role of risk perceptions in health-related behavioural decision making. It concludes by outlining the policy implications for what risk research can tell us about health-related behaviours and decision making.

2.   THEORETICAL CONTEXT OF RISK PERCEPTIONS RESEARCH

Acknowledging the importance of psychology in economics is not novel. Camerer and Loewenstein (2004) note that many of the pre-eminent individuals from the emergence of economics as a distinct discipline incorporated psychological behaviour into their findings. For example, Adam Smith's *Theory of Moral Sentiments* discusses individual behaviour with an understanding of how psychology plays a role in it (Camerer and Loewenstein, 2004).

Individuals have questioned the bounds of humans' rationality as depicted by neoclassical economics for some time. For example, the work of Allais (1953) and Ellsberg (1961) pointed out a series of anomalies in neoclassical economists' depictions of decision making, bringing these issues to the forefront of decision research and holding important policy implications for information provision. The critique of expected utility theory examines economists' normative assumptions and predictions about human decision making.

Standard classical decision-making theory states that individuals make decisions based on the goal of maximizing their expected utility and therefore weight the costs and benefits of alternative courses of action based on their respective probabilities of occurrence (von Neumann and Morgenstern, 1944). The assumption that individuals have independent, continuous and complete preferences underlies this theory.

Savage's work brought together the concepts of expected utility and expected probabilities (1954). This work states that individuals make decisions based upon the utility attached to possible outcomes and that the choices one makes depend upon what one believes the subjective probability of each outcome occurring is likely to be. Subjective expected utility then becomes one's expected value of utility. An individual chooses one decision over another based upon whether the subjective expected utility of that choice is higher. Therefore individuals make decisions depending on their own set of beliefs about the likelihood of each possible outcome. Savage's theory requires that preferences be independent at the moment of decision making (1954), which was demonstrated by Allais (1953) not to be the case.

Evidence from a remarkable number of studies demonstrates that individuals' decision making does not necessarily follow all of the axioms that form part of von Neumann and Morgenstern's (1944) or Savage's (1954) work, suggesting that expected utility theory does not appear representatively valid (Bleichrodt and Pinto, 2002; Gonzalez-Vallejo and Wallsten, 1992; Holt, 1986; Lichtenstein and Slovic, 1973; Tversky and Kahneman, 1981). Individuals do not perceive risks in what would appear to be an ordered decision-making process, instead using mental strategies, or heuristics, to inject certainty around decisions about which the mind is unsure (Hurley and Shogren, 2005; Tversky and Kahneman, 1974; Viscusi, 1992a). This understanding of the realities of decision making has led to the development of prospect reference theory and the application of Bayesian decision-making frameworks to explain how individuals make decisions under uncertainty (Kahneman and Tversky, 1979; Viscusi, 1989; Viscusi and Evans, 2006).

2.1   Relevance of Prospect Theory and Subsequent Developments

Kahneman and Tversky (1979) developed prospect theory to explain the series of anomalies in human decision making violating expected utility theory. Kahneman and Tversky ran a series of experiments to test loss aversion and found individuals' responses to be inconsistent across gambles and to demonstrate a propensity towards loss aversion. In other words, the disutility of losing an outcome of value y appeared greater than the utility attached to gaining an outcome of value y.

Work prior to and following the development of prospect theory demonstrated that any model allowing for the violation of dominance could be entirely flawed. Individuals violate dominance when they fail to prefer unambiguously better outcomes to unambiguously poorer outcomes in decision-making contexts.

Tversky and Kahneman (1992) expanded their work on prospect theory to cumulative prospect theory, which no longer permitted the violation of dominance by borrowing from rank-dependent theory to adjust probability weighting for dominant outcomes. Rank-dependent expected utility theory allows for preferences to be non-linear in probability (Quiggin, 1982). Therefore individuals can overweight only those outcomes for which they perceive the probability of occurrence to be very low as compared to the probability of all outcomes. Cumulative prospect theory allows for the weighting of individual probabilities cumulatively based upon the utility attached to each type of outcome (gain or loss) and further supported prior findings on loss aversion and diminishing sensitivity.

Viscusi (1989) developed prospective reference theory as a variation on expected utility theory and found that individuals use risk information alongside prior beliefs in a Bayesian manner, attaching utilities to alternative courses of action. Viscusi further developed Kahneman and Tversky's model, suggesting that when probabilities are identical for all outcomes, individuals employ biases and affective heuristics such as overweighting low-probability events to make decisions.

Other amendments to expected utility theory have been proposed. For example, Yaari's (1987) dual theory of choice under risk replaces the axiom of independence with the axiom of dual independence. Dual independence under Yaari's construct means that an agent would elect one choice given two options with different risks attached, while an agent operating under expected utility theory would diversify by taking two options of differing degrees of risk (Hadar and Kun Seo, 1995). The dual theory allows for separation in terms of agents' views on risk versus views on related outcomes of that risk, such as wealth if talking about a financial investment choice (Demers and Demers, 1990) or, in the case of health-related risks, utility attached to having a tan and relaxation from smoking.

Prospect theory and its further incarnations find importance when examining risk perceptions about health behaviours because they highlight how people might make decisions when weighing the risks and benefits of courses of action. Time-related elements become especially important in some health-related decisions. For many behaviours such as smoking and drinking, individuals receive the benefits immediately but experience costs in the future. This characteristic suggests that those individuals who choose to undertake behaviours such as smoking weigh benefits in the near term more heavily than future costs or have higher discount rates than those who do not smoke (Khwaja et al., 2006). Therefore individuals make choices based upon perceived utility today as opposed to how this choice might impact the utility gained from activities in the future (Rabin, 1998).

The development of prospect theory demonstrates that risk perceptions are sometimes inconsistent with objective risk information. There are several potential justifications in the literature for the seeming mismatch between available information and preferences. These include the presence of cognitive biases or affect heuristics and information failures in formulating risk perceptions.

2.2   Risk Assessment with Intuitive Feelings (Cognitive Biases or Affect Heuristics)

A wide range of evidence supports claims that individuals use affect heuristics or cognitive biases in decision making where outcomes and/or information seem unclear. The term 'heuristic' describes the thought processes or cognitive biases individuals employ in order to understand potential courses of action about which they do not feel fully informed (Kahneman et al., 1982). These biases can lead to systematic misjudgements such as overestimation or underestimation of risks or the incorporation of biased information sources as fact.

The means by which individuals process information to mould risk perceptions comes in two differing forms: one is more intuitive and feeling-related; the other takes an analytical or rational approach (Epstein, 1994). The psychology literature argues that individuals make decisions based more upon affect and association than on analytical processes (Dake, 1991; Loewenstein et al., 2001). While, in many decisions, both analytical and affective reasoning play crucial roles, across decisional contexts, affect-related variables appear to trump analytics in their influence on risk perceptions (Barrett and Salovey, 2002; Holtgrave and Weber, 1993; Johnson and Tversky, 1983; Loewenstein, 1996; Slovic et al., 2002). For example, value-laden elements dominate individuals' decision-making structures in situations where individuals express non-decisiveness about an issue and the issue evokes emotive responses, such as an environmental topic (Blamey, 1998). Gender has also been found to provide some explanation for differences in perceived risk, with women generally having higher risk perceptions with regard to risks across a range of issues, including health, safety and finance (Slovic, 1987; Flynn et al., 1994).

The phenomenon of incorporating 'affect' or feelings into decisions appears with particular prevalence in risk contexts (Finucane et al., 2000). The mind's interpretation of intuitive feelings varies depending on risk type, the level of understanding about the risk and availability of information at the time of decision making (Slovic et al., 2004). Familiarity and/or experience with a risk such as daily exposure have been shown to influence risk perceptions and resultant behaviours related to that risk (Fischhoff et al., 1978; Hertwig et al., 2004). For example, when looking at an adolescent's decision to smoke, the act of experimenting with smoking is accompanied by little evaluation of risks and instead is driven primarily by affect. When Slovic (2001) asked smokers, 'If you had to do it all over again, would you start smoking?', 85 per cent of adults and 80 per cent of adolescents (14–22 years) responded 'no'.

The extent to which affect or rational decision making matters in risk perceptions development is dependent partly on the availability of information, trust in information sources and knowledge gained from those information sources.

3. THE ROLE OF INFORMATION IN DEVELOPING AND UPDATING RISK PERCEPTIONS

3.1 Injection of Information into Decision-making Frameworks

Information about a risk can be gleaned directly through personal experience and/or informational uptake from exogenous sources such as public health messages or a visit to the doctor. However, without much prior experience with a risky behaviour, individuals lean heavily on indirect experience gleaned from others and information delivered through exogenous sources. Indirect experience provides a different kind of sensory feedback as the reactions to experience can vary on the individual level, ranging from fear to cognitive dissonance (indirect experience and knowledge are discussed in Johnson, 1993).

Those with whom individuals have already established relationships, especially where some level of trust is involved, would be the most likely candidates to exogenously influence perceptions. The extent of this informational asymmetry regarding behavioural risks depends on many factors, including age, knowledge and education. For adolescents, adult figures such as parents, teachers and medical professionals are likely to have more information about a risk than the adolescent himself or herself. Because of this informational asymmetry, adolescents would rely on these agents to provide information to varying degrees, depending on the extent of trust in the relationship and credibility given to that individual as an information source.

Parents can provide information through their own behaviours, directly discussing behavioural risks with their children and also by evidence of health shocks occurring within the household. Previous literature would suggest that health shocks play an important role in altering behaviours and perceptions of risk (Sloan et al., 2003). These health events would contribute to how parents disseminate information to their children, as even if adolescents have already started undertaking a risky behaviour such as smoking, they are unlikely to have had a resulting health shock or even related negative health outcome such as shortness of breath.

Individuals can use information to support either rational or irrational decisions. The rational use of information in a risk perceptions model predicts that as individuals become more knowledgeable about a risk, their behavioural decisions will emerge from the weighting of costs and benefits of a decision given the stock of information presented. Akerlof and Dickens's (1982) theory of cognitive dissonance supports the existence of irrationality in decision-making processes. When individuals are cognitively dissonant, they express a belief that they would like to be true with limited regard to exogenously procured information even in the face of perhaps knowing that alternatives not chosen may have positive attributes (Fishbein and Ajzen, 1975). For adults and risky behaviours, existing beliefs would be subject to cognitive dissonance because of years of personal experience and exposure to information about risks and benefits related to these behaviours. In the case of adolescents and risky behaviours, cognitive dissonance is a more limited concern because of less personal experience with smoking, illicit drugs, binge drinking and risky sexual behaviours, and thus minimal likelihood of attempting to defend held views since existing views are limited.

Rational irrationality differs from rational ignorance in that an ignorant decision maker does not have an opinion about alternative choices. A rationally ignorant decision maker perceives the benefits of gaining new information as minimal and thus employs minimal amounts of information in his formulation of perceptions (Downs, 1957). Caplan (2001) describes some religious believers as rationally ignorant because of their limited desire to acquire more information about their religion or that of others, but maintaining strong beliefs regardless.

Theories of bounded rationality, rational addiction and any other approaches to decision making where individuals weigh the risks and benefits associated with alternative actions implicitly require adequate information to make these assessments. In many cases, however, as discussed above with evidence about the use of affective heuristics, decision making takes place in the absence of full or unbiased information. Viscusi (1997) finds that alarmist decisions and thus overreaction to risks can arise due to government and industry methods of excessively weighting worst-case scenarios and over-advertising certain risks. Similarly, media coverage of an event can have major implications for the risk profile individuals attach to that event (Lichtenstein et al., 1978; Razum et al., 2003; Washer, 2004). Although information proves integral for decision making, the potential benefits of increased levels of information do not always generate more soundly made decisions. Even in the presence of information about a risk, individuals may still develop inaccurate risk perceptions holding implications from a policy perspective.

3.2   Inaccurate Risk Estimation in a Setting of Available and Accessible Information

A wide range of literature has concluded that people overestimate low-probability risks and underestimate high-probability risks (Hurley and Shogren, 2005; Kahneman and Tversky, 1979; Viscusi, 1992a). Armantier (2006) found this to be the case for risks ranging as widely as infectious diseases such as cholera to fireworks, floods, lightning, childbirth, firearms accidents, lung cancer, diabetes and heart disease. There is also evidence of gender-specific nuances to this finding as women overestimate low-probability events by less than men but underestimate those of high-probability by more than men (Hurley and Shogren, 2005).

From a policy standpoint, risk overestimation and underestimation present difficulties. Individuals who overestimate a risk could find themselves needlessly living in a state of heightened concern and thus potentially avoiding transport or going to work in the case of something like flu risks, which has knock-on macroeconomic effects. If, however, information sources such as the government or media overestimate risks, then they lose credibility. Additionally, in a litigious setting, individuals deemed to overestimate the risks of a behaviour perceive themselves as knowledgeable about the risks they have taken and therefore assume liability for the consequences of their actions. Government could also find risk overestimation costly because some measures put in place to mitigate concerns would be unnecessary.

On the other hand, risk underestimation could lead to individuals no longer showing the needed concern over a risky situation and governments and other information sources failing to pay enough attention (Fischhoff et al., 1993). Underestimation also implies lack of knowledge, leading to individuals perhaps undertaking an activity about which they are not fully informed. This situation places more liability on players such as the tobacco, firearms and alcohol industries, producing products carrying risks.

In order to move individuals' risk perceptions to a level of greater accuracy in either direction from under- or overestimation, information sources of many types play a key role. While affect and feelings play a significant role in forming risk perceptions, the availability of adequate information and the way that individuals incorporate this information into their decision-making process remains crucial. One such theoretical model for information uptake that has been successfully used to examine risk perceptions across many subjects (e.g. smoking, skin cancer, traffic accidents) is the Bayesian learning framework (Antoñanzas et al., 2000; Anderson and Lundborg, 2007; Costa-Font and Rovira, 2005; Dickie and Gerking, 1996; Liu and Hsieh, 1995; Lundborg, 2007; Lundborg and Lindgren, 2004; Viscusi, 1990, 1991).

3.3   The Bayesian Learning Framework and Information

The Bayesian learning framework offers a robust construct for explaining how individuals incorporate new information into decision-making processes in order to fill gaps in their current stock of knowledge (Viscusi, 1992b). In a Bayesian learning model the formation of subjective beliefs, according to the different types of information sources individuals face, joins a prior set of beliefs, 'the prior'. The model assumes that information concerning the risks and benefits of a behaviour is constrained by the existence of multiple information channels from which one can distinguish private or individual

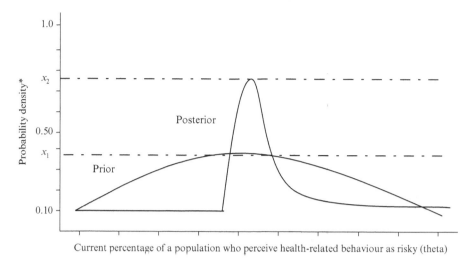

Current percentage of a population who perceive health-related behaviour as risky (theta)

Note: *The probability that theta is equal to x_n.

Figure 17.1   Bayesian approach to how risk perceptions change upon the receipt of new information

(e.g. parents, friends, siblings) and public or collective (e.g. government-related public health efforts, school education programmes, industry advertisements) sources. Due to likely existing information about many health-related risks, individuals mentally form a subjective probability on the likely effects of their behaviour such as smoking or binge drinking. Direct and indirect experiences with risk incorporate such aspects as gender, age, socioeconomic status, risk aversion and time preferences, as these elements can all relate to experience with health-related risk taking.

Depending on the credibility individuals attach to each information source, they update their 'prior' with new information to develop a 'posterior' perception of risk (Viscusi, 1991). Figure 17.1 demonstrates how individuals move towards more certainty about a health-related risk.

The x-axis of this figure measures the accuracy of an individual's perceptions about a risk such as skin cancer rates or likelihood of contracting a sexually transmitted infection, while the y-axis measures the probability density or likelihood that the value of the x-axis is actually equal to the mean. Figure 17.1 assumes that new information gives individuals greater certainty about their perceptions of risks so long as they attach enough credibility to that information source. The variation in perceptions of risk shrinks from the prior position to the posterior position as a result of new information. One would expect that upon the uptake of exogenous information, the variance in adolescents' perceptions of risks would fall more than that of adults. Adolescents would gain greater certainty about risks, whereas adults would feel that they already know more and have less prior uncertainty about risks. Therefore the adults' prior curve may have a sharper spike than that of adolescents, but the change between the prior and the posterior would be greater for adolescents.

In more simple terms but still maintaining the Bayesian learning construct, the risk formulation process looks like the following equation adapted from Viscusi (1991):

$$RISK = \gamma_1 X_1 + \gamma_2 X_2 + \gamma_3 X_3$$

where γ_n represents the weights attached to each type of information source (X), X_1 represents prior risk perception level or what the person thought about the risk prior to gaining new information (endowments), X_2 direct and indirect experience (e.g. seeing parents, friends undertake a risky behaviour) and X_3 exogenous sources of information (e.g. public health classroom lecture or a doctor disseminating risk information). This function for risk perception formulation implies that X_2 and X_3 can only influence *RISK* if the weights attached to them (γ_2 and γ_3) are sufficiently large in comparison to the weight attached to the prior risk perception level (γ_1). As the sizes of γ_2 and γ_3 increase, new sources of information alter risk perceptions to a greater extent than endowments. For a younger population sample, this kind of analysis would assume that $\gamma_2 > \gamma_1$ and $\gamma_3 > t\gamma_1$. Therefore these individuals would enter into the risk development process with limited endowments or prior opinions about the risk and therefore the expectation would be that the weights of direct and indirect experience (γ_2) and exogenous information sources (γ_3) will prove more important in the risk perception development process than prior evaluations of risk perceptions (γ_1).

The Bayesian learning framework garners support in the risk literature since individuals do not look at new information about probabilities as fully informative but add this new information to existing opinions about risks to guide future behavioural choice (Viscusi and Evans, 2006). The Bayesian framework also allows for the presence of cognitive biases. Viscusi (1985) suggests that the employment of cognitive biases in decision making where individuals do not feel fully informed follows this Bayesian learning process. Although decisions formulating risk perceptions may not always be accurate, the way in which individuals employ new information about a risk is predicted within the Bayesian framework (Viscusi, 1985). Viscusi (1997) found, however, that individuals do not follow the Bayesian process in cases where they are not fully informed and place more weight on a source of information that delivers a higher risk assessment given two sources about the same topic. Viscusi (1992a) also suggests that individuals do not fulfil the Bayesian method of processing new information when they fail to understand the meaning of probabilities for possible outcomes.

Where the Bayesian framework fails to accurately depict the uptake of new information, an alternative construct would be useful. However, alternatives to the Bayesian model, such as assuming individuals are completely irrational, would not allow for quantitative testing, instead serving as theoretical background. The Bayesian framework allows for undertaking empirical analysis regarding questions of information uptake and has been shown to suit the analysis of risk perceptions and health-related behaviours (Dickie and Gerking, 1996; Liu and Hsieh, 1995; Lundborg and Lindgren, 2002, 2004; Lundborg, 2007; Viscusi, 1991).

The Bayesian framework does not necessarily reflect exactly how decisions are made in reality, given evidence of the inconsistencies with which individuals make decisions in many contexts such as prospect theory and cumulative prospect theory. Viscusi (1992a) suggests that such violations of expected utility theory as found in prospect theory do not necessarily reflect a lack of rationality in decision making but instead what happens when decisions are made without full information. Expected utility theory used in the Bayesian framework provides a systematic basis for predicting behaviour because of its strict assumptions (Viscusi, 1992a). Savage (1972) also acknowledges how behaviours depart from expected utility theory but without entirely dismissing the theory as it still remains useful as a predictive guide. Experimental findings in both the laboratory and the field demonstrate the failure of individuals to exhibit utility-maximising behaviour. The Bayesian framework, however, offers a stylised framework to which large survey data can be applied in order to answer questions about information uptake under conditions of uncertainty. Understanding the effect of information asymmetries on health-related risk decisions, such as the degree to which principal–agent relationships and spatial proximity matter, is of additional use when examining the theoretical basis for information uptake about health-related risks.

Having discussed some underlying theoretical guidance on information uptake, a guiding conceptual framework for examining decision making around risk-related health behaviours emerges.

4.   CONCEPTUAL FRAMEWORK

Figure 17.2 graphically demonstrates the formulation of risk perceptions by showing the roles of information, credibility effects and cognitive biases throughout this process.

The way in which individuals use information to formulate risk perceptions about risk-related behaviour can be conceptualised as follows. Each individual starts with a set of endowments ('Pre-existing endowments'). These endowments are information the individual knows and characteristics that may influence not only behavioural choices but also the way one perceives new information. One's existing stock of knowledge and opinions can be mediated by demographic and socioeconomic characteristics such as gender, age, household structure, race, education and social class. Previous personal experience with a risk behaviour and/or observation of others' behaviours regarding that risk also act as endowments because of their influence on individuals' stocks of prior knowledge about the risks attached to a behaviour. In addition, one's perceived ability to avoid the negative outcomes associated with the behaviour (exhibiting optimism bias), as well as the extent to which an individual is risk-averse, all inform the set of endowments to which he/she enters into the behavioural decision. An individual's overall attitude towards risks would affect how individuals assess risks about a behavioural choice. Preferences for timing (discount rates) also affect the endowments with which individuals enter into decisions such as smoking, sun tanning and excessive alcohol intake (O'Donoghue and Rabin, 2000).

Individuals then gain and assimilate new information to their set of prior beliefs from a variety of sources according to the Bayesian construct (Viscusi, 1985, 1989). Both endogenous and exogenous factors can act as information sources ('Receive endogenous new information' and 'Receive exogenous new information'). Endogenous new information comes from personal experience of partaking in a behaviour such as smoking or trying smoking for the first time. Exogenous new information comes both from indirect

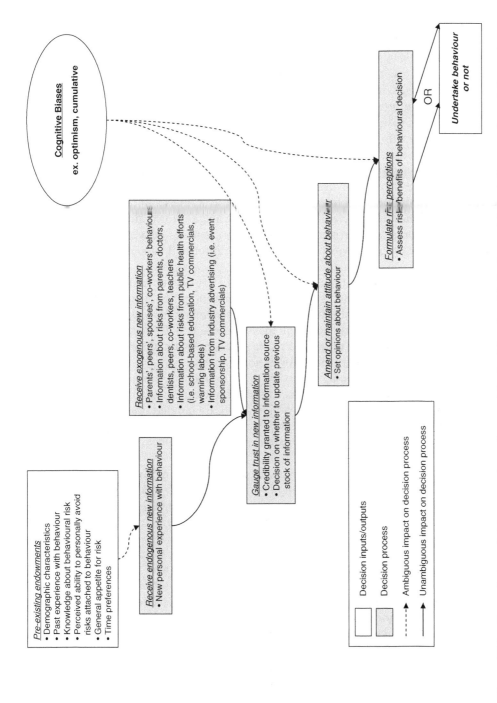

Figure 17.2   Formulation of risk perceptions about a risky health-related behaviour with the influence of new information

experience with the behaviour by seeing behavioural examples of society, parents', siblings', spouse's, roommates' and peers' undertaking the behaviour as well as conveyance of risk information from medical professionals, parents, peers and public-health efforts such as warning labels, school-based educational programmes and television advertisements.

The degree to which each of these information sources alters the way an individual's endowments alone would lead them to perceive risks and then make a behavioural choice depends upon the credibility attached to each of these information sources as well as the extent to which informational asymmetry and spatial proximity play a role in altering credibility levels ('Gauge trust in new information'). The Bayesian learning framework depicts the information uptake process as dependent on the weights attached to each source of information, so the degree to which each is deemed credible limits the level of influence each exerts over risk perceptions (Viscusi, 1985). The strength of any informational asymmetries between exogenous information sources and the individual, such as parents and their adolescent children or medical professionals and their patients, would also probably influence the credibility attached to these information sources (Munro, 1999). In addition, spatial proximity, or the social distances between individuals, may also influence the extent to which individuals trust information sources (Glaeser et al., 2002).

Individuals who display rational ignorance would not take up additional information because of the perception that incremental gains in information would not be of benefit (Downs, 1957). While new information about a behaviour's risks may update individuals' stocks of knowledge, it may not result in individuals actually being more informed as they may either still maintain inaccurate risk estimations (Kahneman and Tversky, 1979; Viscusi, 1992a, 1997) or suffer from information overload.

Upon updating one's previous stock of information, one forms a new attitude about a risky behaviour ('Amend or maintain attitude about behaviour'). This attitude is not entirely new for many risks about which individuals are familiar, but rather an updated version of previous attitudes about the behaviour. In the case where an individual gives no credibility to any additional information acquired, the previous attitude does not change.

These attitudes then inform perceptions of risk by attaching some understanding of the consequences involved with deciding to undertake a risk ('Formulate risk perceptions'). The development of risk perceptions involves some combination of weighing the risks and benefits of a behavioural choice along with the influence of affect and cognitive biases such as optimism and available biases on this process (Arnett, 2000; Finucane et al., 2000; Slovic, 1998; Slovic et al., 2004). Decisions can range from being automatic and entirely based on affect and biases to being more deliberative and cognitively focused.

Based upon attitude and its subsequent contribution to the development of risk perception, an individual decides whether to undertake a behaviour. The relationship between risk perceptions and behaviours has been described as recursive, such that risk perceptions may influence behaviour and behaviour may influence risk perceptions, but the order is unclear. Therefore the process can be depicted as a dynamic one. For this reason, there are two arrows in Figure 17.2, one pointing from risk perceptions to behavioural change and the other pointing in both directions.

Previous literature focusing on adolescents predicts the directionality as risk perceptions influencing behaviours, but behaviours not influencing perceptions after using instruments to control for endogeneity (Lundborg, 2007; Lundborg and Andersson, 2008). For adult populations, the answer would differ as more personal experience with a risk would allow for experience with that behaviour to influence risk perceptions to a greater extent than in the case of adolescents (Viscusi, 1991; Liu and Hsieh, 1995).

At largely any stage of this process, the influence of cognitive biases can be felt in the way individuals interpret numbers, facts and new information (Tversky and Kahneman, 1987; Viscusi, 1985). For example, the way in which risk information may be framed, such as phrasing the risks in terms of likelihood of dying or not dying, may influence the degree to which that information source alters perceptions of risk. In addition, where individuals fail to understand any statistical information given about risks, they would not process new information in the way depicted by the Bayesian learning model, where information sources have little or no credibility attached to them because of a lack of understanding of this new information (Viscusi, 1992a).

5. IMPLICATIONS FOR HEALTH POLICY

Risk perceptions research in general provides policy makers with an evidence base of advice for how to communicate risk information to the public and to understand how the general public will react in the face of different types of risks (Slovic et al., 1982). A better understanding of the development and updating of health-related risk perceptions has implications for public health and risk communication policy. Investigating the cognitive processes individuals use when making decisions about their behaviour augments efforts to correctly inform the public about risks. For many public health challenges such as smoking, drug use, alcohol or sun exposure, much of the population is largely knowledgeable about at least some risks attached to each behaviour. The continuation of such behaviours and sometimes disproportionaley across certain segments of the population means that even with information and knowledge available, it is not equally influencing behaviours across society. Looking at how risk perceptions of these health-related behaviours are formed and updated can be used for achieving public policy aims of reducing preventable exposures to health risks. It provides guidance on how to undertake information campaigns about public health risks by understanding the determinants of risk perceptions. It also aids in targeting populations for specific public health messages by understanding how population sub-groups may develop risk perceptions differently.

For example, countries throughout the developed world are implementing and discussing policies aimed at achieving behavioural goals of improving population eating habits and levels of physical activity. Through meeting such behavioural goals, countries can reduce preventable exposures to cancer, heart disease, diabetes and stroke, thus reducing overall health care expenditure. Risk perceptions research informs such nutrition policy efforts by providing empirical evidence backing up policy proposals. For instance, obesity affects some portions of the population to a greater extent than others, depending on the country. If policy efforts are aimed at specific ethnic minorities, age groups or genders, policy makers have to understand the drivers behind population sub-groups' differing perceptions about the importance of healthy diet and what a healthy diet looks like. Previous research has found sub-group differences based upon gender (Hurley and Shogren, 2005; Lundborg and Andersson, 2008), but further research would help in defining the degree to which ethnicity, age and socioeconomic status play a role in the way individuals update their perceptions of health-related risks such as nutritional choices.

Understanding the decision-making processes (heuristics and cognitive shortcuts) as well as what information sources matter most when individuals make decisions about their behaviour allows for the tailoring of communication policies. As a result, efforts at further public health and preventive health measures will portray risk messages in a complete and useful manner.

Beyond public health policy, risk research has implications for health policy in general when looking at the way individuals interact with a health system and use health-related goods and services. In particular, the use of pharmaceuticals such as medication adherence can be examined under the theoretical framework depicted here. Insurers, health care payers, governments and physicians have to understand the most appropriate way to convey pharmaceutical risks. As important as it is for patients to understand pharmaceutical risks, it is also necessary for them to understand the potential benefits accompanying these risks. It is of financial importance to payers of health care that patients take prescribed medicines appropriately to prevent higher costs in the long term. The same is true for vaccinations, which is both a public health and health care issue.

Improving our understanding of how individuals perceive the risks of medications, vaccinations and treatment options has significant cost implications for health care systems globally. It also falls in line with many health systems' objectives to increase patients' involvement in their own health care decision making. Over the last decade, greater emphasis has been placed on informed choice in health care, which requires understanding individual risk assessment in relation to adherence and consumption patterns. Efforts to increase patient autonomy and personal responsibility as well as cost-containment aims have brought the role of risk perceptions and behavioural patterns to the forefront of discussions about pharmaceutical and health care services consumption.

6.   CONCLUDING REMARKS

Risk-related health decisions are often modelled as ones of expected utility, making the assumption that individuals operate in a rational way by assessing the costs and benefits of a behavioural choice. For example, an adolescent thinking about trying cocaine for the first time might weigh the likelihood of getting caught, the consequences of getting caught, any associated health risks and fear of the unknown against anticipated pleasure associated with cocaine use, looking cool in front of friends and any utility from the thrill associated with partaking in risky activities. The decision-making process of an adolescent thinking about trying cocaine for the first time would probably not be that deliberate and, as the beginning of this chapter explained, the likelihood of someone thinking about this decision within the frame of expected utility is low.

The extensive behavioural economics literature analyses the shortcomings of neoclassical economics. This understanding of how the axioms of neoclassical economics may be violated informs the interpretation of experimental and large-scale survey results.

For example, results regarding different types of questions for eliciting risk perceptions could be interpreted in light of findings about violations of these axioms. This greater understanding of behaviour permits a richer picture of the risk perception development process and, in turn, policy prescriptions to address the resulting behavioural decisions. Some of the biases in decision making are not necessarily associated with irrationality but instead with rational means by which individuals circumvent any informational shortcomings to reach decisions (Viscusi, 1992b).

The theoretical framework set out here should be tested under empirical scrutiny and amended based upon these findings. It offers a way forward for research on health-related risky behaviours, shedding light on how to bring together large-scale empirical research with a rich body of previous research on decision making. Understanding risk perceptions in this way provides empirical evidence to support health policy efforts aimed at reducing preventable exposures to health-related risks and encouragement of appropriate use of pharmaceuticals, vaccines and health services.

REFERENCES

Akerlof, G. and W. Dickens (1982), 'The economic consequences of cognitive dissonance', *American Economic Review*, **72**, 307–19.

Allais, M. (1953), 'Le comportement de l'homme rationnel devant le risque: critique des postulats et axiomes de l'école américaine', *Econometrica*, **21**, 255–83.

Anderson, H. and P. Lundborg (2007), 'Perception of own death risk: an analysis of road-traffic and overall mortality risks', *Journal of Risk and Uncertainty*, **34**(1), 67–84.

Antoñanzas, F., W.K. Viscusi, J. Rovira, F. Brana, F. Portillo and I. Carvalho (2000), 'Smoking risks in Spain: Part I – Perception of risks to the smoker', *Journal of Risk and Uncertainty*, **21**(2–3), 161–86.

Armantier, O. (2006), 'Estimates of own lethal risks and anchoring effects', *Journal of Risk and Uncertainty*, **32**, 37–56.

Armstrong, B.K. and A. Kricker (2001), 'The epidemiology of UV induced skin cancer', *Journal of Photochemistry and Photobiology B: Biology*, **63**(1–3), 8–18.

Arnett, J.J. (2000), 'Optimistic bias in adolescent and adult smokers and nonsmokers', *Addictive Behaviours*, **25**(4), 625–32.

Barrett, L.F. and P. Salovey (eds) (2002), *The Wisdom in Feeling*, New York: Guilford.

Blamey, R.K. (1998), 'Decisiveness, attitude expression and symbolic responses in contingent valuation surveys', *Journal of Economic Behavior & Organization*, **34**, 577–601.

Bleichrodt, H. and J.L. Pinto (2002), 'Loss aversion and scale compatibility in two attribute trade-offs', *Journal of Mathematical Psychology*, **46**, 315–37.

Camerer, C.F. and G. Loewenstein (2004), 'Behavioral economics: past, present and future', in C. Camerer, G. Loewenstein and M. Rabin (eds), *Advances in Behavioral Economics*, Princeton, NJ: Princeton University Press, pp. 3–51.

Caplan, B. (2001), 'Rational ignorance versus rational irrationality', *KYKLOS*, **54**, 3–26.

Costa-Font, J. and J. Rovira (2005), 'When do smokers underestimate smoking related mortality risks?', *Applied Economics Letters*, **12**, 789–94.

Dake, K. (1991), 'Orienting dispositions in the perception of risk: an analysis of contemporary worldviews and cultural biases', *Journal of Cross-Cultural Psychology*, **22**, 61–82.

Demers, Fanny and Michel Demers (1990), 'Price uncertainty, the competitive firm and the dual theory of choice under risk', *European Economic Review*, **34**, 1181–99.

Dickie, M. and S. Gerking (1996), 'Formation of risk beliefs, joint production and willingness to pay to avoid skin cancer', *Review of Economics and Statistics*, **78**(3), 451–63.

Doll, R. and A.B. Hill (1950), 'Smoking and carcinoma of the lung: preliminary report', *British Medical Journal*, **221**(ii), 739–48.

Downs, A. (1957), *An Economic Theory of Democracy*, New York: Harper.

Ellsberg, D. (1961), 'Risk, ambiguity and the Savage axioms', *Quarterly Journal of Economics*, **75**, 643–9.

Elwood, M. and J. Jopson (1997), 'Melanoma and sun exposure: an overview of published studies', *International Journal of Cancer*, **73**, 198–203.

Epstein, S. (1994), 'Integration of the cognitive and the psychodynamic unconscious', *American Psychologist*, **49**, 709–24.

Finucane, M., L. Alhakami, P. Slovic and S.M. Johnson (2000), 'The affect heuristic in judgments of risks and benefits', *Journal of Behavioral Decision Making*, **13**, 1–17.

Fischhoff, B., A. Bostrom and M.J. Quadrel (1993), 'Risk perception and communication', *Annual Review of Public Health*, **14**, 183–203.

Fischhoff, B., P. Slovic, S. Lichtenstein, S. Read and B. Combs (1978), 'How safe is safe enough?: a psychometric study of attitudes towards technological risks and benefits', *Policy Sciences*, **9**, 127–52.

Fishbein, M. and I. Ajzen (1975), *Belief, Attitude, Intention and Behavior: An Introduction to Theory and Research*, Reading, MA and Don Mills, Ontario:Addison-Wesley.

Flynn, J., P. Slovic and C.K. Mertz (1994), 'Gender, race, and perception of environmental health risks', *Risk Analysis*, **14**, 1101–08.

Glaeser, E., D. Laibson and B. Sacerdote (2002), 'An economic approach to social capital', *The Economic Journal*, **112**, 437–58.

Gonzalez-Vallejo, C. and T.S. Wallsten (1992), 'Effects of probability mode on preference reversal', *Journal of Experimental Psychology – Learning, Memory Cognition*, **18**(4), 855–64.

Hadar, J. and T. Kun Seo (1995), 'Asset diversification in Yaari's dual theory', *European Economic Review*, **39**(6), 1171–80.

Hertwig, R., G. Barron, E.U. Weber and I. Erev (2004), 'Decisions from experience and the effect of rare events in risky choice', *Psychological Science*, **15**(8), 534–9.

Holt, C.A. (1986), 'Preference reversals and the independence axiom', *American Economic Review*, **76**(3), 508–15.

Holtgrave, D. and E.U. Weber (1993), 'Dimensions of risk perceptions for financial and health risks', *Risk Analysis*, **13**, 553–8.

Hurley, T.M. and J.F. Shogren (2005), 'An experimental comparison of induced and elicited beliefs', *The Journal of Risk and Uncertainty*, **30**(2), 169–88.

Johnson, B. (1993), 'Advancing understanding of knowledge's role in lay risk perceptions', *RISK: Issues in Health & Safety*, **4**, 189–212.

Johnson, E.J. and A. Tversky (1983), 'Affect, generalization, and the perception of risk', *Journal of Personality and Social Psychology*, **45**, 20–31.

Kahneman, D. and A. Tversky (1979), 'Prospect theory: an analysis of decision under risk', *Econometrica*, **47**(2), 263–92.

Kahneman, D., P. Slovic and A. Tversky (eds) (1982), *Judgment Under Uncertainty: Heuristics and Biases*, New York: Cambridge University Press.

Khwaja, A., F. Sloan and M. Salm (2006), 'Evidence on preferences and subjective beliefs of risk takers: the case of smokers', *International Journal of Industrial Organisation*, **24**, 667–82.

Levin, M.L., H. Goldstein and P.R. Gerhardt (1950), 'Cancer and tobacco smoking', *Journal of the American Medical Association*, **143**, 336–8.

Lichtenstein, S. and P. Slovic (1973), 'Response-induced reversals of preference in gambling: an extended replication in Las Vegas', *Journal of Economic Psychology*, **101**(1), 16–20.

Lichtenstein S., P. Slovic, B. Fischhoff, M. Layman and B. Combs (1978), 'Judged frequency of lethal events', *Journal of Experimental Psychology: Human Learning and Memory*, **4**, 551–78.

Liu, J.T. and C.R. Hsieh (1995), 'Risk perception and smoking behavior: empirical evidence from Taiwan', *Journal of Risk and Uncertainty*, **11**(2), 139–57.

Loewenstein, G.F. (1996), 'Out of control: visceral influences on behavior', *Organizational Behavior and Human Decision Processes*, **65**, 272–92.

Loewenstein, G.F., E.U. Weber, C.K. Hsee and E. Welch (2001), 'Risk as feelings', *Psychological Bulletin*, **127**, 267–86.

Lundborg, P. (2007), 'Smoking, information sources and risk perceptions – new results on Swedish data', *Journal of Risk and Uncertainty*, **34**(3), 217–40.

Lundborg, P. and H. Andersson (2008), 'Gender, risk perceptions, and smoking behavior', *Journal of Health Economics*, **27**(5), 1299–311.

Lundborg, P. and B. Lindgren (2002), 'Risk perceptions and alcohol consumption among young people', *Journal of Risk and Uncertainty*, **25**, 165–83.

Lundborg, P. and B. Lindgren (2004), 'Do they know what they are doing? Risk perceptions and smoking behaviour among Swedish teenagers', *Journal of Risk and Uncertainty*, **28**(3), 261–86.

Mills, C.A. and M.M. Porter (1950), 'Tobacco smoking habits and cancer of the mouth and respiratory system', *Cancer Research*, **10**, 539–42.

Munro, L. (1999), 'A principal–agent analysis of the family: implications for the welfare state', IDPM Working Paper Series, No. 58.

O'Donoghue, T. and M. Rabin (2000), 'Risky behavior among youths: some issues from behavioral economics', Economics Department, University of California, Berkeley, Working Paper E00-285, available at http://repositories.cdlib.org/iber/econ/E00-285/.

Pequignot, G., A.J. Tuyns and J.L. Berta (1978), 'Ascitic cirrhosis in relation to alcohol consumption', *International Journal of Epidemiology*, **7**, 113–20.

Quiggin, J. (1982), 'A theory of anticipated utility', *Journal of Economic Behavior and Organization*, **3**, 323–43.

Rabin, M. (1998), 'Psychology and economics', *Journal of Economic Literature*, **36**, 11–46.

Razum, O., H. Becher, H. Kapaun and T. Junghanss (2003), 'SARS, lay epidemiology, and fear', *The Lancet*, **361**(9370), 1739–40.

Saunders, J.B., J.R.F. Walters, P. Davies and A. Paton (1981), 'A 20-year prospective study of cirrhosis', *British Medical Journal*, **282**, 263–6.

Savage, L.J. (1954), The *Foundations of Statistics*, New York: John Wiley & Sons.

Savage, L. (1972), *The Foundations of Statistics* (2nd edn), New York: Dover.

Schrek, R., L.A. Baker, G.P. Ballard and S. Dolgoff (1950), 'Tobacco smoking as an etiologic actor in disease', *Cancer Research*, **10**, 49–58.

Sloan, F.A., V.K. Smith and D.H. Taylor (2003), *The Smoking Puzzle: Information, Risk Perception, and Choice*, Cambridge, MA: Harvard University Press.

Slovic, P. (1987), 'Perception of risk', *Science*, **236**(4799), 280–85.

Slovic, P. (1998), 'Do adolescent smokers know the risks?', *Duke Law Journal*, **47**, 1133–41.

Slovic, P. (2001), *Smoking: Risk Perception and Policy*, Thousand Oaks, CA: Sage.

Slovic, P., B. Fischhoff and S. Lichtenstein (1982), 'Why study risk perception?', *Risk Analysis*, **2**(2), 83–93.

Slovic, P., M.L. Finucane, E. Peters and D.G. MacGregor (2002), 'The affect heuristic', in T. Gilovich, D. Griffin and D. Kahneman (eds), *Heuristics and Biases: The Psychology of Intuitive Judgment*, New York: Cambridge University Press, pp. 397–420.

Slovic, P., M. Finucane, E. Peters and D.G. MacGregor (2004), 'Risk as analysis and risk as feelings: some thoughts about affect, reason, risk and rationality', *Risk Analysis*, **24**(2), 311–22.

Tversky, A. and D. Kahneman (1974), 'Judgment under uncertainty: heuristics and biases', *Science*, **1985**, 1124–31.

Tversky, A. and D. Kahneman (1981), 'The framing of decisions and the psychology of choice', *Science*, **211**(4481), 453–8.

Tversky, A. and D. Kahneman (1987), 'Rational choice and the framing of decisions', in R. Hogarth and M. Reder (eds), *Rational Choice: The Contrast between Economics and Psychology*, Chicago, IL: University of Chicago Press, pp. 67–84.

Tversky, A. and D. Kahneman (1992), 'Advances in prospect theory: cumulative representation of uncertainty', *Journal of Risk and Uncertainty*, **5**, 297–323.

Viscusi, W.K. (1985), 'A Bayesian perspective on biases in risk perception', *Economic Letters*, **17**, 59–62.

Viscusi, W.K. (1989), 'Prospective reference theory: toward an explanation of the paradoxes', *Journal of Risk and Uncertainty*, **2**(3), 235–64.

Viscusi, W.K. (1990), 'Do smokers underestimate risks?', *Journal of Political Economy*, **98**(6), 1253–69.

Viscusi, W.K. (1991), 'Age variations in risk perceptions and smoking decisions', *The Review of Economics and Statistics*, **73**(4), 577–88.

Viscusi, W.K. (1992a), *Fatal Tradeoffs: Public and Private Responsibilities for Risk*, New York: Oxford University Press.

Viscusi, W.K. (1992b), *Smoking: Making the Risky Decision*, Oxford: Oxford University Press.

Viscusi, W.K. (1997), 'Alarmist decisions with divergent risk information', *The Economic Journal*, **107**, 1657–70.

Viscusi, W.K. and W.N. Evans (2006), 'Behavioral probabilities', *Journal of Risk and Uncertainty*, **32**, 5–15.

Von Neumann, J. and O. Morgenstern (1944), *Theory of Games and Economic Behavior*, Princeton, NJ: Princeton University Press.

Washer, P. (2004), 'Representations of SARS in the UK newspapers', *Social Science & Medicine*, **59**(12), 2561–71.

Wynder, E.L. and E.A. Graham (1950), 'Tobacco smoking as a possible etiologic factor in bronchogenic carcinoma', *Journal of the American Medical Association*, **143**, 329–36.

Yaari, M.E. (1987), 'The dual theory of choice under risk', *Econometrica*, **55**, 95–115.

18 The doctor–patient relationship: a review of the theory and policy implications
Charitini Stavropoulou

1. INTRODUCTION

The doctor–patient relationship remains the cornerstone of medical practice. At the same time it is one of the most complex interactions in health care, which goes beyond consultation and clinical practice and involves aspects that are developed outside the encounter. On the one side of this relationship stands the doctor, whose diagnosing skills, prescribing patterns and referral decisions determine not only health outcomes but also, and to a great extent, health care costs. On the other side stands the patient, who is increasingly empowered to make decisions that concern his health. In many cases he chooses among a number of physicians, he collects information from sources other than the doctor and finally decides whether to adhere to the medical recommendations. These are all decisions that affect his health but also health care utilisation and expenditure.

Health economists and policy makers realise the importance of this relationship on health systems and put great effort into exploring its underlying mechanisms. A number of models have been proposed to understand the elements of the physician's utility function (McGuire, 2000; Scott, 2000), and different payment schemes have been designed in an effort to change physicians' behaviour. The patient's side has received less attention. In health economics the agency relationship that is often used to describe the doctor–patient interaction implies that the doctor acts on the patient's behalf and therefore the majority of the decisions are taken mainly by the former and fewer by the latter.

In recent decades, two trends have challenged this state and call for more attention to be given to the patient's side. The first one is the increasing empowerment of the patient's role in decision making (Kaba and Sooriakumaran, 2007). Patients may require more information during the consultation and are more actively involved in the choice of treatment. Patients have also increased power in choosing the general practitioner or specialist who treats them, with significant consequences for competition, health utilisation and costs.

The second trend is the increasingly high prevalence of chronic illnesses, which has implications in terms of both prevention but also managed care. The majority of these conditions, including cardiovascular diseases, cancer and diabetes, are mostly related to lifestyle choices. In both managing these conditions and ensuring that the patient adheres to the medical recommendations and follows a healthier lifestyle the doctor has a very important role to play.

Understanding the importance of the patient's role in a medical decision is crucial for health economists and policy makers. In that respect health economics may benefit greatly from behavioural sciences, including medical sociology and psychology, which offer elements enabling a better understanding of this interaction.

This chapter reviews the literature on the theory of the doctor–patient relationship, considers the recent research trends and discusses the implications this interaction has for health policy and economics.

The rest of the chapter is organised as follows. Section 2 reviews the theoretical models of the doctor–patient interaction. It begins by exploring the literature of health economics and then reviews models from medical sociology. New insights offered by other fields, such as psychology, are discussed in Section 3. Section 4 explores the implications that various aspects of this relationship have on health policy, while Section 5 summarises and concludes.

2.   REVIEW OF THEORETICAL MODELS OF THE DOCTOR–PATIENT RELATIONSHIP

2.1   Health Economics: An Agency Relationship

In health economics the doctor–patient relationship is often perceived as an agency one. The principal–agent model stresses the information asymmetry between the physician and the patient introduced by Arrow (1963). It states that the doctor acts like an agent maximising the patient's, i.e. the principal's, utility. The doctor holds more information about the patient's health status and the available treatments. The patient has superior knowledge about how these treatments fit with his or her lifestyle and has specific beliefs about medication and illness. The patient communicates these preferences to the doctor, who then acts as an agent for the patient.

In the perfect-agency model, a specific case of the principal–agent theory, the doctor maximises the patient's utility as if it were his own. This model has been extensively used in health economics because of both its conceptual simplicity and the lack of any agreed alternative. Yet this model is not without limitations and criticisms. Empirical evidence has extensively shown that the doctor and the patient bring to the consultation different agendas and that the doctor is very often unable to understand patient needs (Britten et al., 2000). When these needs are not met, the outcomes of the consultation are unsatisfactory and patients may not adhere to the doctor's recommendations. It also seems unrealistic for the perfect-agency model to work in practice as the doctor, apart from the patient's needs, has other constraints that need to be taken into consideration, such as administrative constraints, time issues and personal benefits and costs.

Departing from the perfect-agency model, there is an extensive literature on how physicians can act beyond maximising the patient's utility function only. The doctor wants to improve the patient's health but still has other aspects that he needs to consider. Scott (2000) reviews the model of general practitioners' (GP) behaviour and notes that there is no single common utility function used, but different studies use different arguments in the doctor's utility. The income–leisure framework is common to many models, while workload is another element. The altruistic element is also often found in the models mentioned in the review (Scott, 2000). Some models incorporate this by including patient's utility or welfare in the GP's utility function, while others include patient's economic well-being and the interests of society as arguments in his utility (Blomqvist, 1991).

To put it in other words, economic models allow doctors' behaviour to be driven not only by altruistic elements but also by other aspects such as workload, income, reputation and other non-altruistic factors. Le Grand (2006) describes these two different aspects of doctor behaviour as 'knightly' and 'knavish', and argues that it is perfectly possible that an individual has altruistic motivations for some of his activities and self-interested ones for others. In addition, he has argued that it is not only financial considerations, such as income, that drive self-interested behaviour. Doctors want not only to improve their economic status but also maintain a certain lifestyle, have respectful working relationships with their colleagues and the ability to make clinical decisions without too much interference. That said, a doctor's inability to be entirely empathetic to the patient is not only driven by individualistic elements but also by organisational constraints, such as time pressure and long lists.

The review by McGuire (2000) of the theory and empirical research on physicians' motivation presents three ways a physician can influence the quantity of medical care the patient can buy: non-retradability, which allows quantity setting; choice of non-contractible input; and supply-induced demand. In the first model, doctors influence the quantity of medical care, based on the feature of non-retradability that underlies it. The model assumes complete information about the benefits of medical care; that is, there is no asymmetric information between the two parties. It implies that profit-maximising physicians do not allow patients to choose the utility-maximising quantity given the price the patient pays.

Apart from the quantity, doctors can also influence the quality of care, or effort. This is a key input into health, which, even though observed by patients, may be impossible to verify. This is the second mechanism of physician behaviour as suggested by McGuire (2000). By influencing the quality of care, doctors can control patient demand. The input is observable by the patient; it affects his choice of medical treatment but cannot be influenced by a payer.

Both these mechanisms are based on the assumption of complete information. Yet information asymmetry is a key element of the medical practice that influences their interaction (Arrow, 1963). When patients believe doctors have superior knowledge to them, doctors may be able to persuade patients to demand more or less care. This third mechanism for quantity determination proposed by McGuire (2000) captures the meaning of 'physician-induced demand', as used in the literature. The notion of physician-induced demand has been used widely in the doctor–patient literature and it has been used to explain why doctors lead the patient to consume more than if they had perfect information (Evans, 1974). The model focuses on the supply side of medical care and explains how doctors make patients consume more or less than if they had perfect information about their treatment.

2.2   Medical Sociology: Theory and Empirical Evidence

In medical sociology three main theoretical models have been developed to describe the doctor–patient relationship with regard to decision making. These are paternalism, shared decision making and the informed decision-making model (Charles et al., 1999).

Paternalism

This is the traditional model of the doctor–patient relationship, in which the doctor, as the expert, diagnoses the patient and decides on the appropriate treatment. In this model the patient has a passive role and no active involvement in the decision-making process. Coulter (2002) avoids the term 'paternalistic' and calls this model 'professional choice', arguing that it may be appropriate under some circumstances for the doctor to make decisions without the patient being actively involved. This passive role of the patient in paternalism makes the model similar to that of perfect agency in health economics.

Shared decision model

This model was developed by Charles et al. (1997), who argue that there should be four specific characteristics for shared decision making to be effective:

1. Both the physician and the patient are, to some extent, involved in the treatment decision-making process.
2. Both parties share information.
3. Both take steps to participate in the decision-making process by expressing treatment preferences.
4. A treatment decision is made and both the physician and the patient agree on the treatment to be adopted.

In this framework, both the patient and the doctor are active members in the decision-making process. Evidence on whether this works in practice has not favoured the model. A study by Stevenson et al. (2000) of 62 consultations in the UK, along with interviews with patients and GPs, revealed that there is little evidence that patients and doctors both participate in the consultation in the way described in the model. The study concluded that even the first two of the four components that are necessary for shared decision making to be upheld, that is, for both parties to be involved and exchange information, were not present in the consultations studied.

Informed decision-making model

The informed decision-making model is often presented together with the shared decision model (Britten, 2004), as both indicate a reaction to the model of paternalism. However, Charles et al. (1999) argue that the two models have essential differences that are mainly concerned with the information exchange. In the shared decision model the flow of information is two-sided as both the patient and the doctor exchange information, the latter mainly on the medical level and the former more on the personal level, such as experience and preferences.

In the informed decision-making model the information is mainly one-sided, with the doctor supplying the information to the patient, regarding medical aspects. Also, in the shared decision model the final decision is a common agreement between the two parties, while in the informed model it is the patient who decides.

Towards a holistic theoretical framework

The models of doctor–patient interaction described above focus on a specific aspect of this relationship, that is the decision-making process. This is without doubt very important, especially with regard to understanding non-adherence, and it also helps to narrow down the complexity of the issue. However, it does not offer a holistic perspective of the relationship and therefore it is not sufficient to understand the problem as a whole.

In a review of the literature of the doctor–patient relationship, Ong et al. (1995) proposed a theoretical framework that relates background, process and outcome variables and allows for clear hypotheses regarding these relations. The suggested theoretical framework relates background variables, such as cultural characteristics, to the actual communication during the consultation, to both short-term patient outcomes such as satisfaction, and long-term outcomes such as health status and psychiatric morbidity.

Regardless of the flaws in the framework by Ong et al. (1995), it does provide a systematic and holistic perspective to the doctor–patient relationship and facilitates the understanding of how this relationship affects the patient's decision to adhere to recommendations.

3.   NEW DIRECTIONS FROM PSYCHOLOGY AND ECONOMICS

The argument that physicians' behaviour cannot be explained purely on rational grounds is not new. Arrow (1963) discusses the importance of trust in the doctor–patient relationship. Indeed, a number of emotions that evolve during the consultation have been acknowledged by health economists but have been ignored in their theoretical models of the relationship. In addition, empirical evidence shows that, contrary to what the neoclassical approach would predict, physicians do not always maximise income (Newhouse, 1970; Fuchs, 1978). Significant progress in explaining some of these empirical puzzles has been made by the lately increasing field of behavioural economics. This field, which combines economics and psychology, has resulted in models that offer useful insights into the mechanisms that explain the doctor–patient interaction.

Indeed, Frank (2007) argues there is no area in health economics that 'relies on a vocabulary that is more closely linked to the work of behavioural economics than research on physician behaviour' (Frank, 2007, p. 197). In this section we take Frank's argument one step further. We advocate that behavioural economics is a promising field that allows a better understanding of the mechanisms that underlie not only the doctor's but also the patient's decisions and ultimately will provide a better exploration of the doctor–patient interaction. The rest of this section presents a number of areas where psychology has offered a better insight into the doctor–patient interaction.

3.1   Emotional Agents

An attempt to explore some of the dynamics of the doctor–patient relationship is based on the psychological expected utility theory (henceforth PEU theory) introduced by Caplin and Leahy (2001). The theory is an extension of the expected utility theory of von Neumann–Morgenstern to situations in which agents experience feelings of anticipation regarding future states. It allows for the individual's utility function to depend not only on physical outcomes but also on beliefs about future physical outcomes.

The PEU theory has been used to explain how anxiety may lead patients to avoid visiting the doctor (Köszegi, 2003). Köszegi (2004) has also proposed a model describing the doctor–patient relationship where the doctor makes choices of actions taking into consideration the patient's emotions. The model identifies a number of complications in the doctor–patient interaction that are attributed to anxiety, such as the paradox of emotional patients getting less useful information, which is the opposite of what the neo-classical approach would predict.

Caplin and Leahy (2004) have also applied the PEU theory in a model describing doctor–patient interaction but in a way different to the one presented by Köszegi. They explore the optimal procedure for supplying information to a patient who experiences anticipatory emotions regarding a future health status, after he has sent a signal regarding his emotional status. Finally, in previous work we have shown, using the PEU theory, that different information preferences individuals have may explain why patients do not adhere to the recommendation when the doctor fails to pass on the right information (Stavropoulou and Glycopantis, 2009).

3.2   Heuristic Norms

The complexity of medical decisions has led researchers to propose models of physician behaviour that are based on heuristic norms. Frank and Zeckhauser (2007) argue that physicians do not always tailor their therapeutic treatment to the patients' specific needs but instead they often use 'ready-to-wear' treatments, that is, norms that apply to broad classes of patients. That means they often fail to optimise on a patient-by-patient basis. In some cases, when the associated costs of customised treatment are high, it may be sensible for physicians to use norms. These are described as four types of costs, that is, communication, cognition, coordination and capability costs.

The empirical evidence of the Frank and Zeckhauser study partly supports this argument, that is, that norms may be a sensible response to a complex decision-making environment, confirming previous studies by Chandra and Staiger (2007) and Sommers et al. (2007). However, the results also show that ready-to-wear treatment may also be based on idiosyncratic individual behaviour of the physicians or severe biases in the application of heuristics. This type of bias in ready-to-wear treatment has been supported by previous studies in depression and primary care (Tai-Seale et al., 2007) and can lead to highly suboptimal therapeutic treatments.

3.3   Alternatives to Profit Maximisation

Physicians' behaviour has been a great puzzle for health economists, and a number of studies have been conducted to understand its underlying mechanisms. Empirical evidence has shown a clear departure from the competitive model. Indeed, econometric studies by Feldstein (1970), Newhouse (1970) and Fuchs and Kramer (1972) observe a positive partial correlation between the number of physicians in the market and physician prices. As it turns out that neither the competitive model nor a monopolistic one have been supported by empirical evidence, a number of alternative explanations have been explored. Feldstein (1970) argues that markets experience persistent excess demand, Simon's (1958) satisficing model has also been explored, while the theory of target income has been proposed as a possible alternative to the competitive model. However, these models have also been criticised. Therefore there is no commonly acceptable, behavioural model alternative to that of profit maximisation (McGuire, 2000). This is because of the number of economic but also social and psychological dimensions of the issues considered, which make it difficult for one model to incorporate all aspects.

4.   DOCTOR–PATIENT RELATIONSHIP AND POLICY IMPLICATIONS

Having presented the modelling of the doctor–patient relationship, we consider in this section its policy implications, focusing on three aspects. First, we consider the impact physicians' incentives have on the actual doctor–patient relationship. Second, we discuss the importance of the doctor–patient relationship on satisfaction with health services and choice of physician. Finally, we discuss how this relationship affects the patient's decision, in particular non-adherence to recommendations.

4.1   Physician's Incentives and the Doctor–Patient Relationship

Incentives given to doctors may include financial rewards, payment on the basis of increasing quality of care or even a combination of the two. A number of studies have been conducted to examine the impact of incentives on physicians' behaviour and consequently on health outcomes, cost containment and control of expenditure. These implications have received considerable attention from health economists and are extensively and systematically reviewed in other chapters of this volume. In this section, we review in particular the impact these schemes have on the doctor–patient relationship.

A study by Chaix-Couturier et al. (2000) reviewing the related literature shows that financial incentives clearly affect doctors' behaviour in many ways; they may help reduce the use of health care resources, improve compliance with guidelines and achieve health targets. On the other hand, they may have a negative impact on the doctor–patient relationship because, as the authors argue, motivating doctors with financial rewards increases the conflict of interests between the doctors and the patients, putting their relationship in danger. The authors therefore suggest that they may be better used in combination with other incentives in order to be more effective.

The UK system has provided a fruitful environment for discussing incentives and physicians' behaviour through a number of different schemes that have been implemented in the last two decades. Between 1991 and 1998, GPs in the UK were given the option to hold budgets for prescribing and elective secondary care. Budgets were calculated on the basis of the services consumed by patients before the practice had become a fundholder. Practices participating in the scheme were given the autonomy to retain any surplus that they could then use on additional services to patients or to improve facilities in their practices. The scheme generated incentives to the physicians to reduce unnecessary expenditure and benefit from the surplus that they could allocate as they wished.

Indeed, there is evidence that practices participating in this scheme reduced pharmaceutical cost (Goodwin, 1998), managed to reduce readmissions relatively to the non-fundholders (Dusheiko et al., 2006) and reduced waiting times for their patients

(Propper et al., 2002). Yet administrative and time costs associated with the scheme generated concerns that GPs might divert from patient care, and evidence on this issue has been mixed (Howie et al., 1995; Corney, 1999). A study by Dusheiko et al. (2007) showed that patients in fundholding practices were overall less satisfied than those in non-fundholding ones. In particular, they expressed dissatisfaction with opening hours, GPs' knowledge of their medical history, referrals to specialists and GPs' concern to keep costs down. However, there was no effect on self-reported health outcomes.

The findings also provide some evidence on the strength of the doctor–patient agency relationship. It was possible for GPs to benefit financially from fundholding. GPs who place high weight on the welfare of patients relative to their own will only opt to hold a budget if their patients are thereby made better off. Thus the finding that patients in fundholding practices were less satisfied than those in non-fundholding practices suggests that the agency relationship is weak.

Another major experiment of incentives and physicians' behaviour in the UK is the implementation of the Quality and Outcomes Framework (QOF). The scheme was implemented in April 2004 as part of the new contracts for primary care services in the UK. It is an annual programme that awards achievement points for clinical and organisational indicators as well as patient experience and additional services (such as contraceptive services and child health). Its aim is to incentivise the delivery of quality care (Department of Health, 2004). It was anticipated that the scheme would improve health outcomes of the conditions under the scheme, but on the other hand it generated fears that quality of care for conditions not included would be reduced (Roland, 2004).

A recent study by Campbell et al. (2007) yields some interesting results, using data from primary care in the UK before and after the implementation of the QOF. The study found no strong evidence of the impact of the programme on clinical indicators.

Further evidence shows that the vast majority of the GPs achieved markedly higher quality than was required to maximise their financial rewards, suggesting that they were partially altruistic (Gravelle et al., 2008). Similarly, they also showed that quality delivered to patients was higher in larger practices and in practices with less deprived populations and with a smaller ethnic minority population. This increases considerations for issues of equity in health care.

4.2 Doctor–Patient Relationship, Satisfaction with Consultation and Choice of Provider

The quality of the doctor–patient relationship affects to a great degree the overall satisfaction with the consultation and the experience patients have with the health care system. Indeed, a review of 139 studies provided consistent evidence across different settings that this relationship is the most important factor affecting general satisfaction with health care (Crow et al., 2002). This has significant policy implications, especially with respect to choice of physicians, an issue that is considered widely in many countries, including the UK.

Exploring in more depth the heart of the consultation, a study using data from the English National Health Service (NHS) showed that confidence and trust in the doctor are the two most important factors in explaining the variation in overall patient satisfaction, over and above any other aspects of the GP experience, such as waiting times (Robertson et al., 2008). The authors argue that this may also have implications if the system of choice is extended in England at the GP level in the UK. They suggest that choice would be expected to be driven by the quality of the doctor–patient relationship. In the long term, however, the authors argue that once a good relationship is established, it will then be unlikely for the patient to change practice.

4.3   Doctor–Patient Relationship and Adherence to Recommendations

Adherence to medical recommendations has received an increasing amount of attention recently. Initially, it was perceived as the patient's obedience to the doctor's medical decision, and the term 'compliance' was mainly used (Haynes et al., 1979). In that respect, the paternalistic model presented above was related to the concept of compliance. Determinants of non-compliance were considered to be sociodemographic factors, such as older age and low education.

However, research in the area has evolved and evidence suggests an approach to the issue that attributes less blame to the patient. This change has also been reflected in the term used, where 'adherence' has been preferred by most researchers and policy makers. In that sense, the informed model is closer to the concept of adherence as it gives an active role to the patient, who, being well informed by the doctor, can decide whether to follow the recommendations or not.

The evidence suggests that various factors affect a patient's perception of the doctor–patient relationship and consequently adherence. Farber et al. (2003) conducted telephone interviews with parents of asthmatic children in the Medicaid programme in the USA and reported that misunderstanding of medication was associated with reduced adherence. The risk of misunderstanding was lower if the patient had seen a specialist. Berman et al. (1997) showed that the physician's gender as well as his/her specialty was associated with non-adherence. Confidence in the physician and the health care system as a whole led to better adherence in the study by Kjellgren et al. (1998) in Sweden. Physicians' follow-up communication style and client satisfaction were both predictors of better adherence in the USA (Bultman and Svarstad, 2000).

In a study of 24 countries participating in the European Social Survey, general perceptions that people have about their doctor affected their decision to follow prescribed medication (Stavropoulou, 2011). Individuals' decision to adhere to recommendations depended significantly on whether they felt they were involved in the decision-making process and they were treated as equals by their doctors.

In a qualitative study by Barry et al. (2000) in England, doctors and patients were interviewed to examine their level of communication during consultation. Indeed, it was shown that most of the patients' desires were not met during the consultation and this led to poor adherence. Analysis of the same qualitative study by Berman et al. (1997) showed that misunderstandings between patients and doctors have potential or actual adverse consequences, leading to non-adherence.

Jenkins et al. (2003) interviewed both patients and GPs to correlate their expectations and potential non-adherence. They found that patients had high expectations for communication and participation in the consultation, and that unnecessary prescribing and problems in communication may lead to poor outcomes in terms of non-adherence.

To sum up, the empirical evidence is vast; it is increasing and it clearly shows the importance of the doctor–patient relationship for patients' decision to adhere to the medical recommendations.

5. DISCUSSION

This chapter has reviewed the theories of the doctor–patient relationship and considered some of their policy implications. It identified four main theoretical models. From the field of health economics the relationship is perceived as an agency one, while the medical sociology literature identifies three models: paternalism, shared decision and informed decision model. All models are in agreement in one regard: the complex and multifaceted nature of the doctor–patient relationship. The models acknowledge that there is no single, commonly accepted theory that captures all aspects of this relationship, and all are attempting to understand some of its components.

The review of the health economic literature reveals that there has been a great effort in understanding the physician's behaviour and how he responds to different types of incentives. A number of models have been proposed, and numerous empirical studies have been conducted. The same effort has not been put into exploring the impact on the patient's side. The realisation that the patient is an empowered individual who is allowed to choose the physician he wants, can reject his advice and may make lifestyle choices that lead to reduced health outcomes and increased costs, will force health economists to place more attention on the patient characteristics and understand the drivers of their decisions.

In the future, we believe that there will be a research tendency to explore in more depth the patient's role in the decision-making model. We also anticipate the need for a more interdisciplinary approach to the doctor–patient relationship as it is more commonly accepted that the decisions of the two parties cannot be explained purely on rational grounds. In that respect, literature from medical sociology and psychology is useful, as it provides a more holistic picture of the relationship and gives a significant importance to the patient's role. The potential of combining economics with psychology, despite its great potential in health economics and policy, remains largely unexplored. In this chapter we have reviewed areas of the doctor–patient relationship where psychology has enriched economic concepts to better explain behaviours of the two parties. We argue that there is still great potential in this field to explain some of the empirical puzzles to which the neoclassical approaches have offered a limited solution.

The impact of the above discussion on policy is also important. Policy schemes have been implemented as a way of changing physicians' behaviour, forcing them to better use available resources. A number of interesting cases are presented in the UK. The majority of the evidence has shown that indeed physicians respond to incentives given by different schemes. The impact on costs and savings is more tangible and obvious. What is less clear is the impact of these incentives on the doctor–patient relationship and patients' behaviour. There is evidence suggesting that financial schemes may jeopardise the relationship between the two parties as the physician may put emphasis on financial considerations and overlook personal aspects. In the light of new policies, such as the recent NHS reform that empowers GPs with commissioning roles (Department of Health, 2010), it is extremely important to understand how incentives affect not only the physician's behaviour but also the patient's decisions.

Indeed, there is plenty of evidence to suggest that the doctor–patient relationship affects patients' decisions to follow recommendations. It clearly suggests that any intervention aiming at improving patients' adherence needs to be developed on the basis of a strong doctor–patient relationship. Involvement in the decision-making process, provision of adequate information and generally meeting patients' needs have been shown to be effective ways to a better doctor–patient relationship and to lead to improvement of adherence.

To conclude, we call for a more holistic approach to the issue of the doctor–patient relationship, as it seems that one side, the doctor, has been explored more than the other, the patient. Yet policy makers and health economists understand that patients are now more empowered and take important decisions as to which doctor to choose or whether to follow his/her recommendations. Individuals' lifestyle options have been shown to be a great determinant of chronic conditions, which consequently influence health outcomes and increase health care costs. The role of the doctor in influencing patients' decision is vital.

REFERENCES

Arrow, K. (1963), 'Uncertainty and the welfare economics of medical care', *American Economic Review*, **53**(5), 941–73.

Barry, C.A., C.P. Bradley, N. Britten, F. Stevenson and N. Barber (2000), 'Patients' unvoiced agendas in general practice consultations: qualitative study', *British Medical Journal*, **320**(7244), 1246–50.

Berman, R.S., R.S. Epstein and E. Lydick (1997), 'Risk factors associated with women's compliance with estrogen replacement therapy', *Journal of Women's Health*, **6**(2), 219–26.

Blomqvist, A. (1991), 'The utilisation of health services. Sequences of visits to general practitioners', *Social Science and Medicine*, **16**, 2065–72.

Britten, Nicky (2004), 'What is concordance?', in Christine Bond (ed.), *Concordance: A Partnership in Medicine-taking*, London, Pharmaceutical Press, pp. 9–28.

Britten, N., F.A. Stevenson, C.A. Barry, N. Barber and C.P. Bradley (2000), 'Misunderstandings in prescribing decisions in general practice: qualitative study', *British Medical Journal*, **320**(7233), 484–8.

Bultman, D.C. and B.L. Svarstad (2000), 'Effects of physician communication style on client medication beliefs and adherence with antidepressant treatment', *Patient Education and Counselling*, **40**(2), 173–85.

Campbell, S., D. Reeves, E. Kontopantelis, E. Middleton, B. Sibbald and M. Roland (2007), 'Quality of primary care in England with the introduction of pay for performance', *The New England Journal of Medicine*, **357**(2), 181–90.

Caplin, A. and J. Leahy (2001), 'The psychological expected utility theory and anticipatory feelings', *The Quarterly Journal of Economics*, **116**, 55–79.

Caplin, A. and J. Leahy (2004), 'The supply of information by a concerned expert', *The Economic Journal*, **114**, 487–505.

Chaix-Couturier, C., I. Durand-Zaleski, D. Jolly and P. Durieux (2000), 'Effects of financial incentives on medical practice: results from a systematic review of the literature and methodological issues', *International Journal for Quality in Health Care*, **12**, 133–42.

Chandra, A. and D.O. Staiger (2007), 'Productivity spillovers in health care: evidence from treatments of heart attacks', *Journal of Political Economy*, **115**(1), 103–40.

Charles, C., A. Gafni and T. Whelan (1997), 'Shared decision-making in the medical encounter: what does it mean? (or it takes at least two to tango)', *Social Science and Medicine*, **44**, 681–92.

Charles, C., A. Gafni and T. Whelan (1999), 'Decision making in the physician–patient encounter: revisiting the shared treatment decision-making model', *Social Science and Medicine*, **49**, 651–61.

Corney, R.H. (1999), 'Changes in patient satisfaction and experience in primary and secondary care: the effect of general practice fundholding', *British Journal of General Practice*, **49**, 27–30.

Coulter, Angela (2002), *The Autonomous Patient: Ending Paternalism in Medical Care*, London, UK: Stationery Office (for the Nuffield Trust).

Crow, R., H. Gage, S. Hampson, J. Hart, L. Storey and H. Thomas (2002), 'The measurement of satisfaction with healthcare: implications for practice from a systematic review of the literature', *Health Technology Assessment*, **6**(32), 1–244.

Department of Health (2004), *QOF Guidance*, London: HMSO.

Department of Health (2010), *Equity and Excellence: Liberating the NHS*, Cmd 7881.

Dusheiko, M., H. Gravelle, R. Jacobs and P.C. Smith (2006), 'The effect of financial incentives on gatekeeping doctors: evidence from a natural experiment', *Journal of Health Economics*, **25**, 449–78.

Dusheiko, M., H. Gravelle, N. Yu and S. Campbell (2007), 'The effect of budgets for gatekeeping physicians on patient satisfaction: evidence from fundholding', *Journal of Health Economics*, **26**(4), 242–62.

Evans, Robert G. (1974), 'Supplier-induced demand: some empirical evidence and implications', in Mark Perlman (ed.), *The Economics of Health and Medical Care*, New York: John Wiley & Sons, pp. 162–73.

Farber, H.J., A.M. Capra, J.A. Finkelstein, P. Lozano, C.P. Quesenberry, N.G. Jensvold, F.W. Chi and T.A. Lieu (2003), 'Misunderstanding of asthma controller medications: association with nonadherence', *Journal of Asthma*, **40**(1), 17–25.

Feldstein, M.S. (1970), 'The rising price of physicians' services', *Review of Economics and Statistics*, **51**, 121–33.

Frank, Richard G. (2007), 'Behavioural economics and health economics', in Peter Diamond and Hannu Vartiainen (eds), *Behavioural Economics and its Applications*, Princeton, NJ: Princeton University Press, pp. 195–234.

Frank, R.G. and R. Zeckhauser (2007), 'Custom-made versus ready-to-wear treatments: behavioral propensities in physicians' choices', *Journal of Health Economics*, **26**(6), 1101–27.

Fuchs, V.R. (1978), 'The supply of surgeons and the demand for operations', *Journal of Human Resources*, **13**, 35–55.

Fuchs, Victor R. and Marcia J. Kramer (1972), *Determinants of Expenditure for Physician Services in the United States*, Washington, DC: National Center for Health Services Research.

Goodwin, Nick (1998), 'GP fundholding', in Julian Le Grand, Nick Mays and Jo-Ann Mulligan (eds), *Learning from the NHS Internal Market: A Review of the Evidence*, London: King's Fund Publishing, pp. 43–68.

Gravelle, H., M. Sutton and A. Ma (2008), 'Doctor behaviour under a pay for performance contract: further evidence from the quality and outcomes framework', Centre for Health Economics, University of York CHE Research Paper 34.

Haynes, Brian R., Wayne D. Taylor and David L. Sackett (eds) (1979), *Compliance in Health Care*, Baltimore, MD: Johns Hopkins University Press.

Howie, J.G.R., D.J. Heaney and M. Maxwell (1995), 'Care of patients with selected health problems in fundholding practices in Scotland in 1990 and 1992: needs, process and outcome', *British Journal of General Practice*, **45**, 121–6.

Jenkins, L., N. Britten, F. Stevenson, N. Barber and C. Bradley (2003), 'Developing and using quantitative instruments for measuring doctor–patient communication about drugs', *Patient Education and Counselling*, **50**(3), 273–8.

Kaba, R. and P. Sooriakumaran (2007), 'The evolution of the doctor–patient relationship', *International Journal of Surgery*, **5**(1), 57–65.

Kjellgren, K.I., S. Svensson, J. Ahlner and R. Säljo (1998), 'Antihypertensive medication in clinical encounters', *International Journal of Cardiology*, **64**(2), 161–9.

Köszegi, B. (2003), 'Health anxiety and patient behavior', *Journal of Health Economics*, **22**, 1073–84.

Köszegi, B. (2004), 'Emotional agency: the case of the doctor–patient relationship', mimeo, University of Berkeley, CA.

Le Grand, Julian (2006), *Motivation, Agency and Public Policy: Of Knights and Knaves, Pawns and Queens*, Oxford: Oxford University Press.

McGuire, Thomas G. (2000), 'Physician agency', in Anthony J. Culyer and Joseph P. Newhouse (eds), *Handbook of Health Economics*, Amsterdam: Elsevier Science, pp. 461–536.

Newhouse, J.P. (1970), 'A model for physician pricing', *Southern Economic Journal*, **37**, 174–83.

Ong, L.M., J.C. de Haes, A.M. Hoos and F.B. Lammes (1995), 'Doctor–patient communication: a review of the literature', *Social Science and Medicine*, **40**(7), 903–18.

Propper, C., B. Croxson and A. Shearer (2002), 'Waiting times for hospital admissions: the impact of GP fundholding', *Journal of Health Economics*, **21**, 227–52.

Robertson, R., A. Dixon and J. Le Grand (2008), 'Patient choice in general practice: the implications of patient satisfaction surveys', *Journal of Health Services Research and Policy*, **13**(2), 67–72.

Roland, M. (2004), 'Linking physicians' pay to the quality of care–a major experiment in the United Kingdom', *New English Journal of Medicine*, **351**(14), 1448–54.

Scott, Anthony (2000), 'Economics of general practice', in Anthony J. Culyer and Joseph P. Newhouse (eds), *Handbook of Health Economics*, Amsterdam: Elsevier Science, pp. 1175–200.

Simon, M. (1958), 'Theories of decision making in economics and behaviour science', *American Economic Review*, **49**, 253–83.

Sommers, B.D., C.J. Beard, A.V. D'Amico, D. Dahl, I. Kaplan, J.P. Richie and R.J. Zeckhauser (2007), 'Decision analysis using individual patient preferences to determine optimal treatment for localized prostate cancer', *Cancer*, **110**(10), 2210–17.

Stavropoulou, C. (2011), 'Non-adherence and doctor–patient relationship: evidence from a European survey', *Patient Education and Counselling*, **83**(1), 7–13.

Stavropoulou, C. and D. Glycopantis (2009), 'The doctor–patient relationship under general conditions of uncertainty', Imperial Business School Discussion Paper Series, Discussion Paper No. 2009/06.

Stevenson, F.A., C.A. Barry, N. Britten, N. Barber and C.P. Bradley (2000), 'Doctor–patient communication about drugs: the evidence for shared decision making', *Social Science and Medicine*, **50**(6), 829–40.

Tai-Seale, M., T.G. McGuire and W. Zhang (2007), 'Time allocation in primary care office visits', *Health Services Research*, **42**(5), 1871–94.

Index

absolute-income hypothesis 5, 15
access to health care xi–xii
    ACSH rates as measure of 55–8, 60
    factors affecting 113–14
    generic, in USA 209
    potential policy action 14
    and social services 233, 240, 242–3, 252
    and socioeconomic status 35–46
    unmet need/forgone care 115–23
ACCORD scheme 169
acute ACSCs 54
acute care
    costs and proximity to death 221–5, 227–8
    NHS responsibility for 234–5
acute myocardial infarction (AMI) studies
    89–90, 141
Adams Dudley, R. 148, 149, 150, 152
Aday, L. 113, 114
administrative barriers 233–4, 246, 249–50
adverse selection 151, 152, 167, 262–3
affect heuristics 300–301
ageing population 136–7, 221–2, 225, 229, 263
Agency for Healthcare Research and Quality
    (AHRQ) 53, 55
Allais, M. 298, 299
Allin, S. 114, 120
Alma-Ata Declaration 20, 21–2, 31–2
Alvarez-Rosete, A. 104, 106
Alzheimer's disease 289–92
ambulatory care xii
    definition 50–51
    measuring quality of 51–3
ambulatory care sensitive conditions (ACSCs)
    conceptual framework for 57
    definitions 53
    factors associated with 56–60
    hospitalisations for 53–5
    summary of studies 64–75
    use by policy makers 60–61
Andersen, R.M. 36–7, 44, 56, 57, 113, 114, 130
Andersson, H. 303, 309, 310
Ansari, Z. 53, 54, 55, 56, 60, 68–9
Appleby, J. 97, 99, 101, 104, 106, 108
Armour, B.S. 147, 154
Arrow, K.J. 85, 107, 315, 316, 318
Association of British Insurers 259, 261
Atkinson, A. 13, 113
Audit Commission 237, 245

autonomy and choice 81–2
avoidable mortality 54
avoided waiting value 107–8

Baker, G. 146, 147
Baker, L.C. 186, 190
Banks, J. 9, 102
Barr, D.A. 90, 91
Barr, N. 260, 261, 263, 272, 274, 276
Barron, P. 22, 23
Barros, P.P. 141, 221
Basu, J. 56, 57
Batljan, I. 223, 225, 228
Baumol effect 136
Baumol, W. 134, 135
Bayesian learning framework 184, 187, 303–6,
    308
Beaulieu, N.D. 148, 149, 150, 153
bed blockers 101, 237
behavioural economics 273, 310, 318
Bell, D. 242, 243, 252
Benham, L. 44, 131
Bennett, S. 163, 168, 170
Benyamini, Y. 8, 114
Berthiaume, J.T. 147, 149, 154
Berwick, D.M. 144, 185
Bevan, G. 79, 83, 88, 98, 99, 105, 106, 108
Beveridge model of health care 87–8, 95–6
Billings, J. 53, 54
Bindman, A.B. 65, 73–4
biomarkers 9–10
Birrell, D. 246, 250, 253
Bismarck model of health care 88
Bokhour, B.G. 144, 146, 147
Booth, H. 292, 293
Bound, J. 5, 9
Bowes, A. 242, 249
Breyer, F. 182, 183, 223, 228
Bridgen, P. 236, 237
Britten, N. 315, 317
Brock, A. 284, 286
Brockmann, H. 222, 229
Brodsky, J. 239, 240
Brown, J.R. 259, 262–6, 269–70, 274–5
Busse, R. 164, 165

Cabiedes, L. 79, 86, 88
Cameron, A. 247, 249